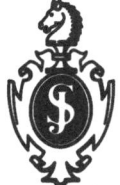

Since 1973 the Royal College of Obstetricians and Gynaecologists has regularly convened Study Groups to address important growth areas within obstetrics and gynaecology. An international group of eminent scientists and clinicians from various disciplines is invited to present the results of recent research and take part in in-depth discussion. The resulting volume containing the papers presented and also edited transcripts of the discussions is published within a few months of the meeting and provides a summary of the subject that is both authoritative and up to date.

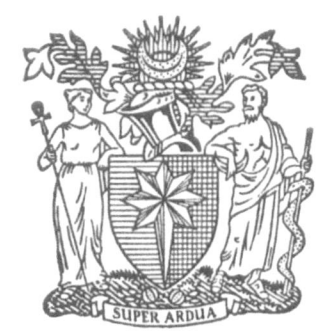

Previous Study Group publications available from Springer-Verlag:

Early Pregnancy Loss
Edited by R. W. Beard and F. Sharp

AIDS in Obstetrics and Gynaecology
Edited by C. N. Hudson and F. Sharp

Fetal Growth
Edited by F. Sharp, R. B. Fraser and R. D. G. Milner

Micturition
Edited by J. O. Drife, P. Hilton and S. L. Stanton

HRT and Osteoporosis
Edited by J. O. Drife and J. W. W. Studd

Antenatal Diagnosis of Fetal Abnormalities
Edited by J. O. Drife and D. Donnai

The Royal College of Obstetricians and Gynaecologists gratefully acknowledge the sponsorship of the Study Group: Organon Laboratories Limited; Schering Health Care Limited; Upjohn Limited

Prostaglandins and the Uterus

Edited by
J. O. Drife and A. A. Calder

With 55 Figures

Springer-Verlag
London Berlin Heidelberg New York
Paris Tokyo Hong Kong
Barcelona Budapest

James O. Drife MD, FRCSEd, FRCOG
Professor of Obstetrics, Department of Obstetrics and Gynaecology,
Clarendon Wing, Leeds General Infirmary, Belmont Grove, Leeds
LS2 9NS, UK

Andrew A. Calder MD, FRCP(Glas), FRCOG
Professor of Obstetrics, Department of Obstetrics and Gynaecology,
The University of Edinburgh, Centre for Reproductive Biology,
37 Chalmers Street, Edinburgh EH3 9EW, UK

ISBN-13: 978-1-4471-1933-3   e-ISBN-13: 978-1-4471-1931-9

DOI: 10.1007/978-1-4471-1931-9

British Library Cataloguing in Publication Data
Prostaglandins and the Uterus. – (Royal College of Obstetricians & Gynaecologists
Study Group Series)
I. Drife, J. O.   II. Calder, A. A.   III. Series
618.2

Library of Congress Data available

Typeset by Wilmaset Ltd, Birkenhead, Wirral

2128/3830-543210   Printed on acid-free paper

Preface

The introduction of prostaglandins into clinical practice has been one of the most important advances in obstetrics and gynaecology in recent years. During the last decade obstetricians have become familiar with these drugs for inducing labour and for terminating second-trimester pregnancy. Within the last year their use has been extended, in association with antiprogestin, to first-trimester termination. Although the effectiveness of prostaglandins in these pharmacological roles is clear, their full potential has still to be explored, and much remains to be learned about their physiology.

Prostaglandins play a central role in the initiation of labour. Further clarification of this role could lead to improvements in preventing or treating preterm labour, which still remains the most important cause of perinatal mortality in this country. Prostaglandins are also intimately involved in the mechanism of menstruation. More detailed understanding of this role should lead to more effective treatments for menorrhagia and dysmenorrhoea. These substances also play a part in the mechanism of implantation, and further research in this area may lead to more effective therapy for infertility.

The Scientific Advisory Committee of the RCOG felt that it was timely to review the current status of prostaglandins and to discuss their future. Prostaglandins were therefore made the subject of the College's 24th Study Group on 30–31 October 1991. An international panel of leading researchers, including clinicians, scientists, and animal physiologists, was invited to participate in a two-day workshop, with time for in-depth discussion as well as the presentation of papers. The workshop was divided into four sessions covering menstruation, early pregnancy, parturition and preterm labour, and represented a rare opportunity for researchers in these disparate areas of prostaglandin research to exchange ideas.

Professor D. T. Baird, Chairman of the Scientific Advisory Committee of the RCOG, was the moving spirit behind the programme planning. Miss Sally Barber, the College Postgraduate Education

Secretary, played an essential part in the organisation of the Study Group and the rapid publication of its proceedings. The Editors wish to thank her for her delightful efficiency and good humour in co-ordinating this project. We also wish to thank the participants who willingly gave up their time for this meeting, met our deadlines for the submission of manuscripts and participated so articulately in the discussion sessions. The chapters in this book and the frank discussions are an up-to-date and authoritative overview for clinicians and will, we hope, provide a stimulus to further research in this exciting field.

December 1991
J. O. Drife
A. A. Calder

Contents

SECTION III: PARTURITION

SECTION IV: PRETERM LABOUR

Participants

Professor J. J. Amy
Department of Gynaecology, Andrology and Obstetrics, Academisch
Ziekenhuis – V.U.B., Laarbeeklaan 101, B-1090 Brussels, Belgium

Professor A. A. Calder
Department of Obstetrics and Gynaecology, The University of
Edinburgh, Centre for Reproductive Biology, 37 Chalmers Street,
Edinburgh EH3 9EW, UK

Dr I. T. Cameron
University Lecturer and Consultant, Department of Obstetrics and
Gynaecology, The Rosie Maternity Hospital, Robinson Way, Cam-
bridge CB2 2SW, UK

Professor J. O. Drife
Department of Obstetrics and Gynaecology, D Floor, Clarendon
Wing, Leeds General Infirmary, Belmont Grove, Leeds LS2 9NS, UK

Professor M. G. Elder
Institute of Obstetrics and Gynaecology, Royal Postgraduate Medical
School, Du Cane Road, London W12 0NN, UK

Associate Professor I. S. Fraser
Department of Obstetrics and Gynaecology, University of Sydney,
New South Wales 2006, Australia

Professor I. A. Greer
Department of Obstetrics and Gynaecology, Glasgow Royal Infirmary, 10 Alexandra Parade, Glasgow G31 3ER, UK

Dr P. Husslein
Associate Professor, 1 Universitätsfrauenklinik Wien, Spitalgasse 23, 1090 Wien, Austria

Dr R. W. Kelly
MRC Senior Scientist, University of Edinburgh, MRC Reproductive Biology Unit, 37 Chalmers Street, Edinburgh EH3 9EW, UK

Professor M. J. N. C. Keirse
Department of Obstetrics, Gynaecology and Reproduction, Leiden University Hospital, Rijnsburgerweg 10, 2333 AA Leiden, The Netherlands

Dr A. López Bernal
Senior Research Fellow, Nuffield Department of Obstetrics and Gynaecology, John Radcliffe Hospital, Headington, Oxford OX3 9DU, UK

Dr M-A. Lumsden
Senior Registrar, Department of Obstetrics and Gynaecology, The Royal Infirmary, Lauriston Place, Edinburgh EH3 9EF, UK

Mr I. Z. MacKenzie
Clinical Reader in Obstetrics and Gynaecology, University of Oxford, Nuffield Department of Obstetrics and Gynaecology, John Radcliffe Maternity Hospital, Oxford OX3 9DU, UK

Professor P. W. N. Nathanielsz
Director, Laboratory for Pregnancy and Newborn Research, Cornell University, College of Veterinary Medicine, 816 VRT, Ithaca, New York 14853, USA

Dr J. E. Norman
Lecturer, Department of Obstetrics and Gynaecology, University of Edinburgh, Centre for Reproductive Biology, 37 Chalmers Street, Edinburgh EH3 9EW, UK

Dr D. M. Olson
Professor, Department of Obstetrics and Gynaecology, Pediatrics and Physiology; Director, Centre for Research in Maternal, Fetal and Newborn Health, 660 Heritage Medical Research Centre, University of Alberta, Canada T6G 2S2

Dr A. Rådestad
Department of Obstetrics and Gynaecology, Karolinska Hospital, S-10401 Stockholm, Sweden

Miss C. M. P. Rees
Parke Davis Lecturer, Nuffield Department of Obstetrics and Gynaecology, John Radcliffe Hospital, Headington, Oxford OX3 9DU, UK

Professor S. K. Smith
Department of Obstetrics and Gynaecology, The Rosie Maternity
Hospital, Robinson Way, Cambridge CB2 2SW, UK

Additional Contributors

Professor D. T. Baird
MRC Clinical Research Professor, Department of Obstetrics and
Gynaecology, University of Edinburgh, Centre for Reproductive
Biology, 37 Chalmers Street, Edinburgh EH3 9EW, UK

Ms S. L. Brown
Department of Physiology, University of Western Ontario, Lawson
Research Institute, St Joseph's Health Centre, London, Ontario,
Canada

Dr H. Cammu
Consultant Obstetrician and Gynaecologist, Department of Gynae-
cology, Andrology and Obstetrics, Academisch Ziekenhuis – V.U.B.,
Laarbeeklaan, 101, B-1090 Brussels, Belgium

Dr L. Cheng
MRC Reproductive Biology Unit, University of Edinburgh, Centre
for Reproductive Biology, 37 Chalmers Street, Edinburgh EH3 9EW,
UK

M. B. O. M. Honnebier
Laboratory for Pregnancy and New Born Research, Department of
Physiology, College of Veterinary Medicine, Cornell University,
Ithaca, NY 14850, USA

Miss E. A. MacLeod
Research Technician, The Centre for Research in Maternal, Fetal and
Newborn Health, 660 Heritage Medical Research Centre, University
of Alberta, Edmonton, Alberta, Canada T6G 2S2

Mrs Z. Smieja
Department of Physiology, University of Western Ontario, Lawson
Research Institute, St Joseph's Health Centre, London, Ontario,
Canada

Dr K. J. Thong
Research Fellow, Department of Obstetrics and Gynaecology,
University of Edinburgh, Centre for Reproductive Biology,
37 Chalmers Street, Edinburgh EH3 9EW, UK

Dr S. P. Watson
Royal Society University Research Fellow, Department of Pharmacology, South Parks Road, Oxford OX1 3QT, UK

Dr E. L. Yong
Lecturer, Department of Obstetrics and Gynaecology, University of Edinburgh, Centre for Reproductive Biology, 37 Chalmers Street, Edinburgh EH3 9EW, UK

Dr T. Zakar
Research Associate, Centre for Research in Maternal, Fetal and Newborn Health, 660 Heritage Medical Research Centre, University of Alberta, Edmonton, Alberta, Canada T6G 2S2

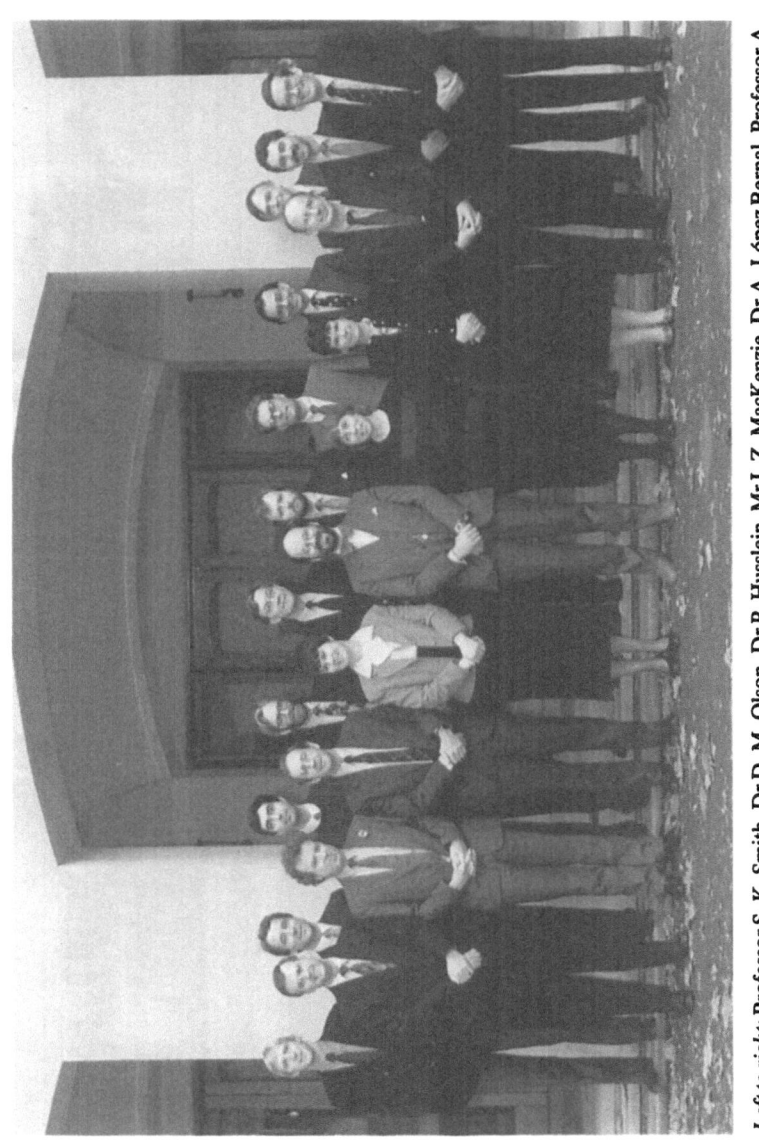

Left to right: Professor S. K. Smith, Dr D. M. Olson, Dr P. Husslein, Mr I. Z. MacKenzie, Dr A. López Bernal, Professor A. A. Calder, Professor I. S. Fraser, Dr J. E. Norman, Professor M. J. N. C. Keirse, Professor J. O. Drife, Professor I. A. Greer, Miss C. M. P. Rees, Dr A. Rådestad, Dr M-A. Lumsden, Professor P. W. N. Nathanielsz, Professor J. J. Amy, Dr R. W. Kelly, Dr I. T. Cameron, Professor M. G. Elder.

Section I

Menstruation

Chapter 1

Synthesis and Metabolism of Uterine Prostaglandins

R. W. Kelly, L. Cheng, J. Thong, E. L. Yong and D. T. Baird

Introduction

Prostaglandins (Fig. 1.1) are paracrine regulators derived mainly from arachidonic acid. They usually act locally and as such can be effective only if tissue levels respond rapidly to changes in synthesis and degradation. The balance of these two processes will determine the effective local concentration and thus relay the signal from other mediators. Within the non-pregnant uterus the endometrium is the main source of prostaglandin whereas in the gravid uterus the amnion, decidua and placenta all have a high synthetic capacity. It is well known that prostaglandins can be synthesised by many white blood cells including platelets, macrophages, neutrophils, mast cells and some T cells [1] and there is a growing awareness of the lymphoid nature of many of the cells in reproductive tissues [2–4].

Inflammatory Mechanisms in the Uterus: Cellular Origin of Prostaglandins

Prostaglandin production in human endometrium has revealed the hormone dependency of both prostaglandin synthetase and prostaglandin dehydrogenase (the enzymes responsible for biosynthesis and inactivation) but the definition of the cell types generating the prostaglandin is still uncertain. Using a monoclonal against CD45 (a marker of lymphoid cells) Tabibzadeh [5] has shown that non-

Arachidonic acid cascade

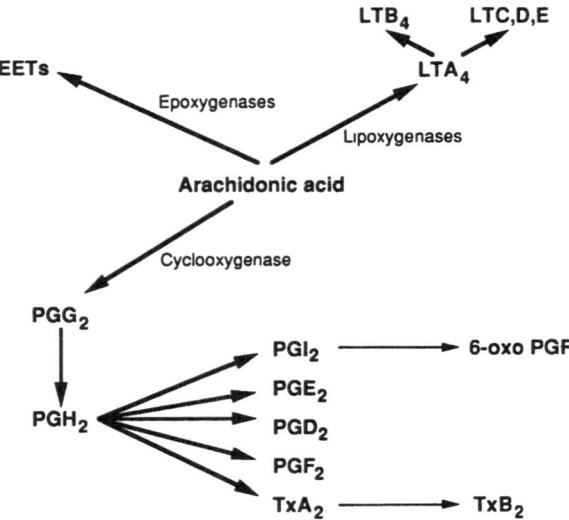

Fig. 1.1. The pathways of metabolism of arachidonic acid.

lymphoid cells proliferate slowly in comparison with lymphoid cells and that CD11+ve (macrophage marker) and CD3+ve (T cell marker) cells contribute to the overall proliferation within the endometrium. At least some of the lymphoid cells (including the T cells) express oestrogen receptors but the T cells do not express the IL-2 receptors which are involved in the normal process of clonal proliferation. In view of the known production of prostaglandins by such cells, the increased proliferation of the CD45+ve cells in the secretary phase could account for a significant amount of prostaglandin production.

The contribution of lymphoid cells to prostaglandin production is difficult to assess for several reasons.

1. In vitro experiments are done in the absence of blood cells
2. In vivo experiments are difficult because of the highly local nature of prostaglandin production and inactivation
3. Because of the problems of intervention without disturbing the system
4. Because of the necessity of identifying cell types retrospectively by employing panels of monoclonal antibodies.

Prostaglandin production and catabolism within the uterus are partly governed by ovarian hormones and this is clearly seen in the non-pregnant uterus where levels in biopsy samples are dependent on the stage of the ovarian cycle [6,7]. Experiments in vitro have determined the steroid dependency showing oestrogen stimulating production and progesterone inhibiting, with glucocorticoids having little effect [8,9]. In the pregnant uterus steroid dependency is also likely but the hormonal dependency is more difficult to establish.

During pregnancy, prostaglandin production must be kept low to maintain a quiescent uterus and progesterone must play a dominant role in this process since progesterone withdrawal leads to eventual abortion. However, in vitro experiments using amnion cells have implicated a range of cytokines and growth factors that stimulate synthesis even in the presence of progesterone and thus a complex interplay may exist between prostaglandins, progesterone and the processes of inflammation [10]. Cytokines are peptides that modulate the immune and inflammatory systems, but they are pleiotropic and thus affect many other cell types. Lymphoid cells are not confined to the pregnant uterus at parturition since early pregnancy decidua contains large granular lymphocytes which have natural killer (NK)-like features [11]. It is known that prostaglandin E is a potent physiological inhibitor of NK cell function [12] and decidual prostaglandin production may thus be involved in the maintenance of the homeostasis of pregnancy.

Endometrium is also a source of cytokine production and action [2]. Endometrial glands possess interleukin-1 (IL-1) receptors and IL-1 increases the production of prostaglandin E from these glands tenfold when explants are cultured with this agent for 24 h [13].

Prostaglandin Catabolism

Although the lungs have been thought of as the main organs of catabolism, many intrauterine tissues have prominent inactivating enzymes. Using the non-pregnant uterus as an example, the critical interplay between production and catabolism can be seen. The importance of catabolic activity is that prostaglandins generated, for instance by mechanical trauma, will be quickly inactivated and prevented from stimulating other inflammatory stages.

The ability of the endometrium to produce prostaglandin rises during the secretory phase of the ovarian cycle. This is clear from the high levels of prostaglandins produced in biopsy samples [6,7] and from immunocytochemistry studies showing the presence of the cyclo-oxygenase enzyme. Evidence from cultured explants, however, suggests that the high progesterone levels repress synthesis [8,9]. Around the midsecretory phase of the cycle when progesterone levels in blood are highest, catabolism in the endometrium is also greatest [14]. Only when progesterone levels fall is synthesis of prostaglandin possible and at the same time the catabolic activity is reduced, allowing effective local prostaglandin $F_{2\alpha}$ concentrations to participate in menstruation. In contrast to the endometrium the myometrium contains sustained high levels of prostaglandin dehydrogenase throughout the mentrual cycle [15].

The hormonal control of prostaglandin dehydrogenase (Fig. 1.2) is not fully understood, the experiments measuring enzyme activity during the cycle suggest that progesterone controls activity [14,15] and there is evidence of reduced prostaglandin dehydrogenase activity during progesterone treatment or parturition [16,17] but there is little supporting evidence for such control. We have examined the effects of the antiprogestin RU486 on catabolism in the uterine tissues of the pregnant guinea pig. The effect of the antagonist was to reduce catabolism in the myometrium, membranes and decidua with a 9-fold reduction

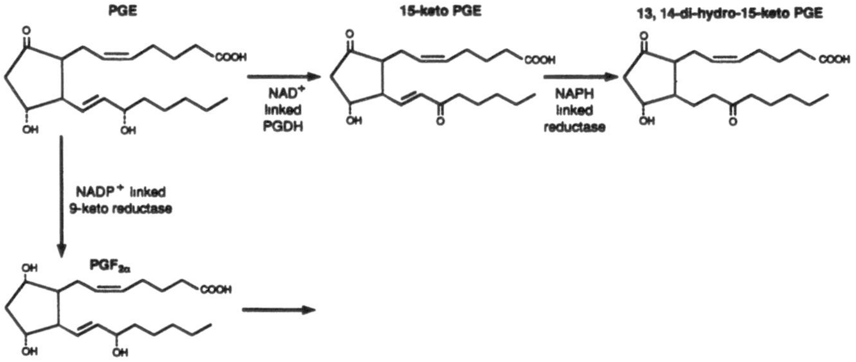

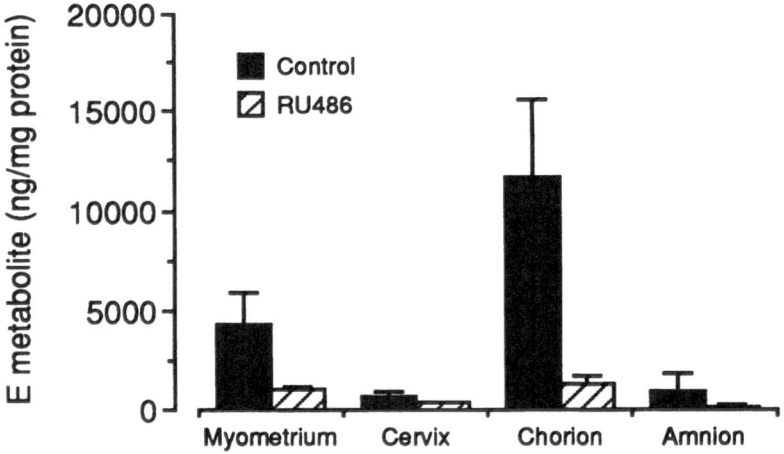

Fig. 1.2. The metabolism of prostaglandin E_2 (as an example). The first step in the deactivation, the oxidation of the 15-hydroxy group by prostaglandin dehydrogenase, removes over 90% of the biological activity as measured in bioassays.

Fig. 1.3. The metabolic capacity of uterine tissues from guinea pigs treated either with vehicle ▨ or with RU486 (10 mg) ■ for 24 h prior to tissue harvesting. Tissue was homogenised and incubated with a large excess (500 ng) PGE and 0.5 mM-NAD as cofactor. Prostaglandin E metabolite (15-keto prostaglandin E_2) was then measured by radioimmunoassay in the incubate. Redrawn from [18].

in the catabolic activity seen in the chorion tissue (Fig. 1.3) [18]. This result provides a partial explanation for the effects of antiprogestins in the guinea-pig model since previous work has shown that the guinea pig responds to antiprogestin treatment with little if any stimulation of myometrial activity but with a greatly enhanced sensitivity of the uterus to exogenous prostaglandin [19,20]. Such a combination could be accounted for by a decrease in effective prostaglandin breakdown induced by RU486. The largest decrease in catabolism was observed in chorion tissue [18] which has the largest prostaglandin dehydrogenase activity and this may reflect the protective role of this membrane which lies between the amnion, the main site of prostaglandin synthesis, and the presumptive target organ, the myometrium. Experiments using cultured human tissue have shown that administration of RU486 in vivo reduces metabolism to some extent in tissues cultured in vitro [21] but co-administration of indomethacin although reducing prostaglandin production did not prevent uterine contractions [22].

Such experiments, although giving a biochemical explanation for the high sensitivity towards prostaglandin associated with a quiescent uterus, do not necessarily prove that the catabolic capacity is progesterone dependent. Recent studies by Chwalisz et al. have shown that antiprogestins can counteract oestradiol-induced glandular proliferation in the rabbit uterus [23] and that this effect can be counteracted with added progesterone [23]. These results have been interpreted as a facilitatory effect of the unoccupied progesterone receptors but also suggest that the antiprogestins can exhibit effective antioestrogenic action although they do not appear to bind to the oestrogen receptor.

Since the chorion could play a major protective role during pregnancy several experiments have investigated whether prostaglandin can pass more readily through the chorion during labour [24,25]. The results of these studies have been equivocal, which suggests that the difference in metabolism if present may be marginal. Since the chorion contains such massive catabolising activity and since it has been shown that the prostaglandin dehydrogenase enzyme is non-uniformly distributed in human chorion [26] an alternative explanation could be proposed. The amnion is an avascular tissue but the chorion is well vascularised and it is possible that prostaglandin E produced by the amnion may have a hitherto

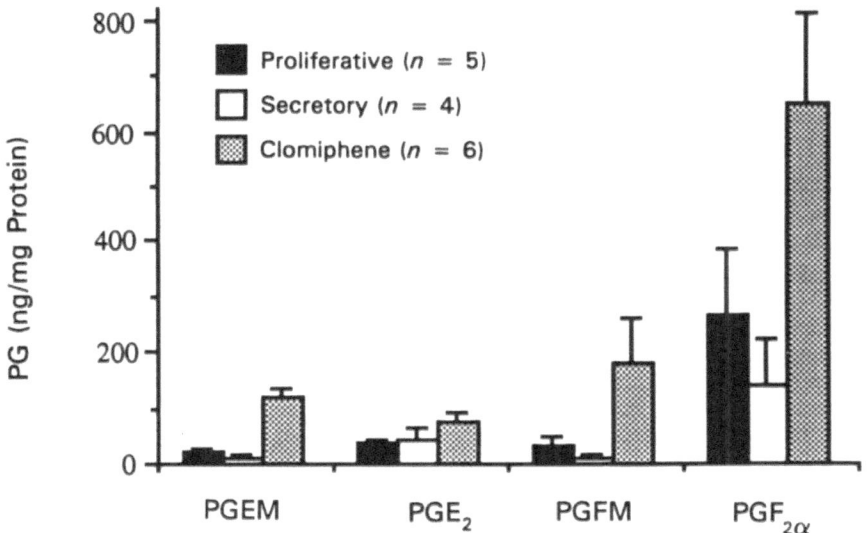

Fig. 1.4. Production of prostaglandin and metabolites from endometrium from women undergoing elective laparoscopic sterilisation and egg donation. Women were given norethisterone from day 21 of the cycle for five days. Seven days after stopping the progestin they were given Clomid (50 mg/day) for 5 days. Laparoscopy and curettage were performed 6 days after finishing the Clomid. Proliferative endometria (days 7–14) and secretory endometria (days 21–26) were obtained from women undergoing D&C.

neglected role in encouraging white cell influx into uterine tissues by acting on the vasculature in the chorio-decidual region.

We have recently examined the catabolic activity of endometrium obtained from women undergoing oocyte recovery who have been given clomiphene for five days early in the menstrual cycle. Although clomiphene is essentially an antioestrogen, the stimulation of FSH early in the cycle results in multiple follicular development which leads to raised oestrogen levels towards midcycle. Endometrium from this group of women showed extensive metabolic activity when maintained in organ culture (Fig. 1.4). In addition immunocytochemistry showed that in the late proliferative stage of the cycle prostaglandin dehydrogenase was evident in the larger more mature glands which presumably are a feature of the exposure to high oestradiol levels in vivo prior to curettage. Small glands did not show positive staining for prostaglandin dehydrogenase. These data suggest that prostaglandin dehydrogenase may be induced in reproductive tissues after prolonged exposure to oestradiol.

Prostaglandin Synthesis

Prostaglandin E plays an important role in the pregnant uterus. Both PGE and its synthetic analogues are effective in inducing labour, ripening the cervix and inducing abortion in early pregnancy. The main source of PGE in the pregnant uterus is the amnion and many agents have been shown to stimulate production of PGE by the amnion (Table 1.1). It seems likely that the control of parturition involves cytokines which are known to be coordinators of the inflammatory response and known to be responsible for the stimulation of prostaglandin synthesis [37]. Since fetal maturation is likely to be the deciding factor in the timing of parturition it seems logical that a fetal product will initiate labour. Thus the demonstration that fetal urine stimulates PGE production [27] may lead to the identification of the responsible compound, though no such agent has yet been found.

Romero et al. [30] have shown that infection and allergic reactions can lead to premature labour. This may be because IL-1 or some other cytokine produced as a result of the infection leads to prostaglandin production which prematurely

Table 1.1. Factors affecting PGE production by human amnion cells in culture

Stimulant	Reference	Inhibitor	Reference
Fetal urine	27	EIPS[a]	34
Bacterial products	28	Gravidin	35,36
Activated granulocyte products	29		
IL-1	28,30		
Protein kinase C (PMA etc.)	31		
EGF	32		
Dexamethasone	33		
Tumour necrosis factor	33		

[a] EIPS = endogenous inhibitor of prostaglandin synthesis.

triggers the physiological cascade of normal parturition. IL-1 may also be produced by the placenta since production by syncytiotrophoblast cells of IL-1α and IL-1β has been demonstrated [38] and it has been shown that this synthesis increases with exposure to microbial products [40].

The search for agents which hold prostaglandin synthesis in check until the time of parturition has been less successful: an endogenous inhibitor of prostaglandin synthesis (EIPS) has been reported but not fully identified [34]. A compound termed gravidin, that is found in amniotic fluid and is thought to be produced by the chorion [35,36], has recently been identified as the secretory component of IgA [39]. Thus, apart from the possible interaction of the inflammatory/immune system with the stimulation of parturition, it seems possible that immune secretions might play a role in maintaining the homeostasis of pregnancy.

When amnion cells in culture are stimulated with the phosphatase inhibitor okadaic acid, large amounts of PGE are produced (Fig. 1.5). In -short-term cultures the protein kinase C stimulant phorbol myristoyl acetate (PMA) is less effective although this appears to be in part through lack of free arachidonic acid (AA) since when AA is added to cultures containing PMA, maximal production of PCE is seen (Fig. 1.5). Okadaic acid has a potent stimulatory effect on endometrial explants maintained in culture (Fig. 1.6). The ratio of cyclo-oxygenase products remains unchanged which again suggests the effect is on the availability of AA. The mechanism by which the phosphatase inhibitor functions is not clear although the phosphatase inhibited is probably of the PP1 type as judged by its sensitivity [40]. Since the liberation of free AA is probably involved it is tempting to speculate that some inhibitory protein that was inactive in its phosphorylated form was being maintained in that form by the okadaic acid. Such

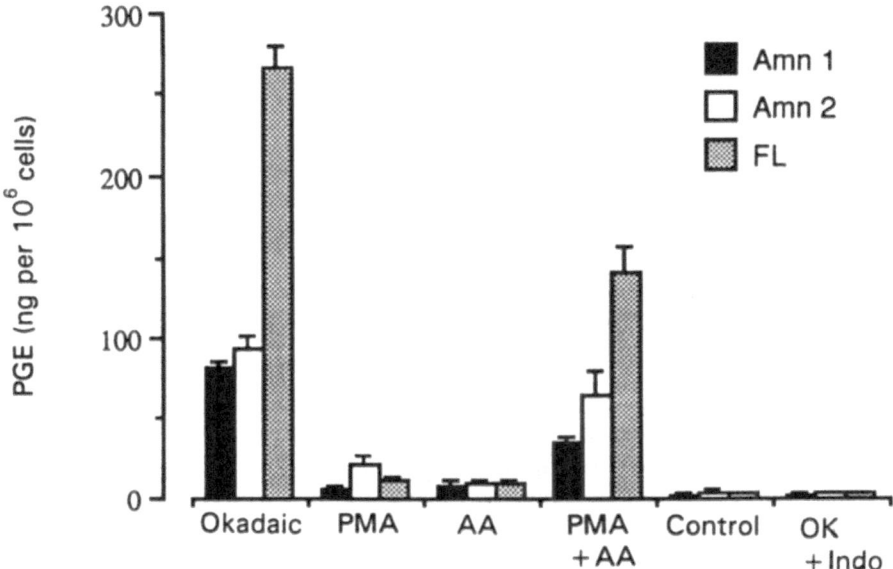

Fig. 1.5. PGE production from amnion cells (cultured for 48 h prior to experiment) from women undergoing elective caesarean section. The amnion cell line FL was purchased from Flow. PGE$_2$ was measured by radioimmunoassay. PMA, phorbol myristoyl acetate; AA, arachidonic acid, OK, okadaic acid; Indo, indomethacin.

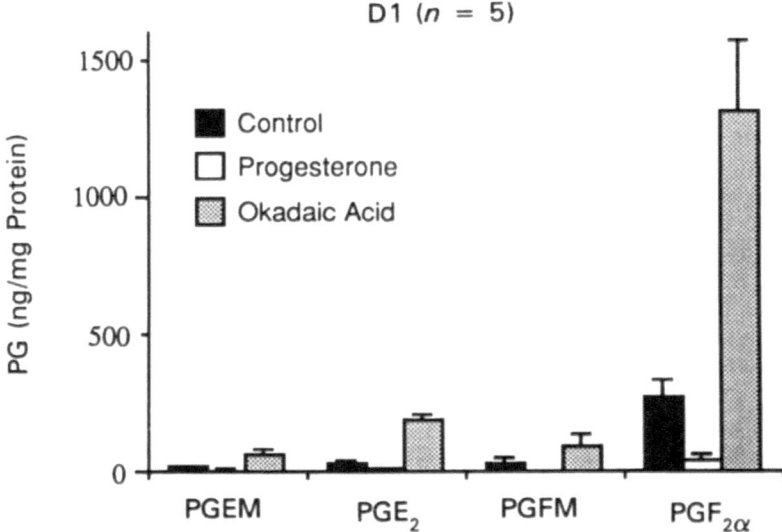

Fig. 1.6. PG production from endometrial explants from proliferative phase (see Fig. 1.4 for details) cultured with medium containing oestradiol (10 nM) and either progesterone (1 μM) or okadaic acid (250 nM)

proteins, now known as lipocortins/annexins [41], have been described although their inactivation by phosphorylation is controversial [42]. The high capacity of the amnion to produce prostaglandin E in response to cytokines and other stimuli may be a part of a negative feedback pathway since PGE inhibits both the production of IL-1 [43], tumour necrosis factor (TNF) [44] and IL-6 [45], another acute-phase cytokine. Thus the initiation of labour may be more dependent on the production of cytokines and the ensuing influx of white cells than on prostaglandin production as such. We have recently investigated the production of an interleukin directly implicated in the recruitment and inactivation of neutrophils which will result in further eicosanoid synthesis.

Recruitment of Prostaglandin Synthesising Cells

There is extensive evidence that parturition is associated with an influx of neutrophils and other white blood cells. Liggins [46] has likened parturition to an inflammatory process and this concept is supported by several disparate pieces of evidence. Studies in sheep show that progesterone withdrawal leads to an invasion of lymphocytes (mainly neutrophils) into the endometrium (both caruncular and intercaruncular) in early pregnancy [47]. RU486 produces a similar effect in monkeys at a later stage of pregnancy (>160 days gestation) where despite a variable response to RU486 there was clear evidence of PMN leukocyte infiltration in the placenta with normal and degenerate placental areas separated by a distinct zone of leukocytosis [48]. Administration of antiprogestins to the pregnant guinea pig also results in the appearance of neutrophils, activated macrophages and mast cells within the uterus. Rath et al. [49] have shown that one of the main agents responsible for cervical ripening is neutrophil collagenase. The experiments of Markee (reviewed in reference 50) show that the period of shrinkage of the *functionalis* layer of the endometrium, which precedes menstrual bleeding, is associated with increased presence of white cells. Activation of these cells could adequately account for the tissue changes associated with this stage of menstruation. The analogy between menstruation and the inflammatory response has recently been reiterated [2]. Thus there is good reason to suppose that the mechanisms of both menstruation and parturition may depend on the recruitment or activation of lymphoid cells. In mammalian pregnancy the tenuous accommodation of the fetal allograft by the maternal host normally extends to term when some, yet to be elucidated, chain of events removes the protection and allows rejection by the immune system. Thus parturition can be viewed as a co-option of the effector arm of the immune system using the normal inflammatory processes. Removal of the protection or activation of the immune system prematurely, would thus lead to abortion or premature labour. Such ideas have been proposed before [46] but our knowledge of the initiation of the inflammatory response has been incomplete and progress in that field will add to our understanding of parturition and menstruation.

The interleukins have been implicated in the initiation of parturiton since interleukin-1 leads to an increase of prostaglandin E production by amnion [28,30] and fibroblasts of the cervix. We have been examining the production of interleukin-8 by the fetal membranes and decidua. Interleukin-8, monocyte-derived chemotactic factor (MDCF), or neutrophil activating peptide-1 (NAP-1) (for a review see reference 51) is a small (72 amino acid) cytokine known to be produced by monocytes, fibroblasts and epithelial cells. The cytokine induces accumulation of neutrophils at inflammatory lesions by chemotaxis, increased neutrophil adhesion to vascular endothelium and an associated transepithelial migration [52]. Interactions between circulating neutrophils and vascular endothelium are greatly enhanced in instances of acute inflammation [53] and the release of a chemotactic factor by the fetal membranes or by the decidua could result in the mounting of a sterile inflammatory reaction sufficient to cause further prostaglandin production, myometrial activity and expulsion of the conceptus. Prostacyclin would have an opposite effect in that it would prevent neutrophil adhesion and thus prevent the essential step preliminary to neutrophil diapedesis. Whether inappropriate enhancement of IL-8 contributes to preeclampsia remains to be seen.

IL-8 is a more potent chemotactic factor than LTB4 or PAF [54] although it may function in part by the stimulation of LTB4 synthesis [54]. Recent findings suggest that IL-8 may exert its chemotactic action indirectly by interacting with mast cells [55]. In addition to the ability of IL-8 to induce neutrophil immigration into tissue it can also activate neutrophils and cause exocytosis [56,57] and as such is a very powerful agent in inducing tissue remodelling.

We have measured IL-8 production by a two-site enzyme immunoassay and have demonstrated that production occurs in both amnion and chorion/decidua. An amnion cell line (FL) can be stimulated to produce elevated IL-8 levels by either okadaic acid or PMA: chorion/decidua produces around 200 ng ml^{-1} per 10^6 cells in 24 h of culture and thus membranes and decidua could be a major source of neutrophil chemotactic signal. Experiments that examined neutrophil accumulation and plasma leakage in rabbit skin have shown that coinjection of prostaglandin E reduced the threshold of IL-8 action by a factor of 100 [58]. Thus PGE and interleukin-8 have a synergistic action and the effects of PGE in inducing abortion, cervical ripening, and labour may in part be due to this synergy with IL-8. Early studies clearly showed that administration of PGE alone was sufficient for an inflammatory response [59]. This may also be due to synergy with IL-8 or other chemotactic peptides. Since IL-8 production can be induced by IL-1 and TNF [51], the action of these compounds as intermediates can be envisaged.

Conclusions

Undoubtedly endometrium possesses a high capacity for prostaglandin production in the secretory phase of the menstrual cycle but this is the time of maximum prostaglandin inactivation by prostaglandin dehydrogenase and therefore it seems preferable that effective concentrations are not reached until progesterone and oestrogen levels decline. There is little doubt that by the time of menstruation prostaglandin levels in menstrual blood are high but this could be caused by the cellular damage. Alternatively, the vasoconstricting action of prostaglandin $F_{2\alpha}$ could be the cause of the ischaemic necrosis involved, and play a major role in the initiation of menstruation. The likening of menstruation and parturition to inflammatory processes suggest that the prostaglandins play a major modulating role in both these processes.

The production of prostaglandins by the non-pregnant and the pregnant uterus may involve lymphoid cells which may be resident or induced by chemotactic factors. In endometrium, lymphoid cells remain in the *basalis* layer and proliferate throughout the menstrual cycle [5]. The pregnant uterus has many lymphoid cells in the decidua and the fetal membranes may play a crucial part in the synthesis of cytokines which leads to parturition. The influx of white cells into the uterus after progesterone withdrawal or antagonism suggests that the anti-inflammatory properties of progesterone may play a crucial role in the maintenance of pregnancy homeostasis. The influence of progesterone on lymphocytes has yet to be fully investigated [60].

At present little is understood about the mechanisms initiating prostaglandin production and parturition but a wider perspective of control mechanisms should lead to an elucidation of these events and the provision of better management of cervical ripening and premature labour.

References

1. Ninnemann JL. Prostaglandins, leukotrienes and the immune response. Cambridge: Cambridge University Press, 1988.
2. Tabibzadeh S. Human endometrium: an active site of cytokine production and action. Endocr Rev 1991; 12:272–90.

3. Adashi EY. The potential relevance of cytokines to ovarian physiology: the emerging role of resident ovarian cells of the white blood cells series. Endocr Rev 1990; 11:454–64.
4. Ito A, Hiro D, Sakyo K, Mori Y. The role of leukocyte factors on uterine cervical ripening and dilatation. Biol Reprod 1987; 37:511–17.
5. Tabibzadeh S. Proliferative activity of lymphoid cells in human endometrium throughout the menstrual cycle. J Clin Enocrinol Metab 1990; 70:437–43.
6. Downie J, Poyser NL, Wunderlich M. Levels of prostaglandins in human endometrium throughout the menstrual cycle. J Physiol (Lond) 1974; 236:465–72.
7. Maathuis JB, Kelly RW. Concentrations of prostaglandin $F_{2\alpha}$ and E_2 in the endometrium throughout the menstrual cycle and after the administration of clomiphene or an oestrogen–progestogen pill and in early pregnancy. J Endocrinol 1978; 77:361–71.
8. Abel MH, Baird DT. The effect of 17β estradiol and progesterone on prostaglandin production by human endometrium maintained in organ culture. Endocrinology 1980; 106:1599–606.
9. Kelly RW, Smith SK. Glucocorticoids do not share with progesterone the potent inhibitory action of prostaglandin synthesis in human proliferative phase endometrium. Prostaglandins 1987; 33:919–29.
10. Manzai M, Liggins GC. Inhibitory effects of dispersed human amnion cells on production rates of prostaglandin E and F by endometrial cells. Prostaglandins 1984; 28:297–307.
11. King A, Loke YW. Uterine large granular lymphocytes: a possible role in embryonic implantation? Am J Obstet Gynecol 1990; 162:308–10.
12. Garcia-Penarrubia P, Bankhurst AD, Koster FT. Prostaglandins from human T suppressor/cytotoxic cells modulate natural killer antibacterial activity. J Exp Med 1989; 170:601–6.
13. Tabibzadeh S, Kaffka KL, Sattaswaroop PG, Kilian PL. Interleukin-1 (IL-1) regulation of human endometrial function: presence of IL-1 receptor correlates with IL-1 stimulated prostaglandin E2 production. J Clin Endocrinol Metab 1990; 70:1000–6.
14. Casey ML, Hemsell DL, Johnston JM, MacDonald PC. NAD dependent 15-hydroxyprostaglandin dehydrogenase activity in human endometrium. Prostaglandins 1980; 19:115–22.
15. Abel MH, Kelly RW. Metabolism of prostaglandins by the non-pregnant human uterus. J Clin Endocrinol Metab 1983; 56:678–85.
16. Bedwani JR, Marley PB. Enhanced inactivation of prostaglandin E_2 by the rabbit lung during pregnancy or progesterone treatment. Br J Pharmacol 1975; 53:547–54.
17. Flower RJ. The role of prostaglandins in parturition with special reference to the rat: "fetus and birth". Amsterdam: Elsevier 1977; 297–318.
18. Kelly RW, Bukman A. Antiprogestagenic inhibition of uterine prostaglandin inactivation: a permissive mechanism for uterine stimulation. J Steroid Biochem 1990; 37:97–101.
19. Elger W, Beier S, Chwalisz K et al. Studies on the mechanisms of action of progesterone antagonists. J Steroid Biochem 1986; 25:835–45.
20. Elger W, Fahnrich M, Beier S, Qing SS, Chwalisz K. Endometrial and myometrial effects of progesterone antagonists in pregnant guinea pigs. Am J Obstet Gynecol 1987; 157:1065–74.
21. Norman JE, Wu WX, Kelly RW, Glasier AF, McNeilly AS, Baird DT. Effects of mifepristone in vivo on decidual prostaglandin synthesis and metabolism. Contraception 1991; 44:89–98.
22. Norman JE, Kelly RW, Baird DT. Uterine activity and decidual prostaglandin production in women in early pregnancy in response to mifepristone with or without indomethacin in vivo. Hum Reprod 1991; 6:740–4.
23. Chwalisz K, Hegele-Hartung C, Fritzemeier K-H, Beier HM, Elger W. Inhibition of estradiol-mediated endometrial gland formation by the antiestrogen onapristone in rabbits: relationship to uterine estrogen receptors. Endocrinology 1991; 129:312–22.
24. Nakla S, Skinner K, Mitchell MD, Challis JRG. Changes in prostaglandin transfer across human fetal membranes obtained after spontaneous labor. Am J Obstet Gynecol 1986; 155:1337–41.
25. Roseblade CK, Sullivan MHF, Khan H, Lumb MR, Elder MG. Limited transfer of prostaglandin E_2 across the fetal membrane before and after labour. Acta Obstet Gynecol Scand 1990; 69:399–403.
26. Cheung PYC, Walton JC, Tai H-H, Riley SC, Challis JRGD. Immunocytochemical distribution and localization of 15-hydroxyprostaglandin dehydrogenase in human fetal membranes, decidua and placenta. Am J Obstet Gynecol 1990; 163:1445–9.
27. Niesert S, Mitchell MD, MacDonald PC, Casey ML. The effect of fetal urine on arachidonic acid metabolism in human amnion cells in monolayer culture. Am J Obstet Gynecol 1986; 155:1310–16.
28. Mitchell MD, Romero RJ, Avila C, Foster JT, Edwin SS. Prostaglandin production by amnion and decidual cells in response to bacterial products. Prostaglandins Leukotrienes Essential Fatty Acids 1991; 42:167–9.

29. Bry K, Hallman M. A product of activated human granulocytes stimulates prostaglandin E_2 synthesis in human amnion cells. Prostaglandins Leukotrienes Essential Fatty Acids 1991; 43:35–42.

30. Romero R, Avila C, Brekus CA, Mazor M. The role of systemic and intrauterine infection in preterm parturition. In: Garfield RE, ed. Uterine contractility: mechanisms of control. Serono Symposia, Norwell, Mass, USA, Serono 1990: 319–53.

31. Sander J, Myatt L. Regulation of prostaglandin E_2 synthesis in human amnion by protein kinase C. Prostaglandins 1990; 39:355–63.

32. Mitchell MD. Epidermal growth factor actions on arachidonic acid metabolism in human amnion cells. Biochim Biophys Acta 1987; 928:240–2.

33. Mitchell MD, Lundin-Schiller S. The regulation of arachidonic acid metabolism in pregnancy. In: Garfield RE ed. Uterine contractility: mechanisms of control. Serono Symposia, Norwell, Mass, USA: Serono 1990: 205–19.

34. Saeed SA, Strickland DM, Young DC, Dang A, Mitchell MD. Inhibition of prostaglandin synthesis by human amniotic fluid: acute reduction in inhibitory activity of amniotic fluid obtained during labour. J Clin Endocrinol Metab 1982; 55:801–3.

35. Wilson T, Aimer GP, Skinner SJM, Liggins GC, Partial purification and characterization of two compounds from amniotic fluid which inhibit phospholipase activity in human endometrial cells. Biochem Biophys Res Commun 1985; 131:22–9.

36. Wilson T, Liggins GC, Joe L. Purification and characterization of a uterine phospholipase inhibitor that loses activity after labor onset in women. Am J Obstet Gynecol 1989; 160:602–6.

37. Arai K, Lee F, Miyajima A, Shoichiro M, Arai N, Yokota T. Cytokines: coordinators of immune and inflammatory responses. Annu Rev Biochem 1990; 59:783–836.

38. Taniguchi T, Matsuzaki N, Kameda T, Shimoya K, Jo T, Saji F, Tanizawa O. The enhanced production of placental interleukin-1 during labor and intrauterine infection. Am J Obstet Gynecol 1991; 165:131–7.

39. Wilson T, Christie DL. Gravidin, an endogenous inhibitor of phospholipase A2 activity is a secretory component of IgA. Biochem Biophys Res Commun 1991; 176:447–52.

40. Cohen P, Holmes CFB, Tsukitani Y. Okadaic acid: a new probe for the study of cellular regulation. Trends Biol Sci 1990; 98–102.

41. Russo-Marie F. Lipocortins: an update. Prostaglandins Leukotrienes Essential Fatty Acids 1991; 42:83–9.

42. Davidson FF, Dennis EA. Biological relevance of lipocortins and related proteins as inhibitors of phospholipase A2. Biochem Pharmacol 1989; 38:3645–51.

43. Kunkel SL, Chensue SW, Phan SH. Prostaglandins as endogenous mediators of interleukin 1 production. J Immunol 1986; 136:186–92.

44. Scales WE, Chensus SW, Otterness I, Kunkel SL. Regulation of monokine gene expression: prostaglandin E2 suppresses tumor necrosis factor but not interleukin-1å or β-mRNA and cell associated bioactivity. J Leukocyte Biol 1989; 45:416–21.

45. Callery MP, Manjino MJ, Kamei T, Flye MW. Interleukin 6 production by endotoxin stimulated Kupffer cells is regulated by prostaglandin E2. J Surg Res 1990; 48:523–7.

46. Liggins GC. Cervical ripening as an inflammatory reaction. In: Ellwood DA, Anderson ABM, eds. The cervix in pregnancy and labour, clinical and biochemical investigations. Edinburgh: Churchill Livingstone, 1981; 1–9.

47. Staples LD, Heap RB, Wooding FBP, King GJ. Migration of leukocytes into the uterus after acute removal of ovarian progesterone during early pregnancy in the sheep. Placenta 1983; 4:339–50.

48. Sinosich MJ, Lee J, Wolf JP, Williams RF, Hodgen GD. RU486 induced suppression of placental neutrophil elastase inhibitor levels. Placenta 1989; 10:569–78.

49. Rath W, Adelmann-Grill BC, Stuhlsatz HW, Severenyi M, Kuhn W. Biophysical and biochemical changes of cervical ripening. In: Egarter C, Husslein P, eds. Prostaglandins for cervical ripening and/or induction of labour. Vienna: Facults-Universitatsverlag. Eicosanoids and Fatty Acids. 1988; 8:32–41.

50. Shaw ST, Roche PC. Menstruation. Reprod Biol 1980; 41:96.

51. Matushima K, Oppenheim JJ. Interleukin 8 and MCAF: novel inflammatory cytokines inducible by IL1 and TNF. Cytokine 1989; 1:2–13.

52. Smith WB, Gamble JR, Clark-Lewis I, Vadas MA. Interleukin-8 induces neutrophil transendothelial migration. Immunology 1991; 72:65–72.

53. Harlan JM. Leukocyte-endothelial interactions. J Am Soc Hematol 1985; 65:513–25.

54. Thomsen MK, Larsen CG, Thomsen HK, Kirstein D, Skak-Niesen T, Ahnfelt-Ronne I, Thestrup-Pedersen K. Recombinant human interleukin-8 is a potent activator of canine

neutrophil aggregation, migration and leukotriene B4 biosynthesis. J Invest Dermatol 1991; 96:260–6.
55. Ribeiro RA, Flores CA, Cunha FQ, Ferreira SH. IL-8 causes in vivo neutrophil migration by a cell dependent mechanism. Immunology 1991; 73:472–7.
56. Elford PR, Cooper PH. Induction of neutrophil mediated cartilage degradation by interleukin-8. Arthritis Rheum 1991; 34:325–32.
57. Masure S. Purification and identification of 91kDa neutrophil gelatinase release by the activating peptide interleukin-8. Eur J Biochem 1991; 198:391–8.
58. Colditz IG. Effect of exogenous prostaglandin E_2 and actinomycin D on plasma leakage induced by neutrophil activating peptide-1/interleukin-8. Immunol Cell Biol 1990; 68:397–403.
59. Kaley G, Weiner R. Prostaglandin E_1: a potential mediator of the inflammatory response. Ann NY Acad Sci 1971; 180:338–50.
60. Szekeres-Bartho J, Chaouat G, Kinsky RA. Progesterone induced blocking factor corrects high resorption rates in mice treated with antiprogesterone. Am J Obstet Gynecol 1990; 163:1320–3.

Chapter 2

Prostaglandins and Menstruation

I. T. Cameron

Disorders of menstruation present a significant burden to health services. Furthermore, hysterectomy, the definitive surgical treatment for menorrhagia, is the most common major operation performed on women of reproductive age in Britain and America [1–3]. Heavy menstrual bleeding may be the result of organic disease such as fibroids, infection or malignancy, but in most cases, no such underlying lesion can be found and the diagnosis of dysfunctional bleeding is made. In some circumstances, and especially at the extremes of the reproductive career, dysfunctional bleeding may be the result of anovulation [4,5]. However, in most women with regular but heavy periods no abnormality of the hypothalamopituitary axis can be demonstrated, and the abnormality is therefore thought to lie at the level of the endometrium itself [6].

The precise mechanisms controlling both normal and abnormal menstruation are not known. This chapter will address aspects of the local control of menstrual bleeding, with emphasis on the involvement of the prostaglandins (PGs). The role of other systems within the endometrium, including the fibrinolytic pathway, has been reviewed elsewhere [7,8].

The Mechanism of Menstruation

In his classical experiments observing the growth and degeneration of endometrial explants in the monkey anterior eye chamber, Markee [9] demonstrated that the onset of menstruation was preceded by a period of rapid regression of the endometrium, followed by intense vasoconstriction of the spiral arterioles, with accompanying vasodilatation of the surrounding iridal vessels. Endometrial regression appeared to be under endocrine control, and could be reproduced by withdrawing oestrogen or gestogen. The intense vasoconstriction was attributed to an unknown pressor agent, released during vascular stasis, and responsible for protection against excessive blood loss.

Endometrial Haemostasis

The haemostatic response to vascular injury has been well characterised in peripheral tissues [10]. Vessel damage reveals subendothelial collagen and is followed rapidly by the cascade of platelet accumulation, fibrin deposition and platelet degranulation and interdigitation, to form the primary haemostatic plug. Over the next few hours the plug is transformed by cellular lysis and further fibrin deposition to form a secondary plug, composed of fibrin and empty platelet remnants.

Haemostatic events in the menstruating uterus are strikingly different. Detailed studies were performed on nine women who had undergone hysterectomy within 72 h of the onset of menstruation [11,12]. In the earliest specimens, stromal disintegration and vessel lesions were seen in the absence of platelet adhesion, despite the exposure of subendothelium to the vessel lumen. Following this, blood extravasation was a prominent feature in the functional endometrium, and the damaged ends of blood vessels were sealed by intrvascular thrombi consisting of various amounts of platelets and fibrin. By 20 h after the onset of bleeding, most of the functional endometrium had been shed, and subsequent haemostasis was achieved not by the deposition of stable platelet–fibrin plugs, but by vasoconstriction of the remaining basal arteriolar fragments.

These studies emphasise the crucial role of a powerful vasoconstrictor in the basal endometrium, both prior to the onset of menstruation, and afterwards to control the degree of blood loss. In addition, the presence of a potent inhibitor of platelet adhesion or aggregation would be suggested.

The Prostaglandins

Six years before the publication of Markee's observations, von Euler [13] had demonstrated a plain muscle stimulant from the male accessory genital glands which he termed "prostaglandin". However, it was not until 1957 that Pickles [14] reported a similar finding in the menstruum, and confirmation of the presence of PGE_2 and $PGF_{2\alpha}$ in menstrual fluid and endometrium not only revealed the nature of the menstrual stimulant, but also provided a candidate for Markee's endometrial vasoconstrictor [15]. Since then, much evidence has accumulated suggesting a role for the PGs in the physiology and pathology of normal and dysfunctional menstruation [16–19].

Biosynthesis and Physiological Actions

The synthesis and metabolism of uterine PGs have been reviewed in detail in Chapter 1. Prostaglandins are not stored in tissues, but are synthesised on

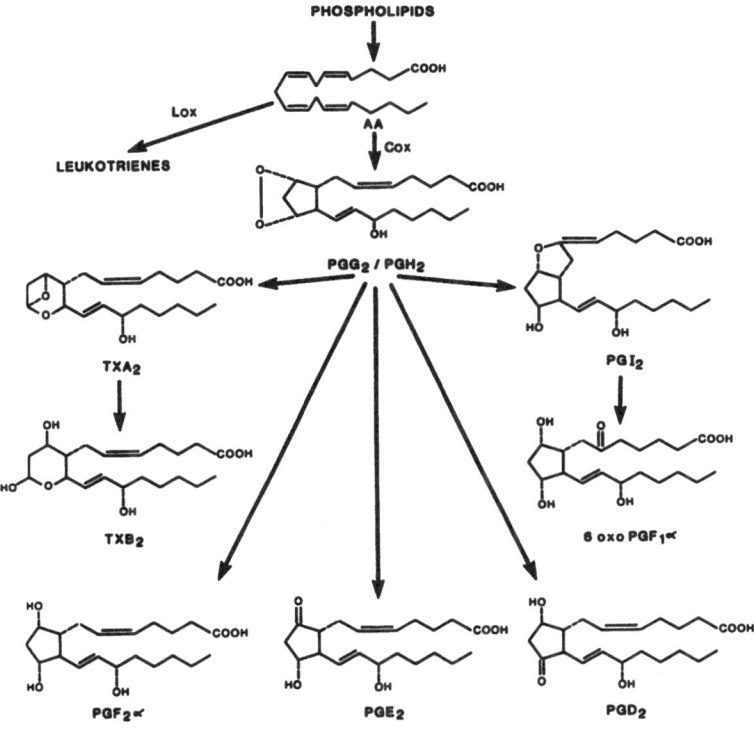

Fig. 2.1. The arachidonic acid cascade, illustrating the major uterine prostaglandin biosynthetic pathways. Lox = lipoxygenase, Cox = cyclo-oxygenase.

demand from precursor arachidonic acid (AA) by the action of specific phospholipases (PLs, Fig. 2.1). Phospholipase A_2 and PLC activity have been demonstrated in human endometrium [20,21], and their action to release membrane-bound AA represents a crucial rate-limiting step in PG biosynthesis [22].

In endometrium, AA is rapidly metabolised via the cyclo-oxygenase pathway to produce the cyclic endoperoxides, PGG_2 and PGH_2, or via lipoxygenase towards leukotriene synthesis. The cyclic endoperoxides are unstable intermediates, and are rapidly converted into the primary PGs (PGD_2, PGE_2 and $PGF_{2\alpha}$), or via thromboxane or prostacyclin synthetase to thromboxane (TX) A_2 and prostacylin (PGI_2) respectively. The latter intermediates have short biological half-lives of 40 s and 3 min, and are converted into their stable products TXB_2 and 6-oxo $PGF_{1\alpha}$. Immunocytochemical studies have demonstrated localisation of cyclo-oxygenase in human endometrium [23]. Intense staining was seen on endometrial surface epithelium throughout the menstrual cycle, with less intense staining on glands and scattered stromal cells.

The physiological response following activation of the AA cascade depends on the relative synthesis of the various PGs, which have different effects on different tissues. Of particular relevance to the uterus are their vascular and smooth muscle-stimulating properties. Thromboxane A_2 is a potent vasoconstrictor and stimulator of platelet aggregation, in contrast to PGI_2 which is a vasodilator and powerful inhibitor of aggregation [24]. Prostaglandin $F_{2\alpha}$ has vasoconstrictor properties, and its myometrial-stimulating action has been implicated in the pathogenesis of primary dysmenorrhoea [15,25–27] and in the generation and maintenance of contractions in the pregnant uterus [28,29]. Prostaglandin E_2 is a vasodilator, with one-sixth of the potentency of PGI_2.

Prostaglandins and the Endometrium

The main endometrium metabolites of AA are PGE_2 and $PGF_{2\alpha}$, and though their production changes throughout the menstrual cycle, the reported pattern of production has varied between studies. A number of groups have suggested an increased PG production in the secretory phase of the cycle in endometrium [30–34], uterine washings [35] and uterine venous blood [36], with the highest concentrations seen at the time of menstruation. Others have demonstrated either no difference [37], or a greater PG production by proliferative rather than secretory tissue in vitro [38–42]. The marked variance in cited data is likely to be due to differences in tissue collection and processing, besides differences in assay techniques between different laboratories. Problems also arise in the extrapolation of in vitro data to the in vivo situation. Prostaglandins are readily produced in response to trauma, and so the process of obtaining tissue will stimulate PG production [43,44]. Specimens obtained by biopsy and subjected to homogenisation probably reflect the potential of the tissue to produce PGs on maximal stimulation. Indeed, tissue concentrations of PGE_2, $PGF_{2\alpha}$ and 6-oxo $PGF_{1\alpha}$, but not broken cell homogenates, accurately reflected the ratio of PG release in vivo, though the absolute measurements were increased by the trauma of tissue handling [45]. The effect of experimental method on the results can be illustrated by studies investigating endometrial PGs and measured menstrual blood loss, for although an association was seen between increased concentrations of PGE, or the ratio of PGE: $PGF_{2\alpha}$, and the degree of blood loss [46,47], such an association was not seen after short-term incubation or superfusion studies [46,48].

Ovarian Control

The observed cyclical pattern of endometrial PG production has suggested a control mechanism mediated by ovarian steroids. In secretory endometrium, oestradiol stimulated release of both PGE_2 and $PGF_{2\alpha}$ [33,39], but no effect was seen in the proliferative phase. This differential response may be attributed to a maximal stimulatory effect of endogenous oestradiol in vivo [18].

Progesterone on the other hand, inhibited PG release in vitro from both proliferative and secretory endometrium in the rhesus monkey and human [33,39,49,50]. This effect of progesterone appeared to be mediated by an indirect inhibition of phospholipase activity [50] analogous to, but different from, the lipocortin-mediated ihibition with glucocorticoids [51]. A paradox therefore exists between those studies suggesting an increased endometrial production in the luteal phase, and those showing an inhibition of PG release by progesterone in vitro. It is likely that the role of progesterone in vivo is to promote the storage of membrane-bound AA. Secretory phase endometrium would therefore have an increased capacity to sythesise PGs from AA; withdrawal of progesterone at luteolysis would remove its inhibitory effect on phospholipase activity and result in a stimulation of PG release prior to the onset of menstruation.

Prostaglandin and Menstrual Bleeding

A role for the PGs in the mechanism underlying menstruation was supported by observations that the administration of $PGF_{2\alpha}$ to women in the luteal phase resulted in the initiation of menstrual bleeding [52,53]. Subsequent studies have suggested an association between the type and quantity of endometrial PG production and the degree of menstrual bleeding. These data will be considered in detail in following chapters. Briefly, however, PGE_2 and $PGF_{2\alpha}$ concentrations were elevated in menstrual fluid of women with menorrhagia [27]. In endometrium, patients with excessive blood loss had either greater levels of total PG ($PGE_2 + PGF_{2\alpha} + PGI_2$), or an increased ratio of the vasodilatory PGE_2 to the vasoconstrictor $PGF_{2\alpha}$ [46,47]. Furthermore, the availability of AA was greater in endometrium of women with menorrhagia than normal controls [54], and reductions in measured menstrual blood loss have been reported after the use of cyclo-oxygenase inhibitors, intrauterine progesterone, and the combined contraceptive pill, all of which impair endometrial prostaglandin production [25,55–57].

A considerable body of data, both direct and circumstantial, has therefore accumulated, implicating the prostaglandins in the initiation and control of menstruation. The crucial role of a powerful endometrial vasoconstrictor has been demonstrated, but its precise nature remains unknown. Although $PGF_{2\alpha}$ has been the best candidate, it is a weak vasoconstrictor, and has failed to show significant constrictor activity on uterine vessels in vitro [58]. The recent description of the endothelins has suggested an alternative to $PGF_{2\alpha}$ as the endometrial vasoconstrictor [59].

Endometrial Endothelins

The endothelins (ETs) comprise a family of peptides with 21 amino acid (Fig. 2.2), cleaved from larger precursor molecules (proETs and preproETs) and similar in structure to the sarafotoxin snake venoms [60,61]. Originally thought to be exclusively of endothelial cell origin, immunoreactive ET has now been demonstrated in human epithelial tissues, including those of lung and the central nervous system. Endothelin-1, the most powerful vasoconstrictor yet discovered, caused a potent long-lasting contraction of human uterine vessels, with a dose–response curve two orders of magnitude to the left of that seen with noradrenaline [62].

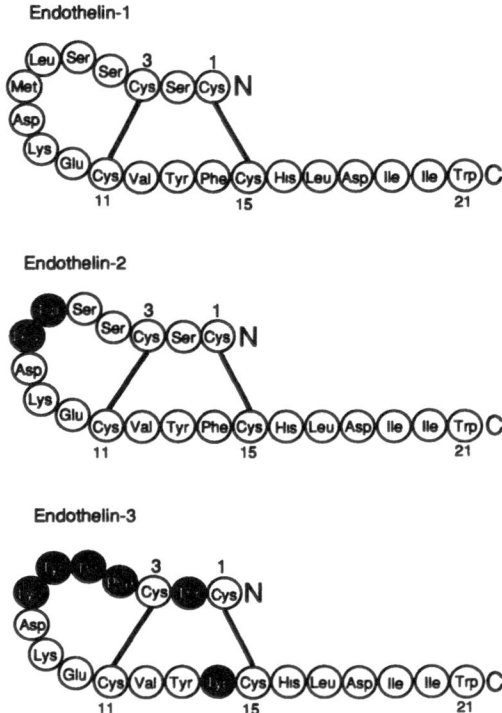

Fig. 2.2. The amino acid sequences of the cleaved human endothelins. The filled circles illustrate the differences in amino acid sequence between endothelin-2 and endothelin-3 and endothelin-1.

Immunocytochemical studies have demonstrated ET-like immunoreactivity (ET-IR) in human endometrium [63]. Using primary antibody raised in rabbits against the C-terminal heptapeptide of ET-1, ET-1R was localised to vascular endothelium in both endometrium and myometrium, and endometrial glandular epithelium, with the greatest intensity of staining at the endometrial–myometrial junction. All gland cells were stained in secretory tissue, but there was a more heterogeneous picture in proliferative tissue.

Antibody directed against the common C-terminus did not allow determination of the precise nature of the endometrial ET-IR because of cross reactivity between the various ET isoforms. Further immunocytochemical studies were therefore performed using antibodies raised against the uncleaved proETs. Immunoreactivity was detected in endometrium using antibodies against proET-1 and proET-3, but not proET-2, and was again confined to vascular endothelium and glandular epithelium, in a pattern similar to that seen with antibodies against the cleaved peptides [64]. The intensity of staining was less with antibodies directed against the proETs than against the cleaved isoforms and these data would suggest that the endometrial ET is ET-1 or ET-3.

The immunocytochemical localisation of endometrial ET-IR was mirrored by the detection of specific binding sites for iodinated ET-1, ET-2 and ET-3 on endometrial glandular epithelium and vascular endothelium [65]. The density of binding sites for each ET isoform was two- to threefold greater in endometrium than myometrium.

Additional evidence for the presence of the ETs in endometrium was provided by the detection of mRNA for both preproET [66], and uncleaved ET (Schofield JP, Jones DSC, Smith SK, unpublished observations) using the polymerase chain reaction. After enzymatic dispersion and growth to confluence, a single species of preproET mRNA was identified by Northern blot analysis, and a time-dependent release of ET-IR was measured in the supernatant of cultured stromal cells. Discrepancies between these data and the immunocytochemical localisation of ET-IR might be accounted for by differences in methodology. In addition, localisation of peptide using immunocytochemistry does not necessarily imply synthesis of peptide by the same cells. Further studies are required to clarify the sites of production of endometrial ET, but the demonstration of extravascular ET in the endometrium would provide a vasoconstrictor which could be available either before or during menstruation, and which would be released from the sloughing tissues, to act on the abluminal aspect of the spiral arterioles to effect a powerful and sustained contraction of vascular smooth muscle.

The ETs may play a role in the local regulation of PG synthesis. Endothelin-1 stimulated the release of $PGF_{2\alpha}$ from explants of human proliferative endometrium [67]. In addition, the increase in $PGF_{2\alpha}$ was attenuated by the PLA_2 inhibitor quinacrine (Fig. 2.3), and ET-1 stimulated accumulation of inositol phosphates, suggesting the additional activation of PLC (Ahmed AA, Cameron IT, unpublished observations).

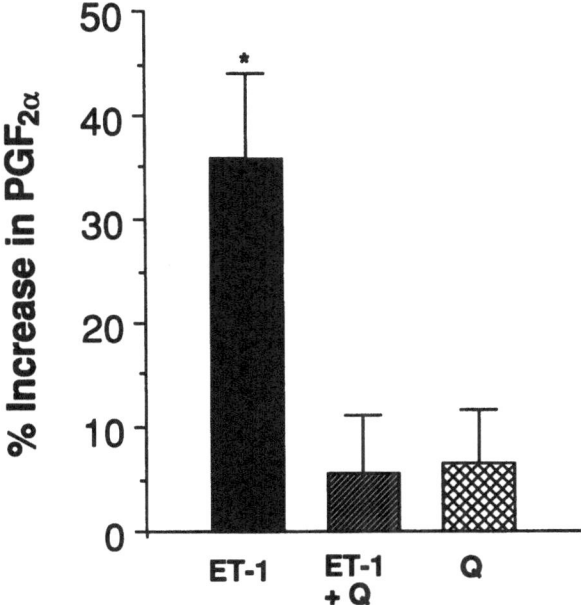

Fig. 2.3. The effect of endothelin-1 (100 nM), either alone, or with the PLA_2 inhibitor quinacrine (Q, 50 μM) on the release of $PGF_{2\alpha}$ from explants of human endometrium in short-term culture. $PGF_{2\alpha}$, measured by radioimmunoassay, is expressed as the percentage increase from control (* $P<0.05$, Mann Whitney U test).

Endometrial Repair

Though vasoconstriction provides the main haemostatic mechanism for the first 24–48 h after the onset of menstruation, blood loss is controlled subsequently by regeneration of the endometrial vessels and surrounding tissues. Prostaglandins may play an important part in endometrial proliferation. In rabbits, inhibition of PG synthesis resulted in an attenuation of DNA turnover, which was reversed by the addition of $PGF_{2\alpha}$, and the stimulation of proliferation by $PGF_{2\alpha}$ was itself inhibited by PGE_2 [68,69].

In addition to a direct role, the PGs have been shown to interact with other mediators of endometrial proliferation. Recent studies have shown that epidermal growth factor (EGF), besides stimulating proliferation in a variety of cell types in vitro, can replace oestradiol in the stimulation of vaginal and uterine growth and differentiation in rat and mouse models [70]. That EGF may play a similar role in the human uterus is supported by the demonstration of mRNA and immunoreactivity for the peptide in endometrium [71,72]. Epidermal growth factor stimulated PGI_2 production by cultured aortic smooth muscle cells [73], whereas in endometrium it augmented the release of PGE_2 [74]. The effect of EGF was further augmented after pretreatment of endometrial cells with oestradiol, and was abolished by the PLA_2 inhibitor lipocortin.

In relation to vascular repair, angiogenin, a 14 kDa protein with sequence homology to pancreatic ribonuclease, stimulated endothelial PGI_2 production by activating PLA_2 [75]. Earlier studies had demonstrated a direct angiogenic action of PGE_1 and PGE_2, but not PGA_2, $PGF_{2\alpha}$, PGI_2 or thromboxane B_2 [76,77]. A role for the PGs in angiogenesis could provide an additional mechanism whereby these compounds could contribute to the control of menstrual loss. However, although the angiogenic activity of adipocytes and sarcoma-producing fibroblasts was dependent on PGs [78], further work is required to determine the precise role of the PGs in endometrial angiogenesis.

Other Paracrine Interactions

The various functions of the endometrium, including the process of menstruation and subsequent tissue regeneration, appear to be controlled by a network of paracrine mechanisms [8,79]. Although this will not be reviewed further here, it should be emphasised that these mechanisms are not independent of one another, but exhibit complex interactions. The relationship between the PGs and the ETs or EGF has been outlined above. Other systems known to interact with AA metabolism in the endometrium include the cytokines, the interferon family and platelet-activating factor [80–83].

Conclusion

Though the morphological events occurring at menstruation have been well characterised, the precise underlying mechanisms are less clearly understood.

There is good evidence that the PGs play an important role in uterine haemostasis, but it is likely that the products of the AA cascade are only one of a variety of paracrine mechanisms affecting this aspect of endometrial function. A better understanding of the factors controlling normal blood loss should lead to improvements in the clinical management of women with disorders of menstruation.

Acknowledgements. I thank Mrs Shashi Rattan for technical assistance, and the East Anglian Regional Health Authority for financial support.

References

1. Office of Population Censuses and Surveys. Hospital in patient statistics, 1985. London: Her Majesty's Stationery Office, 1987; 848.
2. Bunker J, McPherson K, Henneman PL. Elective hysterectomy. In: Bunker J, Barnes BA, Mosteller F, eds. Costs, risks and benefits of surgery. Oxford: Oxford University Press, 1977; 262–76.
3. Dicker RC, Greenspan JR, Strauss LT et al. Complications of abdominal and vaginal hysterectomy among women of reproductive age in the United States. Am J Obstet Gynecol 1982; 144:841–8.
4. Fraser IS, Michie EA, Wide L, Baird DT. Pituitary gonadotrophins and ovarian function in adolescent dysfunctional uterine bleeding. J Clin Endocrinol Metab 1973; 37:407–14.
5. Van Look PFA, Lothian H, Hunter WM, Michie EA, Baird DT. Hypothalamic–pituitary–ovarian function in perimenopausal women. Clin Enocrinol 1977; 7:13–31.
6. Cameron IT, Dysfunctional uterine bleeding. Bailliere's Clinical Obstet Gynaecol 1989; 3:315–27.
7. Hourihan HM, Sheppard BL, Brosens IA. Endometrial hemostasis. In: D'Arcangues C, Fraser IS, Newton JR, Odlind V, eds. Contraception and mechanisms of endometrial bleeding. Cambridge: Cambridge University Press, 1990; 95–116.
8. Findlay JK, Salamonsen LA. Paracrine regulation of implantation and uterine function. Bailliere's Clinical Obstet Gynaecol 1991; 5:117–31.
9. Markee JE. Menstruation in intraocular endometrial transplants in the rhesus monkey. Contrib Embryol 1940; 28:219–308.
10. Wester J, Sixma JJ, Gueze JJ, Van der Veen J. Morphology of the early haemostasis in human skin wounds. Lab Invest 1978; 39:298–311.
11. Christaens GCML, Sixma JJ, Haspels AA. Morphology of haemostasis in menstrual endometrium. Br J Obstet Gynaecol 1980; 87:425–39.
12. Christaens GCML, Sixma JJ, Haspels AA. Haemostasis in menstrual endometrium: a review. Obstet Gynecol Surv 1982; 37:281–303.
13. Von Euler US. Zur kenntis der pharmakologischen wirkungen von nativsekreten und extracten mannlicher accessorischer geschlechtsdrusen. Arch Exp Pathol Pharmacol 1934; 175:78–84.
14. Pickles VR. A plain muscle stimulant in the menstruum. Nature 1957; 180:1198–9.
15. Pickles VR, Hall WJ, Best FA, Smith GN. Prostaglandins in endometrium and menstrual fluid from normal and dysmenorrhoeic subjects. J Obstet Gynaecol Br Cmwlth 1965; 72:185–92.
16. Hagenfeldt K. The role of prostaglandins and allied substances in uterine haemostasis. Contraception 1987; 36:23–35.
17. Smith SK. Prostaglandins and growth factors in the endometrium. Bailliere's Clin Obstet Gynaecol 1989; 3:249–70.
18. Gurpide E, Schatz F, Markiewicz L. Steroid effects on endometrial prostaglandin production. In: D'Arcangues C, Fraser IS, Newton JR, Odlind V, eds. Contraception and mechanisms of endometrial bleeding. Cambridge: Cambridge University Press, 1990; 267–78.
19. Van Eijkeren MA, Christiaens GCML, Sixma JJ, Haspels AA. Menorrhagia: a review. Obstet Gynecol Survey 1989; 44:421–9.

20. Bonney RC. Measurement of phospholipase A_2 activity in human endometrium during the menstrual cycle. J Endocrinol 1985; 107:183–9.
21. Bonney RC, Franks S. Phospholipase C activity in human endometrium: its significance in endometrial pathology. Clin Endocrinol 1987; 27:307–20.
22. Lapetina EG. Regulation of arachidonic acid production: role of phospholipase C and A_2. Trends Pharmacol Sci 1982; 115–18.
23. Van Voorhis BJ, Huetter PC, Clark MR, Hill JA. Immunohistochemical localization of prostaglandin H synthase in the female reproductive tract and endometriosis. Am J Obstet Gynecol 1990; 163:57–62.
24. Ylikorkala O, Makila U-M. Prostacyclin and thromboxane in gynecology and obstetrics. Am J Obstet Gynecol 1985; 152:318–29.
25. Chan WY, Hill JC. Determination of menstrual prostaglandin levels in non-dysmenorrhoeic and dysmenorrhoeic subjects. Prostaglandins 1978; 15:365–75.
26. Lumsden MA, Kelly RW, Baird DT. Is prostaglandin $F_{2\alpha}$ involved in the increased myometrial contractility of primary dysmenorrhoea? Prostaglandins 1983; 25:683–92.
27. Rees MCP, Anderson ABM, Demers LM, Turnbull AC. Prostaglandins in menstrual fluid in menorrhagia and dysmenorrhoea. Br J Obstet Gynaecol 1984; 91:673–80.
28. Csapo AI, Mocsary P, Nagy T, Kaihola HL. The efficacy and acceptability of the "prostaglandin impact" in inducing complete abortion during the second week after the missed menstrual period. Prostaglandins 1973; 3:125–39.
29. Brenneke SP, Castle BM, Demers LM, Turnbull AC. Maternal plasma prostaglandin E_2 metabolite levels during human pregnancy and parturition. Br J Obstet Gynaecol 1985; 92:345–9.
30. Downie J, Poyser NL, Wunderlich M. Levels of prostaglandins in human endometrium during the normal menstrual cycle. J Physiol 1974; 236:465–72.
31. Green K, Hagenfeldt K. Prostaglandins in the human endometrium. Gas chromatographic–mass spectrophotometric quantitation before and after IUD insertion. Am J Obstet Gynecol 1975; 122:611–14.
32. Maathuis JB, Kelly RW. Concentrations of prostaglandin $F_{2\alpha}$ and E_2 in the endometrium throughout the human menstrual cycle, after the administration of clomiphene or an oestrogen–progestogen pill and in early pregnancy. J Endocrinol 1978; 77:361–71.
33. Abel MH, Baird DT. The effect of 17-β-estradiol and progesterone on prostaglandin production by human endometrium maintained in organ culture. Endocrinology 1980; 106:1599–606.
34. Peek MJ, Fraser IS, Phillips CA, Resta TM, Blackwell PM, Markham R. The measurement of human endometrial prostaglandin production. A comparison of two in vitro methods. Prostaglandins 1985; 29:3–18.
35. Demers LM, Halbert DR, Jones DE, Fontana J. Prostaglandin F levels in endometrial jet wash specimens during the normal menstrual cycle. Prostaglandins 1975; 10:1057–65.
36. Jordan VC, Pokoly TB. Steroid and prostaglandin relations during the menstrual cycle. Obstet Gynecol 1977; 49:449–53.
37. Levitt MJ, Tobon H, Josimovich JB. Prostaglandin content of human endometrium. Fertil Steril 1975; 26:296–300.
38. Schatz F, Markiewicz L, Gurpide E. Effects of estriol on $PGF_{2\alpha}$ output by cultures of human endometrium and endometrial cells. J Steroid Biochem 1984; 20:999–1003.
39. Schatz F, Markiewicz L, Barg P, Gurpide E. In-vitro effects of ovarian steroids on prostaglandin $F_{2\alpha}$ output by human endometrium and endometrial epithelial cells. J Clin Endocrinol Metab 1985; 61:361–7.
40. Markiewicz L, Schatz F, Barg P, Gurpide E. Prostaglandin $F_{2\alpha}$ output by human endometrium under superfusion and organ culture conditions. J Steroid Biochem 1985; 22:231–5.
41. Tsang BK, Ooi TC. Prostaglandin secretion by human endometrium in vitro. Am J Obstet Gynecol 1982; 142:626–33.
42. Leaver A, Richmond DH. The effect of oxytocin, estrogen, calcium ionophore A23187 and hydrocortisone on prostaglandin $F_{2\alpha}$ and 6-oxo prostaglandin $F_{1\alpha}$ production by cultured human endometrial and myometrial explants. Prostaglandins Leukotrienes Med 1984; 13:179–96.
43. Green K. Determination of prostaglandins in body fluids and tissues. Acta Obstet Gynaecol Scand 1979; 87(suppl):15–20.
44. Peek MJ, Norman TM, Morgan CC, Fraser IS, Markham R. Trauma-induced human endometrial prostaglandin concentrations. Prostaglandins 1987; 34:919–25.
45. Poyser NL. Tissue levels of prostaglandins and what do they mean? Studies on the guinea-pig uterus. Prostaglandins 1988; 36:645–53.
46. Cameron IT, Leask R, Kelly RW, Baird DT. Endometrial prostaglandins in women with abnormal menstrual bleeding. Prostaglandins Leukotrienes Med 1987; 29:249–57.

47. Smith SK, Abel MH, Kelly RW, Baird DT. Prostaglandin synthesis in the endometrium of women with ovular dysfunctional uterine bleeding. Br J Obstet Gynaecol 1981; 88:434–42.
48. Rees MCP, Anderson ABM, Demers LM, Turnbull AC. Endometrial and myometrial prostaglandin release during the menstrual cycle in relation to menstrual blood loss. J Clin Endocrinol Metab 1984; 58:813–18.
49. Elderling JA, Nay MG, Hobert LM, Longcope C, McCracken JA. Hormonal regulation of prostaglandin production by rhesus monkey endometrium. J Clin Endocrinol Metab 1990; 71:596–604.
50. Wilson T, Liggins GC, Aimer GP, Watkins EJ. The effect of progesterone on the release of arachidonic acid from human endometrial cells stimulated by histamine. Prostaglandins 1986; 31:343–60.
51. Gurpide E, Markiewicz L, Schatz F, Hirata F. Lipocortin output by human endometrium in vitro. J Clin Endocrinol Metab 1986; 63:162–6.
52. Wiqvist N, Bygdeman M, Kirton K. Non-steroidal infertility agents in the female. In: Diczfalusy E, Borell B, eds. Control of human fertility. Nobel symposium 15, 1971; 137–49.
53. Turksoy RN, Safaii HS. Immediate effect of prostaglandin $F_{2\alpha}$ during the luteal phase of the menstrual cycle. Fertil Steril 1975; 26:634–7.
54. Kelly RW, Lumsden MA, Abel MH, Baird DT. The relationship between menstrual blood loss and prostaglandin production in the human: evidence for increased availability of arachidonic acid in women suffering from menorrhagia. Prostaglandins Leukotrienes Med 1984; 16:69–78.
55. Anderson ABM, Haynes PJ, Guillebaud J, Turnbull AC. Reduction of menstrual blood loss by prostaglandin synthetase inhibitors. Lancet 1976; i:774–6.
56. Cameron IT, Leask R, Kelly RW, Baird DT. The effects of danazol, mefenamic acid, norethisterone and a progesterone-impregnated coil, on endometrial prostaglandin concentrations in women with menorrhagia. Prostaglandins 1987; 34:99–110.
57. Bergqvist A, Rybo G. Treatment of menorrhagia with intrauterine release of progesterone. Br J Obstet Gynaecol 1983; 90:255–8.
58. Maigaard S, Forman A, Andersson K-E. Different responses to prostaglandin $F_{2\alpha}$ and E_2 in human extra- and intramyometrial arteries. Prostaglandins 1985; 30:599–607.
59. Cameron IT, Davenport AP. Endothelins in reproduction. Rep Med Review 1992; in press.
60. Yanagisawa M, Kurihara H, Kimura S et al. A novel potent vasoconstrictor peptide produced by vascular endothelial cells. Nature 1988; 332:411–15.
61. Inoue A, Yanagisawa M, Kimura S et al. The human endothelin family: three structurally and pharmacologically distinct isopeptides predicted by three separate genes. Proc Natl Acad Sci USA 1989; 86:2863–7.
62. Fried G, Samuelson U. Endothelin and neuropeptide Y are vasoconstrictors in human uterine blood vessels. Am J Obstet Gynecol 1991; 164:1330–6.
63. van Papendorp CL, Cameron IT, Davenport AP, Brown MJ, Smith SK. Endothelin-like immunoreactivity in human endometrium. J Endocrinol 1991; 129 (suppl):64.
64. van Papendorp CL, Cameron IT, Davenport AP, Brown MJ, Smith SK. Endothelin-like immunoreactivity (ET-IR) in human endometrium. J Reprod Fertil 1991; 7 (abstract series): 40.
65. Davenport AP, Cameron IT, Smith SK, Brown MJ. Binding sites for iodinated endothelin-1, endothelin-2 and endothelin-3 demonstrated on uterine glandular epithelial cells by quantitative high-resolution autoradiography. J Endocrinol 1991; 129:149–54.
66. Economos K, Nagai K, Hersh LB, MacDonald PC, Casey ML. Endothelin expression in the human endometrium: potential role in menstruation. Soc Gynecol Invest 1991; abstract 404:300.
67. Cameron IT, Davenport AP, Brown MJ, Smith SK. Endothelin-1 stimulates prostaglandin $F_{2\alpha}$ release from human endometrium. Prostaglandins Leukotrienes EFA 1991; 42:155–7.
68. Orlicky DJ, Lieberman R, Gerschenson LE. Prostaglandin $F_{2\alpha}$ and E_1 regulation of proliferation in primary cultures of rabbit endometrial cells. J Cell Physiol 1986; 127:55–60.
69. Orlicky DJ, Lieberman R, Williams C, Gerchenson LE. Requirement for prostaglandin $F_{2\alpha}$ in 17β-estradiol stimulation of DNA synthesis in rabbit endometrial cultures. J Cell Physiol 1987; 130:292–300.
70. Nelson KG, Takahashi T, Bossert NL, Walmer DK, McLachlan JA. Epidermal growth factor replaces estrogen in the stimulation of female genital-tract growth and differentiation. Proc Natl Acad Sci USA 1991; 88:21–4.
71. Haining REB, Schofield JP, Jones DSC, Rajput-Williams J, Smith SK. Identification of mRNA for epidermal growth factor and transforming growth factor-α present in low copy number in human endometrium and decidua using reverse transcriptase–polymerase chain reaction. J Mol Endocrinol 1991; 6:207–14.
72. Haining REB, Cameron IT, van Papendorp CL, Davenport AP, Prentice A, Thomas EJ, Smith

SK. Epidermal growth factor in human endometrium: proliferative effects in culture and immunocytochemical localisation in normal and endometriotic tissues. Hum Reprod 1991; 6:1200–5.

73. Blay J, Hollenberg MD. Epidermal growth factor stimulation of prostacylin production by cultured aortic smooth muscle cells: requirement for increased cellular calcium levels. J Cell Physiol 1989; 139:524–30.

74. Ishihara S, Taketani Y, Mizuno M. Effects of epidermal growth factor (EGF) on prostaglandin E_2 synthesis by cultured human endometrial cells. Acta Obstet Gynaecol Jpn 1990; 42:1317–22.

75. Bicknell R, Vallee BL. Angiogenin stimulates endothelial cell prostacyclin secretion by activation of phospholipase A_2. Proc Natl Acad Sci USA 1989; 86:1573–7.

76. Form DM, Auerbach R. PGE_2 and angiogenesis. Proc Soc Exp Biol Med 1983; 172:214–18.

77. Ziche M, Jones J, Gullino P. Role of prostaglandins E_1 and copper in angiogenesis. J Natl Cancer Inst 1982; 69:475–81.

78. Silverman KJ, Lund DP, Zetter BR et al. Angiogenic activity of adipose tissue. Biochem Biophys Res Commun 1988; 153:347–52.

79. Healy DL, Hodgen GD. The endocrinology of human endometrium. Obstet Gynecol Surv 1983; 38:509–30.

80. Tabibzadeh S, Kaffka KL, Satyaswaroop PG, Kilian PL. Interleukin-1 regulation of human endometrial function: presence of IL-1 receptor correlates with IL-1 stimulated prostaglandin E_2 production. J Clin Endocrinol Metab 1990; 70:1000–6.

81. Salamonsen LA, Stuchbery SJ, O'Grady CM, Godkin JD, Findlay JK. Interferon-α mimics effects of ovine trophoblast protein 1 on prostaglandin and protein secretion by ovine endometrial cells in vitro. J Endocrinol 1988; 117:R1–4

82. Mitchell SN, Smith SK. Progesterone and human interferon-α have a different effect on the release of prostaglandin $F_{2\alpha}$ from human endometrium. In: Samuelsson B, Dahlen SE, Fritsch J, Hedqvist P, eds. Advances in prostaglandin, thromboxane, and leukotriene research, vol 21. New York: Raven Press, 1990; 823–6.

83. Alecozay AA, Harper MJK, Schenken RS, Hanahan DJ. Paracrine interactions between platelet-activating factor and prostaglandins in hormonally-treated human luteal phase endometrium in vitro. J Reprod Fertil 1991; 91:301–12.

Discussion

Calder: Menstruation has been described as "the parturition of pregnancy failure" and I think that is an appropriate way of drawing a parallel between this session and later sessions. The man who taught me anatomy described menstruation as "the weeping of the disappointed womb", which is saying much the same thing.

Keirse: Do the prostaglandins that are produced in the amnion have anything whatsoever to do with myometrial contractility?

Kelly: Indirectly yes, but directly perhaps no. They may eventually lead to an increased myometrial contractility by starting off a process of influx of white cells and the changes that they will produce. But actually directly getting through to the myometrium, probably not.

Elder: IL-8 is produced in large amounts by the choriodecidua. Is that under stimulation or is that a basal production?

Kelly: There is a basal production when the cells are put in culture. We suspect this is something to do with the fact that we have disturbed the cells and put them into culture. If they are left in culture for 14 days that basal production drops and production can then be stimulated.

Elder: Can we hear more about the state of knowledge on EIPS?

Kelly: To my knowledge it has not been identified and we still have to bear in mind that it might be some non-specific protein action, which might be mopping up the precursor in the biochemical experiments used to test its activity.

López Bernal: I was interested in the comment about the antioestrogenic effect of RU486. We assayed some placentas we obtained from Ian MacKenzie from women who had received RU486, and P29, an oestrogen-dependent protein, was greatly decreased. What would be the mechanism of action?

Kelly: The mechanism of action is not clear. Challis has recently reported that the endometrial glands in the rabbit respond to an RU-486-like compound – it was a Schering study so it will be a Schering analogue – and this effect is basically on the unoccupied progesterone receptor. The suggestion is that the unoccupied progesterone receptor has itself an action which may be permissive to the role of oestradiol, and occupying that receptor with an antiprogestin removes its permissive action on oestradiol action. So although it is not acting as an antioestrogen its indirect effect is antioestrogenic.

Fraser: A strong case was made for the possible role of interleukins, particularly IL-8, in the release of PGs. Could that be put in perspective with other cytokines that have been tested in this situation, TNF and so forth?

Kelly: TNF and IL-1 are both known to stimulate IL-8 production. Where there is production of IL-1 and TNF, IL-8 would be produced by certain white cell types. It may be an intermediate of the action of IL-1 and TN-F.

I did not mention that in early pregnancy one can get exactly the result one would expect when progesterone is withdrawn. We have evidence that very high levels, 10^{-5}M, will inhibit IL-8 production. High levels may occur within the choriodecidual tissue because progesterone is being produced there and so local concentrations may be very high.

In early studies in the sheep where progesterone was withdrawn by oophorectomy, Staples and co-workers saw an immediate and very marked influx of neutrophils which pervaded through the endometrium of the animal.

Olson: Are there any data describing changes in the IL-8 during gestation or at term?

Kelly: There are no data on IL-8 as far as I know in the reproductive system.

Olson: A question relating to the very interesting work with okadaic acid and the amnion cells. What was the state of those amnion cells? Were they grown in culture to confluence?

Kelly: They were grown to confluence over a period of four or five days.

Olson: We have done biochemical studies on cyclo-oxygenase in amnion cells in culture and find that they lose their cyclo-oxygenase activity with as little as two days of culturing, and in order to make PGs at all from those following that period of time, we have to stimulate cyclo-oxygenase activity. Okadaic acid was not shown in the presence of arachidonic acid. Was it present?

Kelly: It was, but it made no difference. Production was probably maximal with okadaic acid.

Olson: The action of okadaic acid is independent of the presence of free exogenous arachidonic acid?

Kelly: It appears to be in that it is such a massive production. I do not know that production could be higher. It may be saturated in the system, i.e. the production may be maximal. I take the point that it probably has more than one effect.

Olson: Exactly. It must have an effect at the phospholipase and at the cyclo-oxygenase levels.

Kelly: That is right. It would be very nice to know how it could be working on some element in arachidonic acid and on the cyclo-oxygenase.

Olson: Our data with TPA, which are the same as the PMA shown, would suggest that the phorbol ester stimulation of protein kinase C may have a dual action, that is both to release arachidonic acid and to drive the synthesis of cyclo-oxygenase.

I noticed that production of PGs was low in the presence of TPA without arachidonic acid. In our studies – perhaps they were done differently and the time course was different – after a few hours of TPA addition we noticed that there was a slight increase in total PGE output which we attribute to this dual action of the C-kinase.

Kelly: Obviously it does have an effect. In other systems production of PGs is increased in response to TPA, so it must be affecting free arachidonic acid levels as well.

Nathanielsz: To refer to the question about the relevance of fetal membrane PG production, we should not forget that those PGs have access to the fetal endocrine system and there is a lot of interest currently in PG stimulation of fetal pituitary and fetal adrenal.

I for one would slightly disagree with the concept that menstruation is the parturition of the non-pregnant state. There is a fetus there when parturition occurs.

Smith: Can I come back to the question of the antisteroids and how they work and ask about the intracellular roles of the prostaglandins. First, what is the evidence for direct involvement of eicosanoids anywhere in the pathway affecting response elements? Second, there is evidence that both phosphatidic acid and arachidonic acid can affect gut proteins. Is there a view as to how they may explain some of these paradoxes of steroid action when steroid response elements might not be influenced by steroids at all, or are there antisteroids?

Kelly: We unfortunately cannot look for the PGE receptor, or the PGF, or any of the prostaglandin receptors at the moment. If we knew where the receptors were we would know much more about how they worked. However, although we cannot explain what PGF does in several different instances, we can explain its effect on the PI-pathways; it has been shown to stimulate inositol phosphate production.

There is no reason to suggest that PGE acts other than by raising intracellular cyclic AMP levels. I do not think that there is any evidence to suggest otherwise. Certainly, there are those who regard PGE as a paracrine regulator of the white cells, and it may be that a lot of the effects of the prostaglandins are directed towards the white cells. But until we know where the receptors are for these prostaglandins, we are working in the dark.

Lopez-Bernal: A point about the amnion cells. I am not sure whether the FL cells were used. That type of amnion cell does not lose cyclo-oxygenase activity in culture, it retains it almost indefinitely.

Kelly: We did both. We had FL cells and two preparations of amnion from elective sections and the stimulation was there in both, but there was much greater stimulation in the FL cells.

Amy: You discussed the PG metabolism or the potential for PG metabolism in women submitted to C-section before labour, C-section during labour, and women delivering vaginally. Is any conclusion to be drawn from a comparison of these results? I guess these were women that were at a different stage of labour.

I would assume that women delivering vaginally had endometrium taken at delivery, the women who delivered having reached full dilation. Would this mean that the potential for PG metabolism in terms of PG dehydrogenase decreases during labour?

Kelly: It is difficult to say. This tissue, this endometrium, the decidua that has gone through the process of labour, has obviously been subjected to hypoxia and trauma, and so it is possible that the enzyme level would be reduced. That is certainly the suggestion put forward in the paper by Lynette Casey. But I still think that it is possible that there may be some change in dehydrogenase.

John Challis' group (Cheung et al. 1990; reference 26, page 13) have shown that the metabolic capacity within the chorion is regionally distributed, so that it is not all present in one area. So it is possible that there may be a local change in dehydrogenase but it not reflected in the changes we see when we take a big section of tissue and measure its total enzyme content.

Olson: Is there any change in cyclo-oxygenase activity in the endometrium during the cycle?

Cameron: In terms of data looking at immunocytochemical localisation, there was a suggestion that cyclo-oxygenase activity would be greatest in the second half of the cycle. However, one of the problems with using immunocytochemistry quantitatively is that it may not be just that there is less enzyme there, it may be something to do with the binding of the colour itself. It does appear that oestradiol stimulates cyclo-oxygenase activity.

Olson: There is evidence in the sheep – immunocytochemical evidence from about ten years or more ago – showing that there is a change in immunocyto-chemical staining during the luteal phase of the cycle in sheep.

Cameron: The problem with that is that immunocytochemistry cannot be used as a quantitative technique. One must be very careful about implying changes due to something that is purely qualitative.

Olson: I noticed the focus on the phospholipase.

Cameron: That is the crucial enzyme in terms of releasing the arachidonic acid, which can then be transported down the cascade mechanism. If there is a deficiency or a limiting amount of cyclo-oxygenase that would make an important point, but the key enzyme in terms of control is the phospholipase.

Keirse: There was a slide showing PG endoperoxide in the endometrium with an arrow pointing to the myometrium. David Baird has been promoting the idea that endoperoxides could be formed in the endometrium and could then travel into the myometrium, be taken up by cells and utilised by the cyclo-oxygenase system by prostacylcin synthetase. Does Dr Cameron believe that that happens?

Cameron: Whether I believe it happens is immaterial. It is supported by three independent sets of data, from initially Margaret Abel and R. W. Kelly, then work by S. K. Smith looking at women with and without menorrhagia, and then a subsequent study R. W. Kelly and I did together. The data showed that combining endometrium and myometrium seemed to increase the capacity of the myometrium to produce prostacyclin.

Keirse: I have no doubt about that. Mixing all kinds of things together is always supposed to work better. The question is whether in vivo one could envisage a system by which endoperoxides would leave the endometrial cell, travel to the myometrium and would there be taken up and utilised by prostacyclin synthetase. I just do not believe that and I cannot see it.

Cameron: I suppose that this is happening at the time of menstruation when the normal cell barriers are broken down, so I suppose it is a possibility. I do take it that endoperoxides are very short-lived intermediates, and that would be an argument against that concept.

Chapter 3

Prostanoids and Menorrhagia

C. M. P. Rees

Introduction

The volume of menstrual blood lost is important to women's health since excessive bleeding may lead to iron deficiency anaemia and may ultimately necessitate hysterectomy. Menorrhagia accounts for one-third of all hysterectomies performed in England and Wales and is the commonest indication for such surgery [1]. It is one of the commonest reasons for consultations to general practitioners, being in the top ten [2]. It is also the second commonest cause for referral for hospital treatment for all ages and both sexes causing a disproportionate demand on health service resources [3].

Menstrual blood loss (MBL) has a skewed distribution, with a mean of 35 ml and a 90th percentile of 80 ml, as found in the classic study by Hallbert et al. [4]. MBL is considered to be excessive if greater than 80 ml: without treatment such a loss leads to iron deficiency anaemia and constitutes objective menorrhagia. The range of blood loss is vast, varying from as low as 2 ml to as high as 1600 ml (Rees, unpublished observations).

Any examination of MBL control must include objective blood loss measurements. It is a vital assessment since women are unreliable judges of their menstrual blood loss [5]. Only 38% of women complaining of menorrhagia have measured losses greater than 80 ml [6]. MBL can be measured easily by the alkaline haematin method of Hallberg and Nilsson [7].

Although menorrhagia may be due to systemic or pelvic disease, no pathology is found in 50% of cases and most women with menorrhagia have normal ovulatory cycles [5,8]. Therefore in the absence of overt disease, local uterine mechanisms appear to be important in the control of menstrual blood loss [9]. Endometrial arteries of menstruating species are unusual in that they are profusely coiled as they run through the tissue and also that they change during

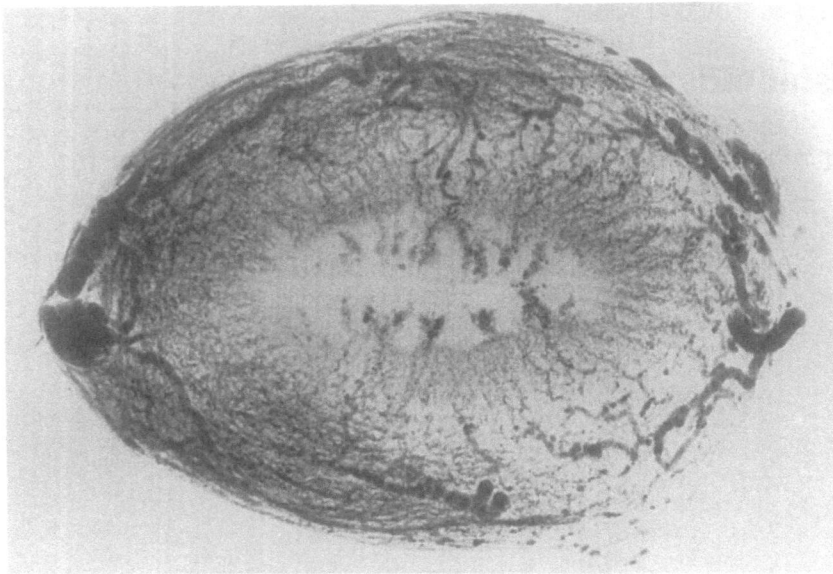

Fig. 3.1. Photomicrograph of an X-ray of a uterine slice where the arterial vasculature has been injected with barium sulphate and gelatine during the luteal phase.

the menstrual cycle. These arterioles undergo profound vasoconstriction which starts 4–24 h before menstruation and lasts until the end of menstrual bleeding. Bleeding results from relaxation of individual arterioles (Fig. 3.1) [10]. Excessive bleeding is probably related to abnormal control of the endometrial vasculature.

Of the pathways thought to play a major role in the process of menstruation the evidence for altered prostaglandin (PG) synthesis is the most compelling. The association of PGs with menstruation was first reported in 1965 by Pickles et al. [11], who found high concentrations of $PGF_{2\alpha}$ and PGE_2 in endometrium and menstrual fluid. Later, Wiqvist et al. [12] demonstrated that administration of $PGF_{2\alpha}$ to women during the luteal phase resulted in menstrual bleeding.

The first suggestion that abnormally increased uterine prostaglandin levels were involved in menorrhagia came from the observation in 1976 that inhibitors of prostaglandin synthesis reduced excessive menstrual bleeding [13]. In the same year Wilman et al. reported elevated endometrial concentrations of both $PGF_{2\alpha}$ and PGE_2 during the menstrual cycle in women complaining of heavy periods [14].

Since then it has been shown that the uterus has a significant capacity to produce prostaglandins and these agents have important effects on haemostasis. Thus prostanoids are thought to play a key role in the aetiology of menorrhagia.

Prostanoids, Synthesis and Haemostasis

Prostanoids are not stored in cells, but are rapidly synthesized once the substrate fatty acid precursor, arachidonic acid, becomes available to the appropriate synthetic enzymes. Arachidonic acid is not present in the free state within cells but is bound in ester linkage to phospholipids: phosphatidylcholine, phosphatidylethanolamine and phosphatidylinositol. Before PG biosynthesis can begin free arachidonic acid must be liberated from cellular phospholipids by the action of phospholipases (A_2, C and D) [15]. Membrane pathways involved in coupling hormone receptors to generation of intracellular signals such as PGs involve the action of a family of GTP-binding proteins, the G-proteins [16–18].

Once released, free arachidonic acid is metabolised through a series of pathways: the cyclo-oxygenase to prostaglandins and 5-lipoxygenase to leukotrienes have both been studied in human uterine tissues [19,20]. The 12-lipoxygenase pathway has been identified but not yet examined in detail [19].

In PG synthesis arachidonic acid is converted into the endoperoxide intermediates PGG_2 and PGH_2 through the action of the cyclo-oxygenase and peroxidase enzymes. Cyclo-oxygenase is present mainly in the superficial and glandular epithelium of the endometrium [21]. PGH_2 and PGG_2 are rapidly converted into the primary prostaglandins $PGF_{2\alpha}$, PGE_2 and PGD_2. PGH_2 is also converted into either thromboxane (TXA_2) or prostacyclin (PGI_2) through the action of thromboxane and prostacyclin synthetase respectively. The principal endometrial PG products are $PGF_{2\alpha}$ and PGE_2 with PGD_2, PGI_2 and TXA_2 in lesser amounts [19,22,23]. Endometrial PG production changes throughout the menstrual cycle being higher in the luteal phase and menstruation than in the follicular phase [23,24]. Myometrial synthetic capacity is less than that of the endometrium: there the main product is PGI_2 and levels do not change during the cycle [19,22,23].

The first step in leukotriene synthesis is oxygenation at C-5 by the 5-lipoxygenase enzyme to form 5-hydroperoxyeicosatetraenoic acid which is then converted into leukotriene A_4 (LTA_4) by dehydration. This unstable allelic epoxide (LTA_4) is either hydrolysed to form leukotriene B_4 (LTB_4) or conjugated with glutathione to form leukotriene C_4 (LTC_4). In turn, LTC_4 is metabolised by γ-glutamyl transpeptidase to leukotriene D_4 (LTD_4) and then by cysteinyl glycinase to leukotriene E_4 (LTE_4). Release of LTC_4, D_4 and E_4 has been detected in human uterine tissues, being higher in endometrium than myometrium [20]. Furthermore, endometrial release varies throughout the menstrual cycle with the highest levels found during the luteal phase and menstruation.

Individual PGs have different effects on haemostasis and thus are differently involved in the control of menstrual bleeding. PGE_2, PGD_2 and PGI_2 cause vasodilatation whereas $PGF_{2\alpha}$ and TXA_2 cause vasoconstriction. Platelet aggregation is promoted by TXA_2 and inhibited by PGD_2 and PGI_2 [25]. Thus PGs are important candidates for the control of menstrual blood loss.

Prostanoid Levels in Menorrhagia

Studies in relation to MBL have examined PGs both in menstrual fluid collected during menstruation and in uterine tissues collected throughout the menstrual cycle. Most include objective MBL measurement.

The levels of PGs in menstrual fluid suggest increased uterine $PGF_{2\alpha}$ and PGE_2 production in menorrhagia during menstruation itself [26]. Studies of endometrial and myometrial PGs have principally used tissues collected at hysterectomy performed mainly at other times during the menstrual cycle. In general PG production by uterine tissues collected throughout the menstrual cycle from menorrhagic women is not increased and does not correlate with MBL [23]. However, in a limited number of samples obtained during the first 2 days of menstruation when the largest volume of menstrual flow occurs, the data are suggestive of a possible relationship between the volume of menstrual blood loss and $PGF_{2\alpha}$, PGE_2 and 6-keto-$PGF_{1\alpha}$ release by endometrium and myometrium [23].

The original proposition of a shift in endometrial synthesising capacity towards PGE_2 in menorrhagic women [27] has not been confirmed subsequently [23,28].

Prostacyclin, the principal myometrial PG product [19,22,23], has also been examined in relation to MBL. Increased production of 6-keto-$PGF_{1\alpha}$ by endometrium and myometrium in menorrhagia has been found only during menstruation [23,29]. However, endometrium from women with menorrhagia appears to be more effective than endometrium from women with normal MBL in enhancing production of the prostacyclin metabolite 6-keto-$PGF_{1\alpha}$ in control preparations of myometrium [30]. In addition prostacyclin is the principal PG product produced by leiomyomas, and may therefore account for the association of these lesions with menorrhagia [31].

The leukotrienes have been examined in relation to menorrhagia, but no correlation was found between leukotriene release in either endometrium or myometrium and menstrual blood loss [20].

Control of Prostanoid Biosynthesis

The increased production of prostaglandin and the suggestion that there may be increased availability of arachidonic acid in uterine tissues from menorrhagic women are leading to studies where control mechanisms are being evaluated [32]. The rate-limiting step in PG biosynthesis is the production of arachidonic acid from phospholipids. The concentration of free arachidonic acid within resting cells is unknown, but is believed to be maintained at low levels. An increase in the release of free arachidonic acid from phospholipids occurs in response to receptor stimulation, but the net concentration attained is unknown. In many tissues, including the uterus, phospholipase activation can involve G proteins and calcium.

The mechanisms usually considered for the control of free arachidonic acid levels within cells involve activation of phospholipase A_2 and the direct generation of arachidonic acid, or activation of phospholipase C and the production of arachidonic acid from diacylglycerol. Arachidonic acid can also be generated by phospholipase A_1 and phospholipase D. Recent work has shown that in several cell types, receptor activation of phospholipase D or of a phosphatidylcholine-specific phospholipase C may be important for the production of diacylglycerol which can then activate protein kinase C and also be metabolised to arachidonic acid. Furthermore, protein kinase C may be involved in the reacylation (reincorporation) of arachidonic acid. It has now been shown that increases in the synthesis of prostaglandins can also occur in some tissues due to metabolism of arachidonic acid produced from low-density lipoproteins following receptor-mediated uptake, but this pathway has received limited attention in the uterus [15].

Finally the molecular control of cyclo-oxygenase can now be studied since its sequence is known [33,34].

G Proteins

The heterotrimic guanine nucleotide-binding proteins (G proteins) act as switches that regulate information-processing circuits connecting cell surface receptors to a variety of effectors. G proteins are present in all cells and control metabolic, humoral, neural and developmental functions. Signal transducing G proteins occur in two forms: the small G proteins that are generally found as single polypeptides composed of about 200 amino acids and the heterotrimic G proteins that are made up of alpha, beta and gamma subunits. The heterotrimic G proteins are associated with signal transduction from cell surface receptors. The alpha subunit binds to guanine nucleotides, and the beta and gamma subunits are always tightly associated. Different G proteins are most readily distinguished by their alpha subunits, though there are also more subtle structural and functional differences in some beta and gamma subunits. G proteins are derived from a large gene family. At present the family is known to contain at least 16 different genes that encode the alpha subunit of the heterotrimer, four that encode beta subunits and multiple genes encoding gamma subunits [16,17].

Receptor G protein-mediated signal transduction involves the following process. Interaction of a G protein with an activated receptor promotes the exchange of GDP, bound to the alpha subunit, for GTP and the subsequent dissociation of the alpha GTP complex with the beta/gamma heterodimer. A single receptor can activate multiple G protein molecules, thus amplifying the ligand binding event. The GTP-bound alpha subunit and probably the free beta/gamma subunit may interact with effector proteins that further amplify the signal. Such effectors include ion channels and enzymes that generate second messengers. Termination of the signal occurs when GTP bound by the alpha subunit is hydrolysed to GDP by GTPase activity of the alpha subunit. The alpha subunit then reassociates with the beta/gamma complex. The situation has recently become more complex as it is becoming evident that G proteins, like receptors, can be an important site for regulation of cellular sensitivity to extracellular signals. Prolonged exposure to agonists for G protein coupled receptors has been shown in some tissues to cause down regulation of G proteins [35].

G proteins and their alpha subunits were initially classified according to their sensitivity to cholera and pertussis toxins [36]. With the advances in cloning and sequencing techniques applied to alpha subunits, they can now be classified according to amino acid sequence similarity [16]. Alpha subunits can now be divided into four classes: G_s, G_1, G_q and G_{12}. It has been known for several years that G proteins are coupled to phospholipases A_2, C and D [37–41], but until recently there was little information about the type of alpha subunit involved. Results within the past year point to the involvement of G_q in pertussis-resistant coupling to phospholipase C activation [18]. A novel 42 kDa protein that activates phospholipase C in a pertussis-resistant manner has been partially purified. The 42 kDa G protein has amino acid sequence identity with the $G\alpha_q$ clone. It specifically activates the beta isotype of phospholipase C but not the gamma or delta forms. Thus G_q is involved in coupling one type of phospholipase C to a specific set of receptor subtypes. At present the type of G protein involved with other phospholipases is not known [16].

G proteins appear to be involved in uterine prostaglandin production. In guinea-pig endometrium, short-term treatment with sodium fluoride stimulated PG production although cholera and pertussis toxins did not [42]. In guinea-pig myometrium, G protein activity is coupled to phosphoinositide phospholipase C [43]. GTP gamma S and sodium fluoride stimulate inositol production and the effect of the former is inhibited by GDP beta S. A G protein responsive system also seems to be present in human uterine tissues and GTP gamma S causes stimulation in a dose-dependent manner (Maslen, Jones and Rees, unpublished observations).

Phospholipases

Phospholipase A_2 and C activity have been detected in uterine tissues [44,45]. Four different types of phospholipase C have been identified by molecular cloning studies in mammalian tissues, all of which are single polypeptides, the products of discrete genes (alpha, beta gamma, delta) [46]. Two novel human endometrial phosphatidylinositol phospholipase C products, probably the result of alternate splicing of the gene have been cloned and sequenced [47]. The sequences are similar to those known for rat phospholipase $C\alpha$. The nucleotide sequence of human non-pancreatic phospholipase A_2 is also known [48,49]. Phospholipase A_2 expression has recently been detected in non-pregnant human uterine tissues (Spencer, Robson and Rees, unpublished observations).

Both phospholipase A_2 and C activity in endometrium have been exmained in relation to menorrhagia. Activity of phospholipase C was found to be increased in women with menorrhagia, whereas that of phospholipase A_2 was not [50].

Cyclo-oxygenase

The nucleotide sequence of cyclo-oxygenase in human and other species (sheep, mouse) is not known [33,34,51,52]. Initially a single mRNA species of 2.8 kb was found. Subsequently other transcripts have been detected: 4.0 kb in sheep tracheal mucosa and 4.1 kb in Rous sarcoma-induced chicken embryo fibroblasts [53,54]. Two transcripts have also recently been described in human endo-metrium [55]. In addition it appears that mRNA for cyclo-oxygenase can occur in two forms: translatable and non-translatable. Conversion into the non-translatable form can be induced by glucocorticoids and reversed by EGF. Therefore, there is a potential to increase understanding of the control of prostaglandin biosynthesis in uterine tissues in menorrhagia [56].

Prostaglandin Receptors

Prostaglandins are thought to act through receptors in the cell membrane. In human uterine tissues, PGE_2 receptors predominate over $PGF_{2\alpha}$ receptors and are found principally in the myometrium [57,58]. Increased concentrations of PGE receptors are present in myometrial specimens obtained from menorrhagic women, and there is a direct correlation between PGE receptor concentration and MBL [57]. Fenamates such as mefenamic acid and sodium meclofenamate are used to reduce menstrual blood loss [13]. Recently, a dual mode of action has been demonstrated for fenamates which is not shared by other inhibitors of PG synthesis. In addition to reducing PG synthesis they also inhibit binding of PGE to its receptor, an effect which may contribute to their efficacy in the treatment of menorrhagia (Fig. 3.2) [59,60]. Furthermore, meclofenamate also affects activation of the PGE receptor in that it inhibits PGE_2-stimulated cAMP generation in human myometrium (Fig. 3.3) [60].

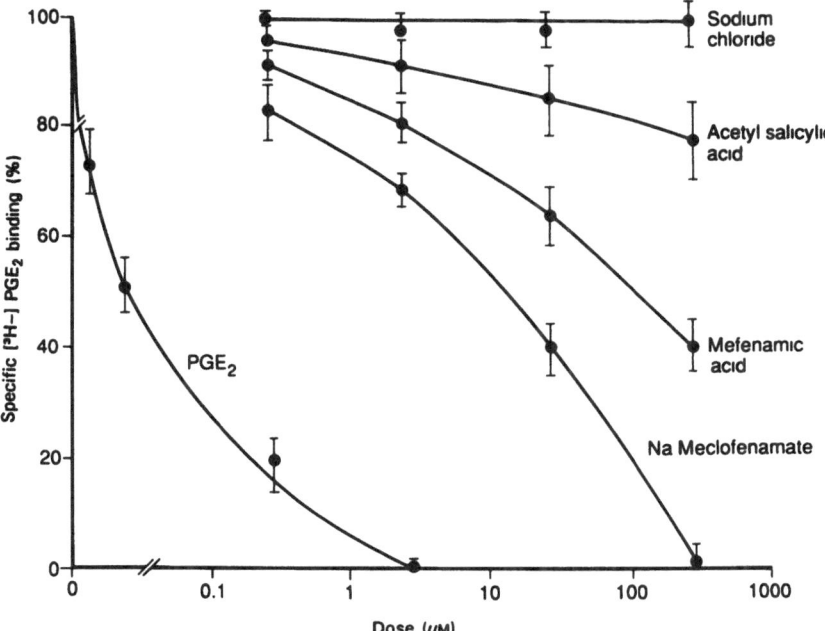

Fig. 3.2. Inhibition of $[^3H]PGE_2$ binding to membrane preparations of human myometrium. Reproduced with permission from Rees et al. [59].

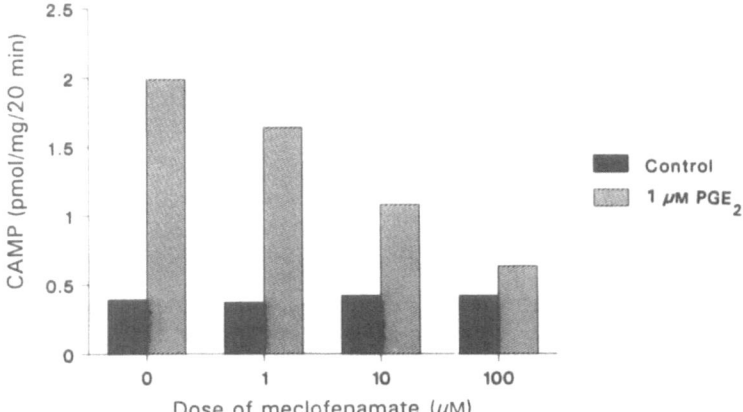

Fig. 3.3. Inhibition of PGE$_2$-stimulated cAMP generation in human myometrium by sodium meclofenamate.

Inhibitors of Prostaglandin Biosynthesis and Menorrhagia

Despite a lack of understanding of detailed biochemical mechanisms, the implication of excessive PG levels in menorrhagia has led to the use of PG synthetase inhibitors in the treatment of this disorder. The effectiveness of these agents was first demonstrated by Anderson et al. in 1976 [13]: mefenamic acid reduced MBL from a pretreatment mean of 119 ml to 60 ml. These findings have been confirmed in other studies [61]. Furthermore, mefenamic acid can be used long term, since follow-up 12–15 months after commencement of treatment showed continued efficacy [61]. Other PG synthetase inhibitors such as ibuprofen also reduce MBL [29].

Conclusions

The recent understanding of the role of prostanoids in menstruation and its disorders has transformed the treatment of women suffering from menorrhagia. New approaches should also be provided by the insights gained through the molecular studies now possible.

References

1. UK Office of Population Censuses and Surveys. Hospital Inpatient Enquiry, Series MB4. Based on a one in ten sample of NHS patients in hospitals in England and Wales. Table P1. London: HMSO, 1985.

2. UK Office of Population Censuses and Surveys. Morbidity statistics from general practice 1981–1982. Series MB5, Table 13. London. HMSO, 1986.
3. Coulter A, Noone A, Goldacre M. General practitioners' referrals to specialist outpatient clinics. Br Med J 1989; 299:304–8.
4. Hallberg L, Hogdahl AM, Nilsson L, Rybo G. Menstrual blood loss – a population study. Acta Obstet Gynecol Scand 1966; 45:320–51.
5. Chimbira TH, Anderson ABM, Turnbull AC. Relation between measured menstrual loss and the patient's subjective assessment of loss, duration of bleeding, number of sanitary towels used, uterine weight and endometrial surface area. Br J Obstet Gynaecol 1980; 87:603–8.
6. Fraser IS, McCarron G, Markham R. A preliminary study of factors influencing perception of menstrual blood loss volume. Am J Obstet Gynaecol 1984; 149:788–93.
7. Hallberg L, Nilsson L. Determination of menstrual blood loss. Scand J Clin Lab Invest 1964; 16:244–8.
8. Haynes PJ, Anderson ABM, Turnbull AC. Patterns of menstrual blood loss in menorrhagia. Res Clin Forums 1979; 1:73–8.
9. Rees MCP. Menorrhagia – an algorithm. Br Med J 1987; 294:759–62.
10. Markee JE. Menstruation in endometrial intraocular transplants in the rhesus monkey. Contrib Embryol Carnegie Inst 1940; 28:219–349.
11. Pickles VR, Hall WJ, Best FA, Smith GN. Prostaglandins in endometrium and menstrual fluid from normal and dysmenorrhoeic subjects. Br J Obstet Gynaecol 1965; 72:185–95.
12. Wiqvist N, Bygdeman M, Kirton K. Nonsteroidal infertility agents in the female. In: Diezfalusy E. Barell V. eds. Nobel symposium 15. Control of human fertility. Stockholm: Almquist and Wiskell, 1965; 137–67.
13. Anderson ABM, Haynes PJ, Guillebaud J, Turnbull AC. Reduction of menstrual blood loss by prostaglandin synthetase inhibition. Lancet 1976; i:774–6.
14. Willman EA, Collins WP, Clayton SG. Studies in the involvement of prostaglandins in uterine symptomatology and pathology. Br J Obstet Gynaecol 1976; 83:337–41.
15. Burgoyne RD, Morgan A. The control of free arachidonic acid levels. Trends Biochem Sci 1990; 15:365–6.
16. Simon MI, Strathman MP, Gautam N. Diversity of G proteins in signal transduction. Science 1991; 252:802–8.
17. Kaziro Y, Itoh H, Kozasa T, Nakafuku M, Satoh T. Structure and function of signal-transducing GTP-binding proteins. Annu Rev Biochem 1991; 60:349–400.
18. Strathmann M, Simon M. G protein diversity: a distinct class of alpha subunits is present in vertebrates and invertebrates. Proc Natl Acad Sci 1990; 87:9113–17.
19. Demers LM, Rees MCP, Turnbull AC. Arachidonic acid metabolism by the nonpregnant human uterus. Prostaglandins Leukotrienes Med 1984; 14:175–80.
20. Rees MCP, Di Marzo V, Tippins JR, Morris HP, Turnbull AC. Leukotriene release by endometrium and myometrium throughout the menstrual cycle in dysmenorrhoea and menorrhagia. J Endocrinol 1987; 113:291–5.
21. Rees MCP, Parry DM, Anderson ABM, Turnbull AC. Immunohistochemical localisation of cyclooxygenase in the human uterus. Prostaglandins 1982; 23:207–21.
22. Abel MH, Kelly RW. Differential production of prostaglandins within the human uterus. Prostaglandins 1979; 18:821–8.
23. Rees MCP, Anderson ABM, Demers LM, Turnbull AC. Endometrial and myometrial prostaglandin release during the menstrual cycle in relation to menstrual blood loss. J Clin Endocrinol Metab 1984; 58:813–18.
24. Downie J, Poyser NL, Wunderlich M. Levels of prostaglandins in human endometrium during the normal menstrual cycle. J Physiol 1974; 236:465–75.
25. Smith BJ. The prostanoids in haemostatsis and thrombosis. Am J Pathol 1980; 99:743–803.
26. Rees MCP, Anderson ABM, Demers LM, Turnbull AC. Prostaglandins in menstrual fluid in menorrhagia and dysmenorrhoea. Br J Obstet Gynaecol 1984; 91:673–80.
27. Smith SK, Abel MH, Kelly RW, Baird DT. Prostaglandin synthesis in the endometrium of women with ovular dysfunction uterine bleeding. Br J Obstet Gynaecol 1981; 88:434–42.
28. Cameron IT, Leask R, Kelly RW, Baird DT. Endometrial prostaglandins in women with abnormal menstrual bleeding. Prostaglandins Leukotrienes Med 1987; 29:249–57.
29. Makarainen L, Ylikorkola O. Primary and myoma associated menorrhagia: role of prostaglandins and effect of ibuprofen. Br J Obstet Gynaecol 1986; 93:974–8.
30. Smith SK, Kelly RW, Abel MH, Baird DT. A role for prostacyclin (PGI$_2$) in excessive menstrual bleeding. Lancet 1981; i:522–4.

31. Rees MCP, Turnbull AC. Leiomyomas release prostaglandins. Prostaglandins Leukotrienes Med 1985; 18:65–8.
32. Kelly RW, Lumsden MA, Abel MH, Baird DT. The relationship between menstrual blood loss and prostaglandin production in the human: evidence for increased availability of arachidonic acid in women suffering from menorrhagia. Prostaglandins Leukotrienes Med 1984; 16:69–75.
33. Yokoyama C, Tanabe T. Cloning of the human gene encoding prostaglandin endoperoxide synthase and primary structure of the enzyme. Biochem Biophys Res Commun 1989; 165:888–94.
34. Bailey JM, Verma M. Identification of a highly conserved 3'UTR in the translationally regulated mRNA for prostaglandin synthase. Prostaglandins 1990; 40:585–90.
35. Milligan G, Green A. Agonist control of G-protein levels. Trends Pharmacol Sci 1991; 12:207–9.
36. Neer EJ, Clapham DE. Roles of G protein subunits in transmembrane signalling. Nature 1988; 333:129–34.
37. Fain JN, Wallace MA, Wojckiewicz JH. Evidence for involvement of guanine nucleotide binding regulatory proteins in the activation of phospholipases by hormones. FASEB J 1988; 2:2569–74.
38. Burch RM, Axelrod J. Dissociation of bradykinin-induced turnover in Swiss 3T3 fibroblasts: evidence for G protein regulation of phospholiase A_2. Proc Natl Acad Sci 1987; 84:6374–8.
39. Cockcroft S, Nielson, Stutchfield J. Is phospholipase A_2 activation regulated by G-proteins? Biochem Soc Trans 1991; 19:334–7.
40. Insel PA, Weiss BA, Slivka SR, Howard MJ, Waite JJ, Godson CA. Regulation of phospholipase A_2 by receptors in MDCK-DI cells. Biochem Soc Trans 1991; 19:330–3.
41. Billah MM, Anthes JC, Mullman TJ. Receptor coupled phospholipase D: regulation and functional significance. Biochem Soc Trans 1991; 19:324–9.
42. Leckie CM, Poyser NL. The effects of cholera toxin, pertussis toxin, sodium fluoride and alpha interferon on prostaglandin production by the guinea-pig endometrium. J Reprod Fertility 1990; 89:325–33.
43. Arkinstall SJ, Jones CT. Pregnancy suppresses G protein coupling to phosphoinositide hydrolysis in guinea pig myometrium. Am J Physiol 1990; 259:E57–E65.
44. Bonney RC. Measurement of phospholipase A_2 activity in human endometrium during the menstrual cycle. J Endocrinol 1985; 107:183–9.
45. Bonney RC, Franks S. Phospholipase C activity in human endometrium: its significance in endometrial pathology. Clin Endocrinol 1987; 27:307–20.
46. Rhee SG. Inositol phospholipid-specific phospholipase C: interaction with the gamma 1 isoform with tyrosine kinase. Trends Biochem Sci 1991; 16:297–301.
47. Jones DSC Smith SK. Human uterine phosphatidylinositol phospholipase C (PI–PLC), its cloning and sequencing. J Reprod Fertil Abstract Series 1991; 7:72.
48. Kramer RM, Hession C, Johansen B et al. Structure and properties of a human non-pancreatic phospholipase A_2. J Biol Chem 1989; 264:5768–75.
49. Seilhamer J, Pruzanski W, Vadas P et al. Cloning and recombinant expression of phospholipase A_2 present in rheumatoid arthritic synovial fluid. J Biol Chem 1989; 264:5335–8.
50. Bonney RC, Higham JM, Watson H, Beesley JS, Shaw RW, Franks S. Phospholipase activity in the endometrium of women with normal menstrual blood loss and women with proven ovulatory menorrhagia. Br J Obstet Gynaecol 1991; 98:363–8.
51. Merlie JP, Fagan D, Mudd J, Needleman P. Isolation and characterisation of the complementary DNA for sheep seminal vesicle prostaglandin endoperoxide synthase (cyclooxygenase). J Biol Chem 1988; 263:3550–3.
52. De Witt DL, El-Harith EA, Kraemer SA et al. The aspirin and heme-binding sites of ovine and murine prostaglandin endoperoxide synthases. J Biol Chem 1990; 265:5192–8.
53. Rosen GD, Birkenmeier TM, Raz A, Holtzman MJ. Identification of a cyclooxygenase related gene and its potential role in prostaglandin formation. Biochem Biophys Res Commun 1989; 164:1358–65.
54. Xie W, Chipman JG, Robertson DL, Erikson RL, Simmons DL. Expression of a mitogen-responsive gene encoding prostaglandin synthase is regulated by mRNA splicing. Proc Natl Acad Sci 1991; 88:2692–6.
55. Spencer M, Robson KJH, Rees M. Changes in the level of cyclooxygenase mRNA transcripts in human endometrium during the menstrual cycle. J Reprod Fertil Abstract Series 1991; 7:72.
56. Bailey MJ, Makheja AN, Pash J, Verma M. Corticosteroids suppress cyclooxygenase messenger RNA levels and prostanoid synthesis in cultured vascular cells. Biochem Biophys Res Commun 1988; 157:1159–63.
57. Adelantado JM, Rees MCP, Lopez Bernal A, Turnbull AC. Increased uterine prostaglandin E receptors in menorrhagic women. Br J Obstet Gynaecol 1988; 95:162–5.
58. Hofman GE, Rao CV, Barrows GH, Sanfilippo JS. Topography of human uterine prostaglandin

E and $F_{2\alpha}$ receptors and their profiles during pathological states. J Clin Endocrinol Metab 1983; 57:360–6.

59. Rees MCP, Canete-Soler R, Lopez-Bernal A, Turnbull AC. Effect of fenamates on prostaglandin E receptor binding. Lancet 1988; ii:541–2.

60. Lopez-Bernal A, Buckley S, Rees CMP, Marshall JM. Meclofenamate inhibits prostaglandin E binding and adenyl cyclase activation in human endometrium. J Endocrinol 1991; 129:439–45.

61. Fraser IS, McCarron G, Markham R, Robinson M, Smyth E. Long term treatment of menorrhagia with mefenamic acid. Obstet Gynecol 1983; 61:109–14.

Chapter 4

Prostaglandins in Dysmenorrhoea and Endometriosis

M. A. Lumsden

Dysmenorrhoea is derived from Greek, meaning difficult monthly flow, but is now usually taken to mean painful menstruation. It may occur secondary to an unrelated group of pelvic pathologies such as pelvic inflammatory disease, uterine abnormality, uterine leiomyomata or endometriosis or it may be idiopathic in origin. Dysmenorrhoea is a symptom complex consisting of cramping lower abdominal pain which is worst at the onset of the menses and is often accompanied by gastrointestinal, cardiovascular and urological symptoms. It may cause incapacity lasting some days particularly if preceded by the premenstrual syndrome. Primary and secondary dysmenorrhoea differ slightly in their symptomatology but it is often difficult to distinguish between the two on history and examination alone. Primary dysmenorrhoea is much commoner in teenagers than that associated with endometriosis which tends to occur around ten to fifteen years later. The pathogenesis of the former has been reasonably well worked out and it is also amenable to treatment. Endometriosis is a complex condition and it is now uncertain that it actually causes the symptoms with which it has been traditionally associated. This problem will be discussed in detail below.

Prostaglandins and Primary Dysmenorrhoea

It was in 1965 that Pickles first suggested that prostaglandins may be involved in primary dysmenorrhoea [1]. He extracted a smooth muscle stimulant from the menstrual fluid which was identified as a mixture of prostaglandins. Since then much evidence has been put forward to confirm that prostaglandins are involved although their mechanism of action is not clear. The properties of the prostaglandins commonly found in endometrium and menstrual fluid which could contribute to the aetiology of dysmenorrhoea are summarised in Table 4.1. Both $PGF_{2\alpha}$ and PGE_2 are present in menstruating endometrium [2–4] and menstrual fluid [1,5,6] in high concentrations. $PGF_{2\alpha}$ has been shown to have strong oxytocic activity both in vitro [7] and in vivo [8]. Its administration in vivo is consistently accompanied by dysmenorrhoea-like pain [9] and even on occasion, menstrual bleeding [10]. $PGF_{2\alpha}$ is also a potent vasoconstrictor, a property which combined with increased myometrial contractility is thought to cause ischaemic pain (Fig. 4.1).

Table 4.1. The properties of prostaglandins which may contribute to the pathogenesis of dysmenorrhoea

1. $PGF_{2\alpha}$ and PGE_2 are found in endometrium and menstrual fluid in high concentrations
2. The synthesis of $PGF_{2\alpha}$ is influenced by the concentration of circulating steroids
3. Infusion of $PGF_{2\alpha}$ into the uterus is always accompanied by pain and, on occasion, menstrual bleeding
4. $PGF_{2\alpha}$ is a vasoconstrictor
5. PGE_2 is known to be hyperalgesic
6. Prostaglandins influence intracellular processes, e.g. the phosphatidylinositol cycle which may influence calcium metabolism and thus myometrial contractility

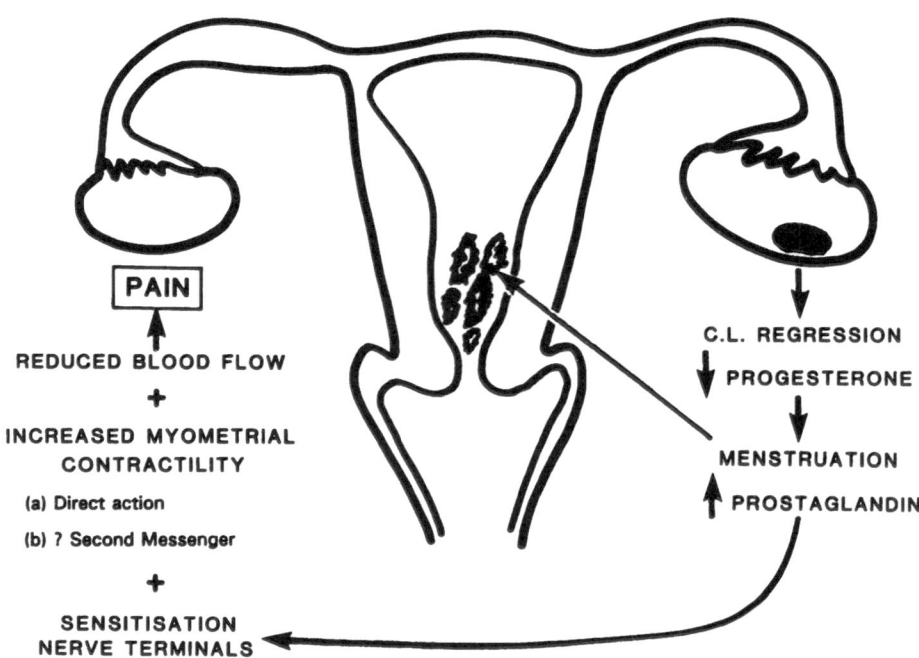

Fig. 4.1. A schematic diagram of the possible role of $PGF_{2\alpha}$ in the induction of the pain of dysmenorrhoea. Prostaglandins are produced at menstruation and the excess $PGF_{2\alpha}$ may produce pain via the mechanisms illustrated.

The role of uterine hyperactivity has received attention in the literature since it was first suggested by Novak and Reynolds in 1932 [11–18]. All agree that hyperactivity is the problem although there is some uncertainty as to whether there are irregular dysrhythmic contractions or simply elevated uterine tone [14,19]. Åkerlund and Anderssen suggest that high amplitude peaks which have been shown to accompany the severe pain are responsible [20] although these have been demonstrated in women in the absence of pain [19,21]. More recently studies have been performed in which the pain is graded continuously using a pen recorder which charts both this and changes in intrauterine pressure at the same time [22] (Fig. 4.2). This demonstrates that although the pain tends to increase in line with the intrauterine pressure there is a delay of about 45 s between the peak of the contraction and that of the pain. The significance of this in relation to blood flow will be discussed later. However, the studies are in overall agreement that the uterine activity is greater in those with dysmenorrhoea than those without and that this is likely to contribute to the pain.

When $PGF_{2\alpha}$ is infused into the uterus it causes dysmenorrhoic-like pain as stated above (Fig. 4.3). This finding is universal although the amount of $PGF_{2\alpha}$ required varies between individuals and at different stages of the menstrual cycle. Although PGE_2 is present in endometrium and menstrual fluid it has a variable effect on uterine contractility and may even lead to relaxation when administered during the menses [23]. However, it has been demonstrated that its administration can increase the sensitivity of nerve endings, a factor which could theoretically increase the pain of dysmenorrhoea [24].

The role of prostaglandins in the increased uterine activity of primary

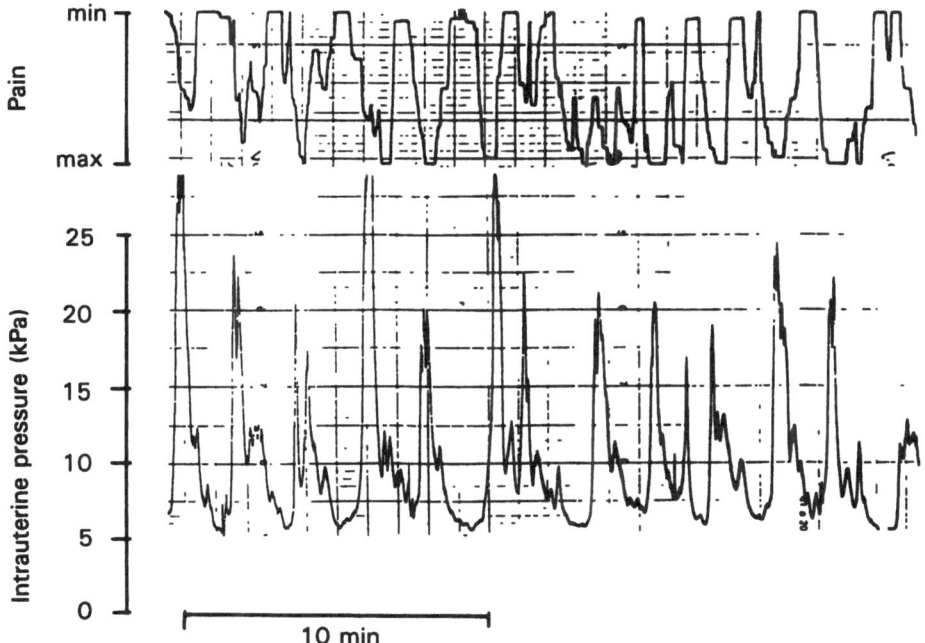

Fig. 4.2. Intrauterine pressure as measured with a microtransducer catheter compared with a recording of the pain experienced by the patient [22].

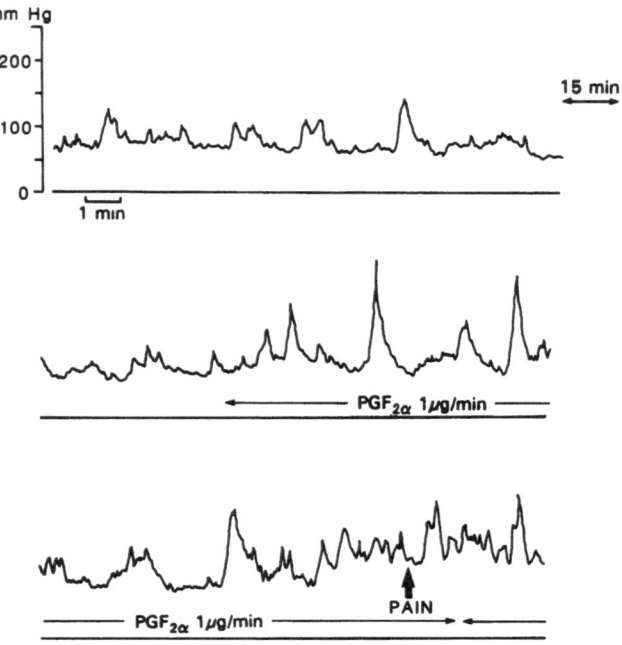

Fig. 4.3. The induction of pain on infusing PGF$_{2\alpha}$ into the uterus which is associated with increased uterine contractility.

dysmenorrhoea was studied in a group of women selected as being likely to have primary dysmenorrhoea. They were all young and nulliparous and infection, endometriosis and uterine abnormality were excluded (by laparoscopy in two cases). Menstrual fluid was collected in a contraceptive diaphragm daily during the menses and the concentration of PGF$_{2\alpha}$ and PGE$_2$ measured after forming the stable methyl oxime derivative. Uterine contractility was measured during the hour immediately following fluid collection and a comparison made of the results to see if the factors were directly related. The prostaglandin concentration was significantly higher in those suffering from dysmenorrhoea when compared with a group of matched controls [25] (Fig. 4.4). This difference was apparent for both PGF$_{2\alpha}$ and PGE$_2$ on days 1 and 2, but was lost by days 3 and 4 when the pain had disappeared in all cases. The increase in concentration was proportionately greater for PGF$_{2\alpha}$ than PGE$_2$ in that in the study group the ratio of PGF$_{2\alpha}$ to PGE$_2$ was 8.4 ± 1.7 ng/ml menstrual fluid on day 1, declining to 2.2 ± 0.5 ng/ml on day 4. This relative increase was not found to the same extent in the control group where the ratio was 4.2 ± 0.8 on day 1 and 1.4 ± 0.5 on day 4. The fact that the concentration of PGF$_{2\alpha}$ declined significantly between days 1 and 2 in the women with dysmenorrhoea but not in the control group suggests that there is either a decline in production or an increase in metabolism of prostaglandins during the menses in all women but occurring to a greater extent in women suffering from dysmenorrhoea. There is possibly a shift in endoperoxide metabolism in favour of PGF$_{2\alpha}$ production suggesting that different mechanisms control the concentrations of the different prostaglandins. It appears that the endometrial synthesis of PGF$_{2\alpha}$ but not PGE$_2$ is under the control of the steroid hormones [2,26]. A

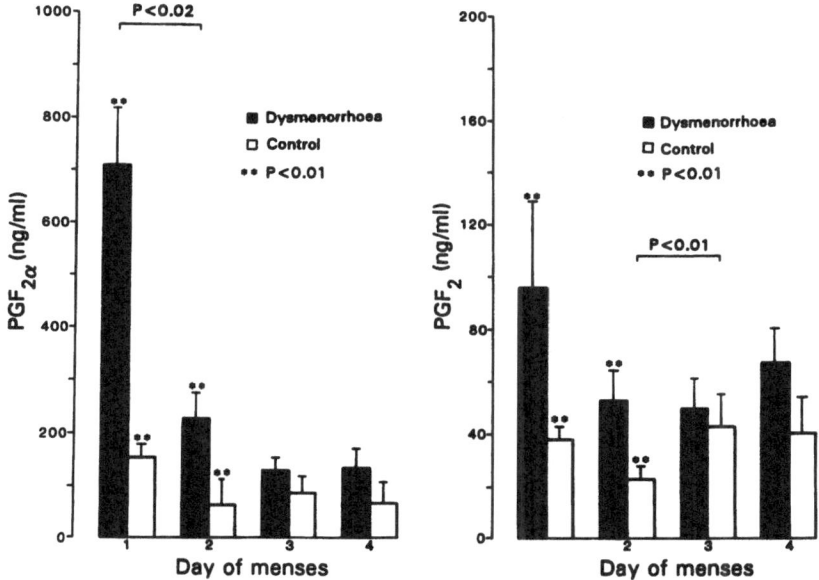

Fig. 4.4. The prostaglandin concentration in menstrual fluid in a group suffering from dysmenorrhoea as compared with pain-free controls [23].

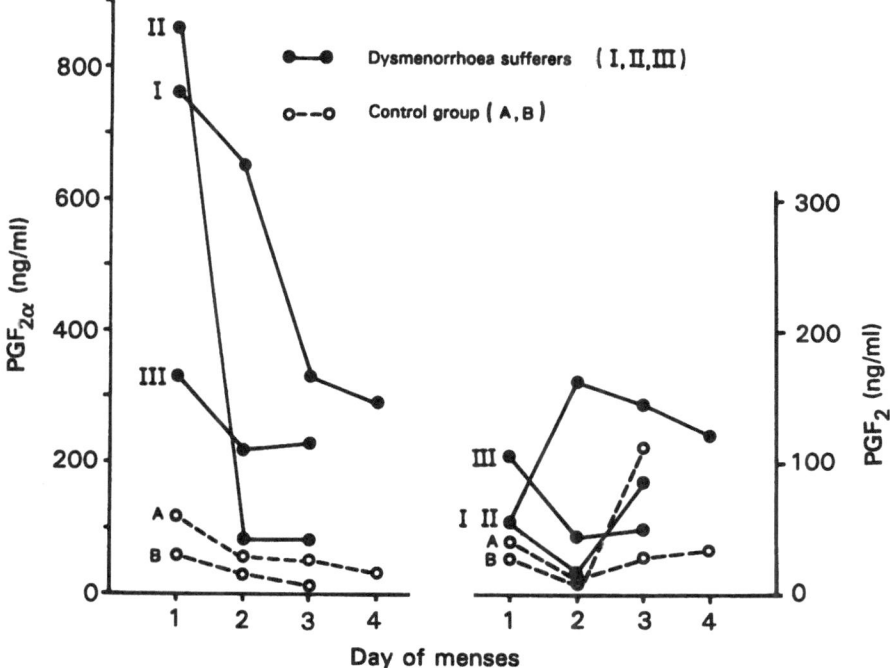

Fig. 4.5. Prostaglandin concentrations in menstrual fluid during the menses in three subjects with and two without pain.

higher concentration of oestradiol in the secretory phase has been demonstrated in those with dysmenorrhoea compared with pain-free controls [27,28]. This may alter both the synthesis and metabolism of the prostaglandins.

There is no overlap in the concentration of prostaglandins between the dysmenorrhoea and control groups on day 1 of the menses (Fig. 4.5). However, there was no correlation with uterine contractility on this day [29]. This may be because the amount lost in the fluid and the amount absorbed by the myometrium are not proportional, or that the two measurements were not made simultaneously. There was a significant co-relation on day 2 between the concentration of $PGF_{2\alpha}$ and uterine work in those with dysmenorrhoea, suggesting that part of its action may be to increase the contractility of the uterus. PGE_2 may also be involved in dysmenorrhoea but probably acts via another mechanism.

Dysmenorrhoea and the Oral Contraceptive Pill

Primary dysmenorrhoea is usually relieved by taking the oral contraceptive pill. This was thought to be due to significant decrease in uterine contractility (Fig. 4.6) and inhibition of ovulation which prevents the rise in prostaglandin production which occurs in the late secretory phase [26]. Although endometrial prostaglandin concentration remains high, it is likely that the overall content is decreasing since the endometrium is thin and atrophic. Prostaglandin metabolite concentrations are also less in women whose dysmenorrhoea is relieved by taking the contraceptive pill [30]. A significant finding is likely to be the decreased baseline uterine activity demonstrated by Ekström et al. [31]. Although there is an apparent decrease in sensitivity to prostaglandin administration while taking the oral contraceptive, the uterine response is in fact unchanged; it is rather that the increase in activity is superimposed on a decreased baseline and thus the pain induced is less.

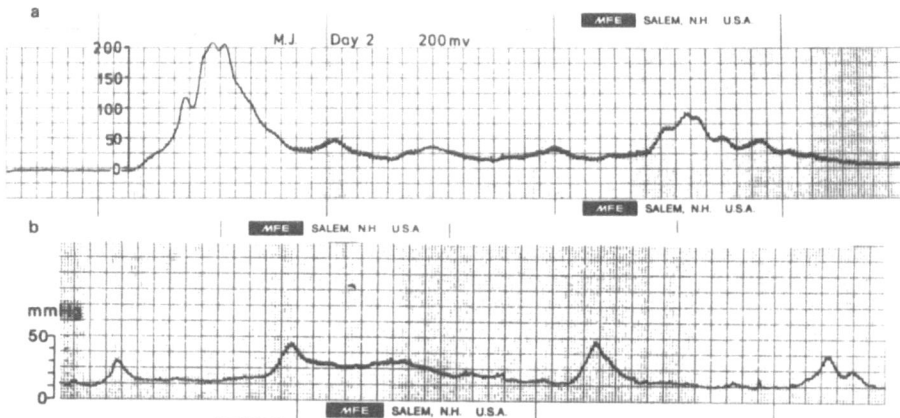

Fig. 4.6. The uterine contractility associated with dysmenorrhoea (a) is decreased by administering an oral contraceptive pill (b) which also relieves the pain.

Prostaglandin Synthetase Inhibitors

The use of these drugs in the treatment of primary dysmenorrhoea has contributed greatly to our understanding of the aetiology of the problem. These drugs inhibit the synthesis of prostaglandins as well as having a direct analgesic effect and are successful in over 75% of patients with primary dysmenorrhoea [32]. They have been shown to decrease the concentration of prostaglandins in menstrual fluid [33] and it has been suggested that some drugs, e.g. ibuprofen, preferentially decrease $PGF_{2\alpha}$ concentrations. They also decrease uterine contractility at the same time as providing pain relief [34–36].

Prostaglandins and Uterine Blood Vessels

It has been suggested that $PGF_{2\alpha}$ may exert part of its effect by causing vasoconstriction of the myometrial vessels. However, studies in vitro in which vessels of different calibres have been removed from different parts of the uterus suggest that this is not the case [37]. Fig. 4.7 illustrates a blood vessel with a decreased diameter as it approaches the endometrial–myometrial junction, the

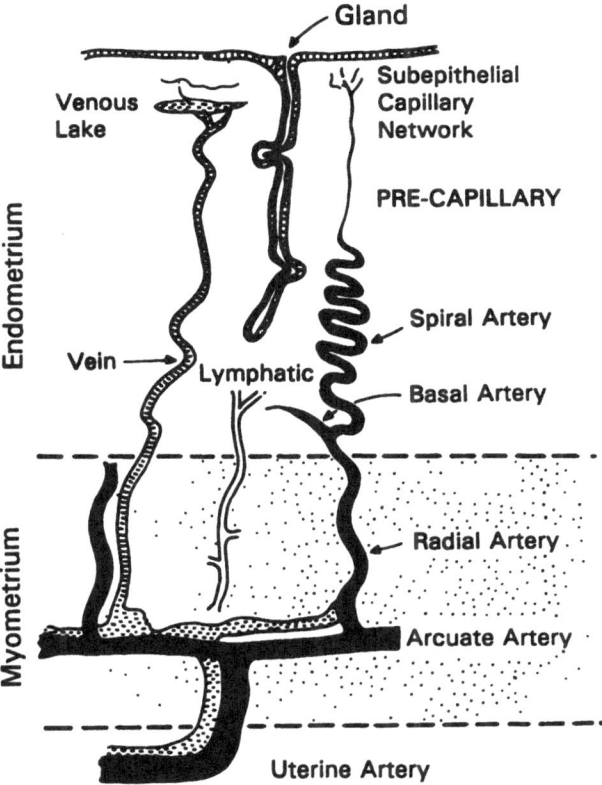

Fig. 4.7. The blood supply to the uterus illustrating the decrease in vessel diameter which occurs. Resistance is provided by the radial and basal arteries.

smaller vessels providing greater resistance. $PGF_{2\alpha}$ is only a weak constrictor at this level as compared with vasopressin or endothelin. The effect of $PGF_{2\alpha}$ on uterine contractility may be more important than its vasoconstrictor effects although it may have an action in decreasing the overall blood supply to the uterus by affecting larger diameter vessels. It is likely that other factors produced locally act with the prostaglandins to produce vasoconstriction particularly at the level of the resistance vessels.

Other Factors of Importance

Not all women respond to prostaglandin synthetase inhibitors which suggests that other factors may be important in the aetiology of the pain. Leukotrienes, produced from arachidonic acid by the action of 5-lipoxygenase, stimulate uterine contractions [38] and are also produced by endometrium [39]. Leukotriene release appears to be greater from uteri from those with dysmenorrhoea than those without [40] although there is a large variability between subjects and all the women studied were likely to have had a menstrual problem since the tissue samples were collected at hysterectomy.

Vasopressin is another factor likely to be of importance in primary dysmenorrhoea. Levels of vasopressin are higher on day 1 of menstruation in those with dysmenorrhoea than those without [41]. It has a potent action when infused into the uterus and causes dysmenorrhoea-like pain. It is possible that some of its action comes from its effect on the prostaglandins although vasopressin still stimulates the uterus in the presence of prostaglandin synthetase inhibitors suggesting a direct action on the uterus. Vasopressin is also a potent vasoconstrictor being particularly active on the small resistance vessels. It may therefore act with $PGF_{2\alpha}$ to produce dysmenorrhoea. Analogues of vasopressin have been shown to decrease uterine contractility and relieve dysmenorrhoea. Unfortunately these drugs are not being developed for this purpose at present.

Endothelin, which has been recently identified in endometrium [42], is the most potent vasoconstrictor known and also stimulates smooth muscle in other systems. It stimulates $PGF_{2\alpha}$ synthesis in vitro although the concentrations required are very high [43]. There is evidence that it may affect PG metabolism. Nothing is yet known about its role in dysmenorrhoea although its properties will make further study of interest.

Endometriosis

Endometriosis is an enigmatic condition occurring in women in their twenties and thirties. It is commonly diagnosed in those undergoing fertility investigation or who have dysmenorrhoea which fails to respond to treatment with prostaglandin synthetase inhibitors or the oral contraceptive pill. In the latter group the age is often less than those presenting with infertility. Out of a group of six women under 25 years with resistant dysmenorrhoea, three had endometriosis, the youngest being 17 years old. Laparoscopy is thus important in this group of patients. It has always been thought that endometriosis is the cause of both the infertility and the menstrual symptoms. However, the severity of the symptoms does not correlate with the extent of the disease and it is uncertain that treatment of mild disease improves pregnancy prospects.

Much attention has centred on the peritoneal fluid since the pelvic organs are bathed in it and volumes may be quite considerable in the secretory phase. It is likely that factors in the peritoneal fluid may affect ovarian function, tubal motility and even uterine contractility. Also, growth-promoting substances could influence the production of chemicals and hormones within the ovaries and uterus. A large number of studies have measured prostaglandins within the peritoneal fluid (Table 4.2) [44–56]. The results are inconsistent; some show an increase in prostaglandin concentration, whereas others are unable to demonstrate any difference from the chosen control group. There is also little agreement as to which prostaglandin is chiefly affected. Prostacyclin, as assessed by measurement of its metabolic 6-oxo-PGF$_{1\alpha}$, has been found in elevated levels in many women with endometriosis. It is likely that much is produced from white cells within the peritoneal cavity, the numbers of these being highly variable. The significance of these results is thus difficult to determine. It is difficult to compare the studies for a number of reasons. The control group chosen may comprise fertile women undergoing laparoscopic sterilisation or women with unexplained infertility but who do not have endometriosis. It is likely that the former group is most useful when establishing a link with infertility but no consistent differences in prostaglandin levels are noted. Some studies measure content rather than concentration whereas others measure both. The volume of peritoneal fluid

Table 4.2. Studies of the PG concentration in peritoneal fluid in those with endometriosis. (This is a simplified summary of the studies since the reported increase is often only significant under certain specified conditions, e.g. stage of cycle)

Reference	6-KF	TxB$_2$	PGF	PGE
Increase				
Drake [44]	+	+		
Badawy [46]			+(PGFM)	
Drake [48]	+	+		
Sgarlata [49]			(+)	(+)
Dawood [50]	+			
Koskimies [51]	+	+		
Ylikorkola [52]	+	+		
Badawy [53]			+	+
DeLeon [55]	+	+	+	+
No increase				
Rock [45]	–		–	–
Halme [47]			–	–
Dawood [50]	–	–	–	–
Mudge [54]	–			
DeLeon [55]	–	–	–	–
Yamaguchi [56][a]	–	–	–	–

[a] This study demonstrated a rise in leukotriene C in adenomyosis. 6-KF, 6-keto-PGF$_1$; TxB$_2$, thromboxane B$_2$ (metabolic products of prostacyclin and thromboxane A$_2$, respectively).

varies during the cycle and consequently the time and ease of collection also vary. None of the quoted studies have standardised their methods to allow meaningful comparison.

Most of the studies are more concerned with infertility than dysmenorrhoea. This is not looked at as a separate symptom although chronic pelvic pain is discussed by Dawood et al. [50]. However, this study did not demonstrate any difference between those with and those without pain in association with endometriosis. The study by Willman et al. [4] suggested that there are higher endometrial levels of prostaglandins in those with pelvic pathology including endometriosis but I am not aware of any carefully controlled studies which have addressed the problem. The effectiveness of the prostaglandin synthetase inhibitors is also debateable. Overall, it is considered that they are much less effective in endometriosis than in primary dysmenorrhoea which suggests that other factors, possibly including those described above, may be of greater importance.

Despite this absence of evidence for a specific cause-and-effect relationship, it is widely believed that the symptoms of endometriosis are a result of ectopic endometrial tissue. To investigate this in women would require longitudinal, controlled, and invasive experiments that would be ethically unacceptable. Accordingly, numerous animal models have been developed to simulate endo-metriosis in women. Surgical transplantation of endometrium into the peritoneal cavity in rats, rabbits and monkeys has consistently resulted in reduced fecundity [57–59]. The monkey is probably the best model because its endocrinological and menstrual cycles are similar to those in women and it also develops spontaneous endometriosis. Schenken and Asch [57] have performed a number of studies in which the surgical implantation of endometrium was controlled by performing similar operations on a second group of monkeys with implantation of ornamen-tal fat tissue. Laparotomy was then performed at a consistent time after the oestradiol peak to allow meaningful comparison between groups. Prostaglandin contents were measured in peritoneal washings as well as in the tissue autografts and the results are presented in Table 4.3 [58]. The concentrations of $PGF_{2\alpha}$ and PGE in peritoneal washings were not significantly altered after adipose tissue implantations although microscopic endometriosis was present in some animals. All monkeys with ectopic endometrial autografts demonstrated increased $PGF_{2\alpha}$ concentrations in peritoneal washings, but this was significant only in monkeys with moderate to severe disease. PGE concentrations were not significantly different. The increased $PGF_{2\alpha}$ content in ectopic endometrium was significantly greater than in adipose autografts. There was a lower incidence of ovulation in those with severe disease due to an increased incidence of luteinised unruptured follicles. There was no difference in the endocrinological profiles of the two groups of monkeys. Thus in this carefully controlled study a difference in $PGF_{2\alpha}$ concentration in peritoneal fluid has been demonstrated. However, it is uncertain if monkeys have menstrual problems.

Factors Influencing Growth and Maintenance of Endometriosis

Endometriosis shares many morphological aspects with the eutopic endometrium but differs in its biological behaviour. Oestrogen is the most important factor involved in the appearance, growth and maintenance of the ectopic tissue. The mechanism of action on the target tissue has not been fully explained. Ectopic and

Table 4.3. Prostaglandin concentrations in (a) peritoneal washings and (b) tissue autografts made by transplanting endometrium into the peritoneal cavity of the monkey. Transplantation of adipose tissue was performed in a control group.

(a) Peritoneal washings

		Concn (ng/ml peritoneal washing)			
		$PGF_{2\alpha}$		PGE	
Group	n	Before	After	Before	After
Control	5	0.20±0.09	0.28±0.08	1.06±0.33	0.07±0.36
Endometriosis					
Mild	5	0.30±0.08	0.58±0.11	1.51±0.47	1.73±0.42
Severe	2	0.18±0.01	0.62±0.05	0.57±0.01	0.55±0.11

After the autografts the $PGF_{2\alpha}$ concentration is significantly greater in monkeys with severe endometriosis ($P<0.05$).

(b) Tissue autografts

		Concn (ng/mg protein)	
Group	n	$PGF_{2\alpha}$	PGE_2
Adipose tissue	5	0.02±0.01	0.06±0.02
Endometriosis			
Mild	5	0.05±0.01	0.08±0.02
Severe	2	0.04±0.01	0.10±0.05

The concentration of PGF_2 is greater in those with both severe and mild endometriosis ($P<0.05$) than in those with adipose tissue grafts.

Values are means ±SEM.
Adapted from Schenken et al. Am J Obstet Gynecol 1984; 150: 349.

eutopic endometrium are not synchronised in their histological changes: ectopic tissue implants present a maturation disorder and it is possible to find glands with different degrees of differentiation and organisation in the same implant [60]. Complete secretory modification is rarely found in endometriosis and this could have an impact on prostaglandin production since levels in normal endometrium are known to vary during the menstrual cycle [2,26]. Oestrogen and progesterone receptors are present in the ectopic endometrium although concentrations are lower than in intrauterine tissue [61]. Cyclical variation has not been observed in the receptor population [62] and there seem to be differences in the way that oestrogen is handled by the endometrium at the two sites [63].

It is now an established fact that some of the action of oestrogen may be mediated by growth factors. One of the most likely of these is epidermal growth factor (EGF). Growth and differentiation of the internal genitalia of the mouse can be induced by EGF in the complete absence of oestradiol [64] and there is evidence that it may mediate some of the effects of oestradiol in the human uterus [65]. EGF is a potent stimulator of proliferation in many cell types including fibroblasts, keratinocytes and epithelial cells [66]. EGF-like immunoreactivity has been demonstrated in both eutopic and ectopic endometrium collected from those with endometriosis [67]. Endometrial EGF receptors have been demonstrated in the human [68] and EGF receptors have been identified in ectopic endometrium using immunohistochemistry and in most cases the concentration was decreased by the standard treatments (Danazol, GnRH agonists) for endometriosis [69]. About 20% of samples were positive for EGF-R but negative for ER suggesting a role in the growth and maintenance of the tissue. EGF is also known to affect prostaglandin production in human amnion cells [70,71]. There are thus two possibilities for symptom production. Either increased PG production may be stimulated within the ectopic endometrium, or the EGF may be transported to the uterus where a local increase in prostaglandin production may occur. This increase in prostaglandin production may be a result of an increased turnover in the phosphatidylinositol cycle which leads not only to further prostaglandin production [72] but also to altered calcium metabolism within the cell. It has been suggested that the inositol phosphates may be important intracellular messengers mediating the effects of EGF [73].

Endometriosis: an Inflammatory Process

Endometriosis provokes a marked inflammatory response in the peritoneum. Factors produced by the ectopic tissue could enhance the recruitment of

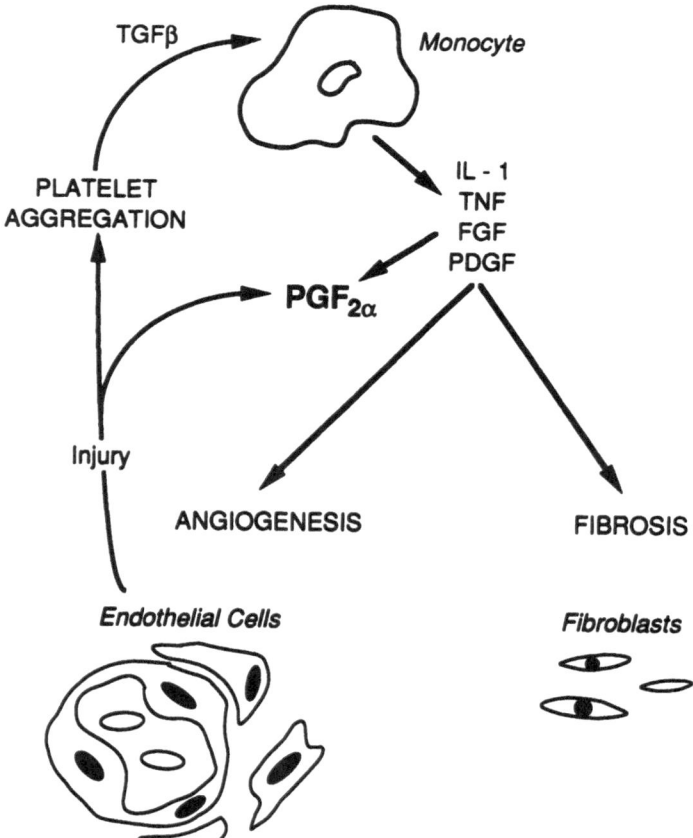

Fig. 4.8. The possible role of the inflammatory response in the production of $PGF_{2\alpha}$ in endometriosis which may be involved in the genesis of dysmenorrhoea and other associated symptoms.

monocytes which then become activated (Fig. 4.8). Activation of phagocytic monocytes (macrophages) is associated with release to the surrounding medium of substances which may have adverse effects on various physiological functions. Interleukin-1 is a product of macrophages and is believed to be a primary mediator of host responses to inflammation and immunological challenges [74] and a possible role for it has been suggested in the infertility associated with endometriosis [75]. One important factor may be the stimulation of PG synthesis [76] which may have a role in the production of the associated symptoms.

Endometriosis and Dysmenorrhoea

Dysmenorrhoea is a symptom resulting from various aetiologies. It seems likely that the pain has a similar final common pathway although initiating factors will vary with the pathology. Other sorts of pain may occur in endometriosis, which complicates the picture since these may not involve prostaglandins. The prostaglandins are likely to be a link in a chain rather than a single important factor and the study of the interactions involved in this pathological process may lead to a better understanding of the basic mechanism of menstruation and its disorders.

References

1. Pickles VR, Hall WJ, Best FA, Smith GN. Prostaglandins in endometrium and menstrual fluid from normal and dysmenorrhoeic subjects. Br J Obstet Gynaecol 1965; 72:185–92.
2. Downie J, Poyser NL, Wunderlich M. Levels of prostaglandins in human endometrium during the normal menstrual cycle. J Physiol 1974; 236:465–72.
3. Singh E, Baccarini I, Zuspan F. Level of prostaglandin $F_{2\alpha}$ and E_2 in human endometrium during the menstrual cycle. Am J Obstet Gynecol 1975; 121:1003–6.
4. Willman E, Collins W, Clayton S. Studies in the involvement of prostaglandins in uterine symptomatology and pathology. Br J Obstet Gynaecol 1976; 83:337–41.
5. Chan WY, Hil JC. Determination of menstrual prostaglandin levels in non-dysmenorrhoeic and dysmenorrhoeic subjects. Prostaglandins 1978; 15:363–75.
6. Pulkkinen MO, Henzl MR, Csapo AT. The effect of naproxen-sodium on the prostaglandin concentration of the menstrual blood and uterine "jet-washings" in dysmenorrhoeic women. Prostaglandins 1978; 15:543–50.
7. Bygdeman M. The effect of different prostaglandins on the human myometrium in vitro. Acta Physiol Scand [Suppl] 1964; 63 242:1–78.
8. Martin JN, Bygdeman M. The effect of locally administered $PGF_{2\alpha}$ on the contractility of the non-pregnant human uterus in vivo. Prostaglandins 1975; 9:243–53.
9. Lundström V. The myometrial response of intra-uterine administration of $PGF_{2\alpha}$ and PGE_2 in dysmenorrhoeic women. Acta Obstet Gynecol Scand 1977; 56:167–72.
10. Karim SM, Hillier K, Somers K, Trussell RR. The effects of prostaglandins E_2 and $F_{2\alpha}$ administered by different routes on uterine activity and the cardiovascular system in pregnant and non-pregnant women. J Obstet Gynecol Br Cmwlth 1971; 78:172–9.
11. Novak E, Reynolds BR. The cause of primary dysmenorrhoea with special reference to hormonal factors. JAMA 1932; 99:1466–72.
12. Wilson L, Kurzrok R. Uterine contractility in functional dysmenorrhoea. Endocrinology 1940; 27:23–8.
13. Woodbury R, Torpin R, Child G, Watson H, Jarber M. Myometrial physiology and its relation to pelvic pain. JAMA 1947; 134:1081–5.
14. Filler W, Hall W. Dysmenorrhoea and its therapy: a uterine contractility study. Am J Obstet Gynecol 1970; 106:104–9.

15. Lundström V, Gréen K, Wiqvist N. Prostaglandins, indomethacin and dysmenorrhoea. Prostaglandins 1976; 11:893–904.
16. Csapo AI, Pulkkinen MO, Henzl MR. The effect of naproxen-sodium on the intruterine pressure and menstrual pain of dysmenorrhoeic patients. Prostaglandins 1977; 13:193–9.
17. Anderssen KE, Ulmsten U. Effects of nifedipine on myometrial activity and lower abdominal pain in women with primary dysmenorrhoea. Br J Obstet Gynaecol 1978; 85:142–8.
18. Åkerlund M. Pathophysiology of dysmenorrhoea. Acta Obstet Gynecol Scand [Suppl] 1979; 87:27–32.
19. Lumsden MA, Baird DT. Intrauterine pressure in dysmenorrhoea. Acta Obstet Gynecol Scand 1985; 64:183–6.
20. Åkerlund M, Anderssen K. Vasopressin response and terbutaline inhibition of the uterus. Obstet Gynecol 1976; 48:528–36.
21. Pulkkinen MO. Suppression of uterine activity by prostaglandin synthetase inhibitors. Acta Obstet Gynecol Scand [Suppl] 1979; 87:39–43.
22. Ekström P, Forsling M, Kindahl H, Åkerlund M. Perception of pain in primary dysmenorrhoea in relation to uterine activity and concentrations of vasopressin and a $PGF_{2\alpha}$-metabolite. J Neuroendocrinol: special issue, 4th International Conference on the Neurohypophysis 1989; 168–71.
23. Martin JN, Bygdeman M. The effect of locally administered PGE_2 on the contractility of the non-pregnant human uterus in vivo. Prostaglandins 1975; 10:253–65.
24. Ferreira S, Nakamura M, Castro M. The hyperalgesic effects of prostacyclin and prostaglandin E_2. Prostaglandins 1978; 16:31–7.
25. Lumsden MA, Kelly RW, Baird DT. Primary dysmenorrhoea: the importance of both prostaglandin E_2 and $F_{2\alpha}$. Br J Obstet Gynaecol 1983; 90:1135–40.
26. Maathuis JB, Kelly RW. Concentrations of prostaglandins $F_{2\alpha}$ and E_2 in the endometrium throughout the human menstrual cycle, after the administration of clomiphene or an oestrogen-progesterone pill and in early pregnancy. J Endocrinol 1978; 77:361–71.
27. Strömberg P, Åkerlund M, Forsling ML, Granström E, Kindahl H. Vasopressin and prostaglandins in premenstrual pain and primary dysmenorrhoea. Acta Obstet Gynecol Scand 1984; 63:533–8.
28. Ylikkorkola O, Puolakka J, Kauppila A. Serum gonadotrophins, prolactin and ovrian steroids in primary dysmenorrhoea. Br J Obstet Gynaecol 1979; 86:648–53.
29. Lumsden MA, Kelly RW, Baird DT. Is prostaglandin $F_{2\alpha}$ involved in the increased myometrial contractility of primary dysmenorrhoea? Prostaglandins 1983; 25:683–92.
30. Hauksson A, Åkerlund M, Forsling M, Kindahl H. Plasma concentrations of vasopressin and a prostaglandin $F_{2\alpha}$ metabolite in women with primary dysmenorrhoea before and during treatment with a combined oral contraceptive. J Endocrinol 1987; 115:355–61.
31. Ekström P, Juchnicka E, Laudanski T, Åkerlund M. Effect of an oral contraceptive in primary dysmenorrhoea – changes in uterine activity and reactivity to agonists. Contraception 1989; 40:39–47.
32. Dingfelder JR. Primary dysmenorrhoea treatment with prostaglandin inhibitors: a review. Am J Obstet Gynecol 1981; 140:874–9.
33. Chan WY, Dawood Y. Prostaglandin levels in menstrual fluid of non-dysmenorrhoeic and of dysmenorrhoeic subjects with and without oral conctraception or ibuprofen. Adv Prostaglandin Thromboxane Leukotriene Res 1980; 8:1443–7.
34. Pulkkinen MO, Csapo AI. The effect of ibuprofen on the intrauterine pressure and menstrual pain of dysmenorrhoeic patients. Prostaglandins 1978; 15:1055–62.
35. Lundström V, Gréen K, Svanberg K. Endogenous prostaglandins in dysmenorrhoea and the effect of prostaglandin synthetase inhibitors (PGSI) on uterine contractility. Acta Obstet Gynecol Scand [Suppl] 1979; 87:51–6.
36. Smith R, Powell J. Intrauterine pressure changes during dysmenorrhoea therapy. Am J Obstet Gynecol 1982; 143:286–9.
37. Maigaard S, Forman R, Andersson KE. Different responses to prostaglandin $F_{2\alpha}$ and E_2 in human extra- and intramyometrial arteries. Prostaglandins 1985; 30:599–608.
38. Weichman BM, Tucker SS. Contraction of the guinea pig uterus by synthetic leukotrienes. Prostaglandins 1982; 24:245–53.
39. Demers LM, Rees MC, Turnbull AC. Arachidonic acid metabolism by the non-pregnant human uterus. Prostaglandins Leukotrienes Med 1984; 14:175–80.
40. Rees MCP, DiMarzo V, Tippins JR, Morris HR, Turnbull AC. Leukotriene release by endometrium and myometrium throughout the menstrual cycle in dysmenorrhoea and menorrhagia. J Endocrinol 1987; 113:291–5.

41. Åkerlund M, Strömberg P, Forsling ML. Primary dysmenorrhoea and vasopressin. Br J Obstet Gynaecol 1979; 86:484–7.
42. Cameron IT, Davenport AP, van Papendorp C et al. Endothelin-like immunoreactivity in human endometrium. J Reprod Fertil 1992: in press.
43. Cameron IT, Davenport AP, Brown MJ, Smith SK. Endothelin-1 stimulates prostaglandin $F_{2\alpha}$ release from human endometrium. Prostaglandins Leukotrienes Med 1991; 42:155–7.
44. Drake TS, Brien WF, Ramwell PW, Metz SA. Peritoneal fluid thromboxane B_2 and 6-keto-prostaglandin F_1 in endometriosis. Am J Obstet Gynecol 1981; 140:401–4.
45. Rock JA, Dublin NH, Ghodeoankar RB, Bergquist CA, Erozan YS, Kimball AW. Cul-de-sac fluid in women with endometriosis: fluid volume and prostanoid concentration during the proliferative phase of the cycle – days 8–12. Fertil Steril 1982; 37:747–50.
46. Badawy SZA, Marshall L, Gabal AA, Nusbaum ML. The concentration of 13,14-dihydro-15-keto prostaglandin $F_{2\alpha}$ and prostaglandin E_2 in peritoneal fluid of infertile patients with and without endometriosis. Fertil Steril 1982; 38:166–70.
47. Halme JS, Becker S, Hammond MG, Raj MHG, Raj S. Increased activation of peritoneal macrophages in infertile women with mild endometriosis. Am J Obstet Gynecol 1983; 145:333.
48. Drake TS, O'Brien WF, Ramwell PW. Peritoneal fluid prostanoids in unexplained infertility. Am J Obstet Gynecol 1983; 147:63.
49. Sgarlata CS, Hertelendy F, Mikhail G. The prostanoid content in peritoneal fluid and plasma of women with endometriosis. Am J Obstet Gynecol 1983; 147:563.
50. Dawood MY, Kahn-Dawood FS, Wilson L. Peritoneal fluid prostaglandins and prostanoids in women with endometriosis, chronic pelvic inflammatory disease and pelvic pain. Am J Obstet Gynecol 1984; 148:391–5.
51. Koskimies AI, Tenhunen A, Ylikorkala O. Peritoneal fluid 6-keto-prostaglandin $F_{1\alpha}$, thromboxane B_2 in endometriosis and unexplained infertility. Acta Obstet Gynecol Scand [Suppl] 1984; 123:19–21.
52. Ylikorkola O, Koskimies A, Laatkainen T, Tenhunen A, Viinikka L. Peritoneal fluid prostaglandins in endometriosis, tubal disorders and unexplained infertility. Obstet Gynecol 1984; 63:616.
53. Badawy SZA, Marshall L, Cuenca V. Peritoneal fluid prostaglandins in various stages of the menstrual cycle: role in infertile patients with endometriosis. Int J Fertil 1985; 30:48.
54. Mudge TJ, James MJ, Jones WR, Walsh JA. Peritoneal fluid 6-keto-prostaglandin $F_{1\alpha}$ levels in women with endometriosis. Am J Obstet Gynecol 1985; 152:901.
55. DeLeon FD, Vijayakumar R, Brown M, Rao CV, Yussman MA, Schultz G. Peritoneal fluid volume, estrogen, progesterone, prostaglandin and epidermal growth factor concentrations in patients with and without endometriosis. Obstet Gynecol 1986; 68:189–94.
56. Yamaguchi M, Mori N. Prostaglandin and leukotriene concentration of the peritoneal fluid of endometriosis and other gynecological disorders in the secretory phase. Prostaglandin Leukotriene Med 1990; 39:43–5.
57. Schenken RS, Asch RH. Surgical induction of endometriosis in the rabbit: effects on fertility and concentrations of peritoneal fluid prostaglandins. Fertil Steril 1980; 34:581–7.
58. Schenken RS, Asch RH, Williams RF, Hodgen GD. Etiology of infertility in monkeys with endometriosis: luteinized unruptured follicles, luteal phase defects, pelvic adhesions and spontaneous abortions. Fertil Steril 1984; 41:122–30.
59. Schenken RS, Williams RF, Hodgen GD. Experimental endometriosis in monkeys. Ann NY Acad Sci 1991; 622:256–65.
60. Lessey BA, Metzeger DA, Haney AF, McCarty KS. Immunohistochemical analysis of estrogen and progesterone receptors in endometriosis: comparison with normal endometrium during the menstrual cycle and the effect of medical therapy. Fertil Steril 1989; 51:409–15.
61. Prakash S, Ulfelder H, Cohen BR. Enzyme-histochemical observation on endometriosis. Am J Obstet Gynecol 1965; 91:990–7.
62. Kauppila A, Vierikko P, Isotalo H, Ronnemberg L. Cytosol estrogen and progestin receptor concentration and 17β-hydroxysteroid dehydrogenase activities in the endometrium and endometriotic tissue: effects of hormonal treatment. Acta Obstet Gynecol Scand [Suppl] 1984; 123:45–52.
63. Vierikko P, Kauppila A, Ronnemberg L, Vihko R. Steroidal regulation of endometriosis tissue: lack of induction of 17β-hydroxysteroid dehydrogenase activity by progesterone, medroxyprogesterone acetate, or danazol. Fertil Steril 1985; 43:218–26.
64. Nelson KG, Takahashi T, Bossert NL, Walmer DK, McLachlan JA. Epidermal growth factor replaces estrogen in the stimulation of female genital-tract growth and differentiation. Proc Natl Acad Sci USA 1991; 88:21–5.
65. Lumsden MA, West CP, Bramley TA, Rumgay L, Baird DT. The binding of epidermal growth

factor to the human uterus and leiomyomata in women rendered hypoiatrogeneic by continuous administration of an LHRH agonist. Br J Obstet Gynaecol 1988; 95:1299–304.

66. Carpenter G, Cohen S. Epidermal growth factor. Annu Rev Biochem 1979; 48:193–236.

67. Haining REB, Schofield JP, Jones DSC, Rajput-Williams J, Smith SK. Identification of mRNA for epidermal growth factor and transforming growth factor present in low copy number in human endometrium and decidua using reverse transcriptase – polymerase chain reaction. J Mol Endocrinol 1991; 6:207–14.

68. Chegini N, Rao CV, Wakim N, Sanfilippo J. Binding of ^{125}I-epidermal growth factor in human uterus. Cell Tissue Res 1986; 246:543–8.

69. Melega C, Balducci M, Bulletti C, Galassi A, Jasonni VM, Flamigni C. Tissue factors influencing growth and maintenance of endometriosis. Ann NY Acad Sci 1991; 622:256–65.

70. Mitchell MD. Epidermal growth factor actions on arachidonic acid metabolism in human amnion cells. Biochim Biophys Acta 1987; 928:240–2.

71. Casey ML, Mitchell MD, MacDonald PC. Epidermal growth factor-stimulated prostaglandin E_2 production in human amnion cells: specificity and nonesterified arachidonic acid dependency. Mol Cell Endocrinol 1987; 53:169–76.

72. Orlicky DJ, Silio M, Williams C, Gordon J, Gerschenson LE. Regulation of inositol phosphate levels by prostaglandins in cultured endometrial cells. J Cell Physiol 1986; 128:105–12.

73. Sawyer ST, Cohen S. Enhancement of calcium uptake and phosphatidylinositol turnover by epidermal growth factor in A-431 cells. Biochemistry 1981; 20:6280–6.

74. Dinarello CA. An update on human interleukin-1: from molecular biology to clinical relevance. J Clin Immunol 1985; 5:287.

75. Fakih H, Baggett B, Holtz G, Tsang K, Lee JC, Williamson HO. Interleukin-1: a possible role in the infertility associated with endometriosis. Fertil Steril 1987; 47:213–17.

76. Rossi V, Breviario F, Ghezzi P, Dejana E, Montovani A. Interleukin-1 induces prostacyclin in vascular cells. Science 1985; 229:174–6.

Discussion

Calder: There does not seem to be any great doubt about the role of $PGF_{2\alpha}$ as a stimulant of myometrial contractility in the non-pregnant uterus, but perhaps there is still some confusion about PGE_2; in one of the slides the PGE_2 both stimulated and inhibited the myometrium. In some of the old data there were variations through the menstrual cycle and differences in vitro and in vivo and so on. Are we any clearer nowadays about how that issue might resolve?

Rees: I do not think we are any clearer than we were several years ago, mainly because dysmenorrhoea has not received much attention in scientific research and so we are still in the in vivo and in vitro situation.

Smith: The problem with dysmenorrhoea is that clinically we essentially have effective treatments.

Lumsden: We do for primary dysmenorrhoea but it is not true for dysmenorrhoea as a result of pathology. There is not a vast amount of evidence but many people would have an anecdotal impression that the prostaglandin synthetase inhibitors are not as effective, and so it is likely that other factors will be involved; or it may be that enough of the drug is just not getting to the right place.

Smith: It was felt many years ago that there was no such thing as primary and secondary dysmenorrhoea, it was just dysmenorrhoea.

Lumsden: And that is fair enough. It is a symptom; it may not have an apparent cause or it may have an apparent cause, such an endometriosis, fibroids or uterine abnormality. But it is likely that the symptom is the same.

Smith: As I see it the purpose here is to discuss the scientific aspects and interplay. In the case of primary dysmenorrhoea, there must be little doubt that non-steroidal anti-inflammatory drugs do reduce the pain of dysmenorrhoea and are widely used in clinical practice and are now widely seen to be effective.

If we look at endometriosis and the developing regimes for medical treatment or even laser surgery for endometriosis, the clear and unequivocal story is that the dysmenorrhoea and the pain of endometriosis are highly significantly improved by these medications.

Maybe if we have to pick an area which has been resolved, this is one where by and large it has been.

Fraser: I would take issue with that. I believe that there is a difference because, from the symptomatology that these women describe, the women who have pain associated with endometriosis have pain which begins very much earlier in the menstrual cycle, it does have different characteristics. They may well complain of a similar type of pain to women with primary dysmenorrhoea on days 1 or 2 of the onset of menstruation, but there must be other mechanisms which contribute at other times, when they have pain in the luteal phase, and perhaps continuing for a longer period during the actual process of menstruation.

In women with dysmenorrhoea which is secondary to recognisable pelvic pathology, there must be other mechanisms which are playing a role as well. Although our evidence on treatment is highly anecdotal, it is, I believe, convincing enough that the women with endometriosis do not get nearly such good results from treatment with prostaglandin inhibitors.

Lumsden: If we look at the treatment failures, I think that clinically one should try the synthetase inhibitors and the pill, and if the woman does not respond, do a laparoscopy. In my small study over the last 10 years about 50% of the patients have endometriosis and they are treatment failures, and so obviously there are more mechanisms. But it may be related to the fact that the ectopic endometrium does not behave exactly the same as the eutopic endometrium in that it does not have the same secretory response; it is not exactly the same tissue. And this may be why they are getting symptoms at a slightly different time of the cycle.

There must be other factors involved, and it may be the importance of, say, EGF stimulating other pathways to come into play.

Smith: Even if that is true, and probably I would agree on that, the treatments that are now available are very effective in reducing the dysmenorrhoea – I am thinking of endometriosis – particularly with the agonists.

Lumsden: To my mind there are two important things. At the moment it is established practice to give agonists and treatments for endometriosis for a limited period of time and quite often on stopping treatment the symptoms will resume very quickly, even before the ectopic endometrium has grown.

But that apart, we can use pathological processes to learn about the physiology and we do not understand the physiology of menstruation. It may be quite useful to look at endometrium in this context to learn about the importance to factors which affect the calibre of blood vessels. All women get vasocontriction at the onset of menstruation otherwise they would not menstruate, but they do not all get pain.

In order to understand the physiology, one often has to look at the pathology.

Lopez-Bernal: To answer the question about the effect of prostaglandins on contractility in the non-pregnant uterus, in vitro it is clear that $PGF_{2\alpha}$ always stimulates contractility. PGE_2 and PGE_1 can be very frustrating because they have a biphasic effect both in time and in dose. The problem with PGE_2 is that on the one hand it increases cyclic AMP that tends to relax, but on the other hand it also releases calcium from the cytoplasmic reticulum which favours contractility.

Another very frustrating aspect is that the human myometrium, as opposed to the myometrium from, say, the rat or the guinea pig, habituates very quickly to prostaglandin and one cannot do sustained dose responses. But generally speaking $PGF_{2\alpha}$ increases contractility by bringing calcium from the outside, and PGE_2 has biphasic effects. Normally the prolonged effect is relaxation because of cyclic AMP stimulation.

Cameron: To refer to the potential role for endothelins in dysmenorrhoea, Dr Lumsden's data are supported by data from Freedman and Simonson showing potent stimulation of uterine vessels with endothelin-1. Also endothelin-1 stimulates not only vascular smooth muscle by myometrial smooth muscle both in rabbits and in humans, so not only would there be a potential role because of vasoconstriction, but also the compounds can stimulate uterine muscle quite potently.

Radestad: We heard that lipoxygenase products such as leukotrienes might play a role in dysmenorrhoea. Since there are no inhibitors available, has anybody had the opportunity to study their effect on the uterus?

Rees: I have not, but I would expect that it will treat the women who have no pathology and who do not respond to prostaglandin synthetase inhibitors. Perhaps 10% of women do not respond to prostaglandin synthetase inhibitor, and since we know that there are higher levels of leukotrienes in endometrium during dysmenorrhoea, we would expect a response. But Abbott, who I think has the only orally active agent at the moment, has not yet attacked that aspect even though from a commerical point of view it would be an enormous market for them.

Kelly: Dr Rees was looking at doses of meclofenamate of about 100 μmol and at about 10 μmol was beginning to get an effect. Could these concentrations, which I would reckon are about 3 mg/kg, be attained in the human after treatment with fenamates?

Rees: With that dose of meclofenamate we get that level; and that has been measured by some studies in which one oral dose of sodium meclofenamate was taken and serum levels were measured afterwards; that level was found after 2 h.

Kelly: Of the 3 mg/kg?

Rees: Yes.

Kelly: And that will be available in the tissue as well as the blood?

Rees: That we do not know. Measurements were only made in the blood.

Nathanielsz: To return to the question about PGE_2. I am not too familiar with this area but it seems to me that with the prostaglandins, in exhibiting the actual agent in vivo or in vitro, we are back in the situation we were in with the catecholamines where it is not really whether we are giving adrenaline or noradrenaline, but whether the alpha- or the beta-receptor is there. There is a lot of new knowledge becoming available – Rod Coleman at Glaxo gave a very good paper at the Strasbourg symposium suggesting that there are changes in the populations of the prostaglandin receptors, and that has been mentioned a couple of times; so far I think only to show that we are very ignorant in this area.

Keirse: I agree. I have been brought up with the idea that primary dysmenorrhoea disappears after a pregnancy yet I have seen a number of exceptions to that rule. But I know of no evidence.

Lumsden: There is some good evidence from observation of the nerve endings in the cervix which shows that these are destroyed by full-term pregnancy.

Something that would be interesting, although I certainly do not know the answer, is whether the cervix has to be fully dilated, or if, say, somebody has a pregnancy and is delivered be elective section, the dysmenorrhoea is relieved in the same way. I am not aware of any data.

Fraser: The epidemiological data suggest that 60% or 70% of women with primary dysmenorrhoea get an apparent significant improvement after one pregnancy and there is also evidence – whether it is the same women or another group – of further improvement after a second pregnancy. But there is no further improvement after that. There is still a group of between 10% and 20% who have significant dysmenorrhoea after one or more pregnancies.

We currently have evidence of two major mechanisms in what might be called ovulatory menorrhagia, that is through disturbances of the arachidonic acid metabolism, which Dr Rees has discussed in great detail, but also through increased tissue plasminogen activator and increased fibrinolytic activity in the endometrium. Most of those are old data but there are some newer data. Are those two completely independent processes with different roles in different women with menorrhagia, or is there some link in which they may be tied in together? I guess my question is leading to some possible therapy. Perhaps by combination therapy between prostaglandin inhibitors and fibrinolytic inhibitors we may get a much better improvement than we do with either on their own.

Rees: I think they are complementing mechanisms and PGs can stimulate TPA production. I have studied the occasional woman who had only a partial response to, say, Ponstan, and then added tranexamic acid and there was a further reduction in blood loss. But it is only a few cases.

Calder: Can I ask about the lady who lost 1.6 litres of blood. Did she make a habit of this and is she still alive?

Rees: She made a habit of it. She was a university lecturer who when we detected that she was losing 1.6 l (and expedited her hysterectomy from a two-year waiting list to a two-week one) said that these periods were very typical for her. The only reason that she could go to work was that her periods started at the weekends, and when she had her preoperative blood transfusion she said it was the first time she had felt well since the menarche. Her haemoglobin used to run at levels of between 8 and 10 and she used to top herself up with iron when she felt "a bit tired". Her GP had thought that she was just tired and perhaps slightly heavier than average.

Calder: Do those at the very top of the scale respond as well to medical measures?

Rees: We have had some at the top of the scale to whom we gave gestrinone and they responded.

Calder: What about mefenamic acid?

Rees: I have not used it at the top end of the scale, but one would expect it to reduce it by between 30% and 50%, which is not what they want. And by the time they come to hospital, they have already gone through that mill.

MacKenzie: The combined contraceptive pill relieves primary spasmodic dysmenorrhoea and it relieves menorrhagia of no organic cause. How does it work and does it work in the same way for both disorders?

Rees: It does induce endometrial atrophy, and although there is some dispute as to the exact prostaglandin concentration in the endometrium overall the prostaglandin concentration will be very low. Certainly in menstrual fluid prostaglandin concentration is very low.

MacKenzie: And is it achieved by reducing endometrial thickening?

Rees: It is a possibility.

MacKenzie: Is there any other explanation?

Smith: That is unlikely. It is unlikely because the principal source of prostaglandins in the endometrium is the glands and as that is a single layer, the changing of the stromal structure will not make any difference.

There are some data showing a significant reduction of PG production from oral contraceptives, so it cannot just be a reduction in the polymorphonucleo-cytes.

MacKenzie: How is that reduction brought about?

Smith: It is the differential effect of the steroids. Synthetic steroids, as opposed to natural steroids, have a different sequence from each other. One requires oestrogen and progesterone cyclically, and not at the same time, and there are all sorts of potential mechanisms.

Rees: There is a study looking at the prostaglandin concentration of endometrium in women on the pill having laparascopic sterilisations in which it was found that the concentration in women on the pill was in fact elevated compared to normal controls.

Kelly: That is right; but the total content of prostaglandin was reduced.
There is evidence in rabbits that the contractility of the myometrium in response to intravenous PGF is greatly reduced after the administration of progesterone. One might expect with the oral contraceptive pill that the effect of progesterone would be to diminish the contractility of the myometrium.

Lumsden: It is not that simple. There have been studies where this has been done in humans and there was one that suggested that this was so, but this has also been refuted and it is not as clearcut as this.
Professor Smith's explanation is too simple. The glands in the endometrium of someone who is on the pill are not the same in structure or function as those in the late or middle-late secretory phase in someone who is not. Let us say the changes that are induced within the endometrium, not just atrophy but the alteration of its function, may well be why it is so effective.

Fraser: It is fair to say also that the oral contraceptives that we use nowadays are predominantly progestogenic and that there is exposure to progesterone from very early in the cycle, which almost certainly is inhibiting the development of a whole series of biochemical processes.
What we have heard during this session is just pointing out how little we know about which mechanisms are most important, how they interrelate, and how we are suppressing them with our very simplistic treatments.

MacKenzie: It is possible, is it not, that with the current enthusiasm for endometrial ablation there must be among the women having that procedure some with spasmodic dysmenorrhoea. They ought to be getting improvement.

Lumsden: They do not.

MacKenzie: That, therefore, questions the whole concept of the prostaglandins, or prostaglandin production being that important.

Lumsden: This may be where growth factors come in. In the majority of cases not all of the endometrium is removed.

Fraser: I would take issue with that. If one gets good results in terms of amenorrhoea, or dramatic reduction in the volume of blood loss with the endometrial ablation procedure, the majority of women with dysmenorrhoea of the primary spasmodic type usually have a dramatic improvement, though not all: we are seeing about 60% who get a dramatic improvement.

Smith: But some of that reduction in pain is from the cessation of the passage of blood clots, which surely induce pain.

MacKenzie: What is the evidence for that? What evidence could there possibly be that the passage of blood clots causes the pain – apart from anecdotal evidence?

Fraser: Women describe events very clearly – at least the women that I have had an opportunity to question in detail about this. Many women with a clear history of menorrhagia describe a feeling of having no pain at some stage even when bleeding is fairly heavy, and then suddenly pain begins, and shortly after that they do pass what to them is a blood clot; we know that these are not true blood clots but they pass this mass of jelly-like substance. They describe very clearly as if this were something that is passing through the cervix, and as soon as it has passed out, or they feel it is filling the vagina, not necessarily coming to the outside, then the pain gets less. So I suspect that the passage of something through the cervix in some of these women with menorrhagia is contributing to their symptoms. And I agree entirely it is anecdotal.

Calder: There is doubt as to whether the blood does clot in the uterus.

Fraser: Blood does clot in the uterus but it is broken down very rapidly. These women are not getting mature fibrin forming in fibrin monomers. But somewhere they are getting aggregations of blood with mucinous proteins that are forming liver-like aggregations which the women describe as clots or tissue.

MacKenzie: That is confirmed at hysterectomy. When one does a hysterectomy on a woman with menorrhagia who is menstruating, and one opens the uterus up, it is not that uncommon to find a clot.

Kelly: The fact of a clot being relieved could be because that clot is full of white cells which are producing cytotoxic and inflammatory agents. It could be the removal of that from the lumen of the uterus that can reduce a lot of the pain directly.

Fraser: It could easily be. We have no idea.

Chapter 5

Treatment of Menorrhagia

I. S. Fraser

Introduction

Menorrhagia is the loss of excessive amounts of blood at the time of menstruation. Definitions are far from precise, and there is little agreement on exact usage among clinicians from different centres. Here the term is used to mean a complaint of excessively heavy bleeding irrespective of its regularity or frequency. Objective confirmation of excessive bleeding in clinical practice is difficult, and numerous studies have demonstrated that there is little correlation between a complaint of heavy bleeding and research measurements of a loss of greater than 80 ml per menstrual period [1–4]. This chapter will attempt to take into account the difference between the broadly accepted clinical diagnosis and the narrower objective research definition.

Assessment, Perception and Tolerance

Before considering the specifics of treatment of menorrhagia, it is necessary to consider why many women who present with a complaint of excessive bleeding do not actually have it! Most studies which have addressed this problem have found that 40%–60% of women presenting with a complaint of excessively heavy bleeding have an objectively measured blood loss of less than 80 ml per menses [3].

Menorrhagia is the doctor's assessment based, at least initially, on the woman's description of her own perception of her menstrual loss [5]. The woman's perception is based on her observations – visual, tactile and olfactory – of the total menstrual loss. It is now well recognised that the menstrual loss contains a substantial amount – 50%–60% – of fluid which cannot be accounted for by whole blood [6], yet the objective verification of menorrhagia in research studies is based solely on measurement of menstrual haemoglobin content. Hence, it appears that the patient and clinician may be assessing different parameters in determining the complaint.

Therefore, menorrhagia is primarily a subjective complaint that a woman is having difficulty coping with the heaviness, or a perceived change in heaviness, of her periods. This may be causing:

1. Iron deficiency or anaemia;
2. Disturbance of her social, occupational or sexual activities;
3. Concern about possible serious underlying disease (specifically cancer);
4. Worsening of an underlying depression associated with poor tolerance of menstruation;
5. Decreased menstrual tolerance after sterilisation.

Each of these presentations may need to be treated differently, and therefore requires precise definition in each individual.

Causes of Menorrhagia

Precise management of menorrhagia depends on a reasonably accurate diagnosis of the underlying condition [5], since therapies may vary considerably depending on cause. Causes fall into three broad categories. They may often be recognised on a careful history and examination alone, although a substantial minority of women require more thorough evaluation.

Pelvic Disease

This is the commonest category of causes of menorrhagia. The mechanism of abnormal bleeding is not clearly understood in any of these, although there is some reason to believe that disturbances of prostaglandin synthesis or metabolism may be involved in some. Those in which a prostaglandin abnormality is most likely to be involved include endometriosis and adenomyosis [7,8], and perhaps rarities like myometrial hypertrophy.

Myomata

Objective measurements of menstrual blood loss confirm that the position of the myoma is clearly related to the degree of menorrhagia, with intrauterine, submucous, intramural and subserous being related in decreasing order of severity [9].

Adenomyosis

There is no dispute that this condition is sometimes related to menorrhagia, but objective measurements of blood loss are few.

Endometriosis

This is a controversial cause of menorrhagia, and many do not believe that it causes excessively heavy bleeding. Although there is good anecdotal evidence that many women with endometriosis do not bleed heavily, some certainly do [9,10]. There is sufficient evidence to accept that the association is causal in some cases, and this may well be mediated through a prostaglandin-related mechanism. A substantial proportion of women with dysmenorrhoea and menorrhagia associated with endometriosis will have their symptoms improved by prostaglandin inhibitors [11].

Endometrial Polyps

These poorly understood lesions are not uncommon and are sometimes associated with menorrhagia. Mechanisms are unknown.

Polycystic Ovarian Disease

This may cause anovulatory dysfunctional uterine bleeding, typically at frequent intervals. Prostaglandins may be involved, but mechanisms are uncertain, since total endometrial prostaglandin synthesis appears to be low with anovulation [12].

Endometrial Carcinoma

This is a rare presenting cause of menorrhagia, but up to 50% of premenopausal women with endometrial adenocarcinomas may have menorrhagia.

Intrauterine Devices

These iatrogenic causes of menorrhagia are included under this heading, although modern copper IUDs do not increase menstrual blood loss as much as the first generation inert devices. It is probable that IUDs cause menorrhagia in a proportion of women through prostaglandin-related mechanisms, although there is suggestive evidence that menorrhagia is often related to major disturbances in the relationship of the IUD to the uterine wall (e.g. embedding, partial perforation and rotation [13].

Other rare causes include myometrial hypertrophy, uterine vascular malformations and perhaps pelvic inflammatory disease and bicornuate uterus.

Systemic Disease

These diseases account for only a very small proportion of cases of menorrhagia, but they should not be forgotten in severe cases or those which do not respond to initial therapy. There is little evidence for a prostaglandin mechanism in these cases unless it is mediated through platelet function in some of the coagulation disorders. Systemic diseases which may be involved in menorrhagia include:

1. Coagulation disorders
2. Hypothyroidism
3. Systemic lupus erythematosus
4. Chronic liver failure
5. Other very rare causes

Dysfunctional Uterine Bleeding (DUB)

This is a diagnosis of exclusion and should only be made after basic investigations have excluded obvious disease as described above. Nevertheless, it is a useful clinical working diagnosis even before investigations have been completed. DUB is a diagnosis which does not necessarily apply only to excessively heavy bleeding, but may also include excessively prolonged and excessively frequent bleeding [5].

Our present understanding of the mechanisms of DUB has been thoroughly discussed in Chapter 3.

Management of Menorrhagia

Management is not confined to the application of medical and surgical therapies, but also includes an individualised approach to each patient to define her condition and to provide sufficient information to motivate her to continue medication according to instructions for as long as is necessary, or to understand the need for surgery.

Investigation

Investigations will depend to some extent on details of the history, but in general should always include a full blood count, office hysteroscopy and endometrial biopsy rather than blind curettage. There is now good evidence that the incidence of false negative results with blind curettage is unacceptably high [9,14,15]. In some cases there will be indications to carry out estimation of serum ferritin or thyroid stimulating hormone (TSH), a partial coagulation screen, a high resolution pelvic ultrasound scan or a diagnostic laparoscopy.

Counselling

Counselling and the provision of information are an essential part of the management of this condition, especially in optimising compliance. This should include clear instructions about drug use and a firm reassurance about the exclusion of serious disease such as cancer. Good counselling, perhaps accompanied by use of a simple menstrual calendar, may allow a substantial improvement in the tolerance of menstruation and even avoid the use of drug or surgical therapy in those without iron deficiency, anaemia or specific disease.

Therapy

Treatment of menorrhagia is often far from logical. With a little more attention to individual complaints it could be made much more precise for the majority of patients, even in our present state of incomplete understanding of mechanisms.

Drug Therapy

The medical literature is replete with drugs which have been proposed for the treatment of menorrhagia down the ages. Most were probably not very effective except as placebos for those women whose menstrual blood loss was actually still within the normal range. It is of interest that Dr H. Beckwith Whitehouse, in his historic Hunterian lecture in 1915 [16], proposed the local application of "thrombokinase in the form of an extract of endometrium or testicle" or if that did not work "fibrin ferment supplied by Messrs Parke, Davis and Co as 'Coagulose' ", although he does not report results in a form which would convince today's sceptics!

Prostaglandin Inhibitors (Non-Steroidal Anti-inflammatory Agents: NSAIDs)

This review will concentrate particularly on the role of prostaglandin inhibitors in the treatment of menorrhagia, but will also try to put their use in context with other established medications. Most prostaglandin inhibitors act predominantly as inhibitors of the cyclo-oxygenase enzyme system (Fig. 5.1) which is responsible for synthesis of prostaglandin endoperoxides and is located in the microsomal fraction of the cell. Some of these agents, such as meclofenamic acid, may also have an inhibitory effect on the lipoxygenase pathway [17]. Additionally, there is evidence that some act as weak end-organ inhibitors. For example, there is evidence that the fenamates inhibit binding of PGE_2, and perhaps other prostaglandins, to their target organs [18,19]. In practice, any differences in mode of action of individual PG inhibitors do not seem to make much difference to overall clinical efficacy, although there are individual women who seem to respond well to one agent but not so well to another. These clinical differences between preparations have not been well explored.

Numerous objective studies have now been reported on menstrual blood loss measurements in women receiving treatment with prostaglandin inhibitors for

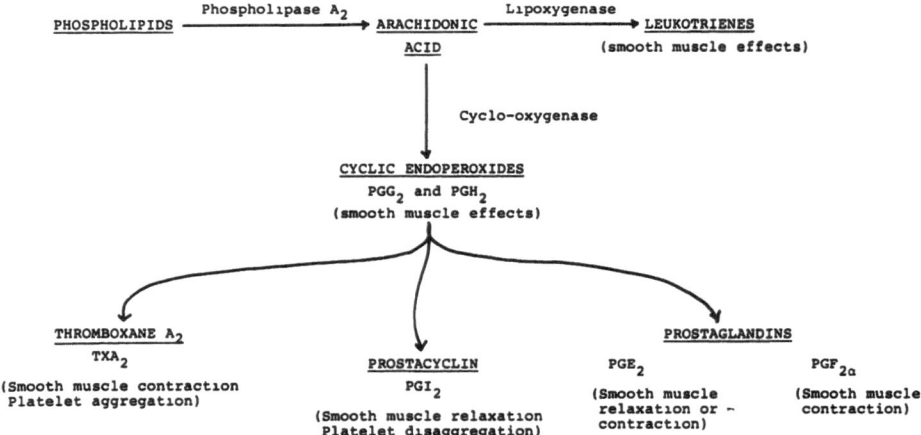

Fig. 5.1. Simplified pathways of arachidonic acid metabolism indicating the main synthetic enzyme systems. Most prostaglandin inhibitors act predominantly as cyclo-oxygenase inhibitors, and some may also inhibit the lipoxygenase system.

menorrhagia due to ovulatory dysfunctional uterine bleeding. Most reports have used mefenamic acid [3,20–30], but some have utilised naproxen or naproxen sodium [26,30–32], meclofenamic acid [33], ibuprofen [34], flufenamic acid [20], diclofenac sodium [35] or flurbiprofen [36]. The overall results seem to be broadly similar although individual studies vary considerably because of relatively small numbers of subjects. There is a wide variation in individual patient response, with the overall mean reduction in measured loss during treatment being of the order of 30%–40%. There is some indication that women with heavier loss experience a greater percentage reduction in loss than those with less heavy bleeding [3,22,37]. For example, Fig. 5.2 shows a mean reduction of 37% in menstrual blood loss in women treated with mefenamic acid when placebo-treatment blood loss was greater than 60 ml, but no mean reduction when blood loss on placebo was less than 40 ml [37]. This is of considerable practical importance because a high proportion of women presenting with menorrhagia do not actually have excessive loss. Meclofenamate sodium is absorbed more rapidly than most other prostaglandin inhibitors and probably has a more potent clinical effect because of greater end-organ binding [19]. Excellent clinical results (in only one study) have been reported with reductions in blood loss of the order of 40%–50% over four cycles of use [33]. It used to be thought that it caused more side effects than other prostaglandin inhibitors, but this has not been borne out by recent experience.

Most investigators have used short-term regimens with the initiation of therapy at the onset of bleeding and intermittent doses until after the usual end of excessively heavy bleeding. Dosage regimens vary greatly according to the preparation, but may need to be individually titrated to the patient's response in order to obtain optimum long-term results. Compliance may be a problem because many women do not like taking regular medication every month and will often wait to see whether the period is going to be a "bad" one or a "good" one before starting medication. Clinical results seem to be much worse in these circumstances. I strongly recommend women to start medication at the very first sign of bleeding and then take successive doses every 4–8 h depending on the

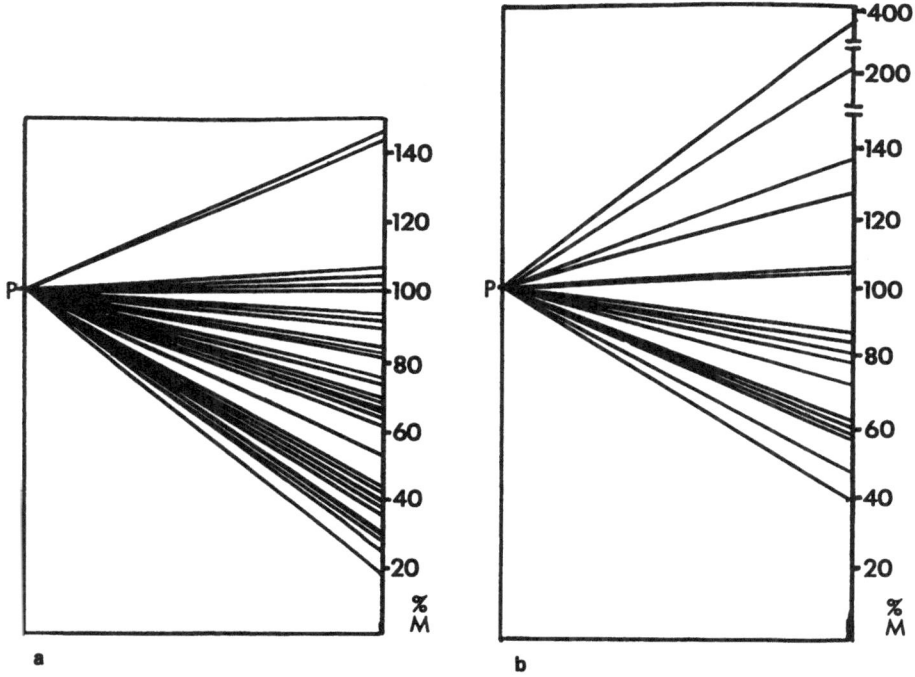

Fig. 5.2. Percentage change in menstrual blood loss (averaged over two cycles) in 69 women with subjective menorrhagia during mefenamic acid (M%) treatment as a percentage of their measured menstrual loss during treatment with placebo (P). **a** Women with placebo loss of greater than 60 ml/cycle; **b** Women with placebo loss of less than 40 ml/cycle. Modified from Fraser [37].

persistence or recurrence of symptoms, and continue this until half a day beyond the time when they would normally have stopped bleeding heavily. It should be noted that a small number of women stop menstruating when a prostaglandin inhibitor is given at the first sign of menstruation [38], and these individuals may need to wait until the period is well established in subsequent cycles.

A significant proportion of women with heavy loss do not obtain benefit from these agents, and a small number actually experience a consistent increase in measured loss during treatment with prostaglandin inhibitors ([30] Fig. 5.3). The mechanism of this unusual response is quite unknown at the present time. The range of individual responses is illustrated in Fig. 5.2 [37], and shows that some fortunate women obtain up to an 80% reduction in loss. Those women with the greatest loss usually gain the greatest benefit. Overall, it appears that 50%–60% of women with objective menorrhagia will gain a sufficient reduction in loss to justify long-term therapy. Most studies now agree that there is also a significant reduction in duration of bleeding during treatment with mefenamic acid [3,28,29].

Many doctors report that their patients find that the initial reduction in menstrual bleeding is not maintained with long-term therapy. However, this is not the finding with objective measurements over time spans of more than one year. We have found persistent reductions of the same order of 25%–35% over 16 months in 34 women [24]. The explanation for most of the failures to maintain a

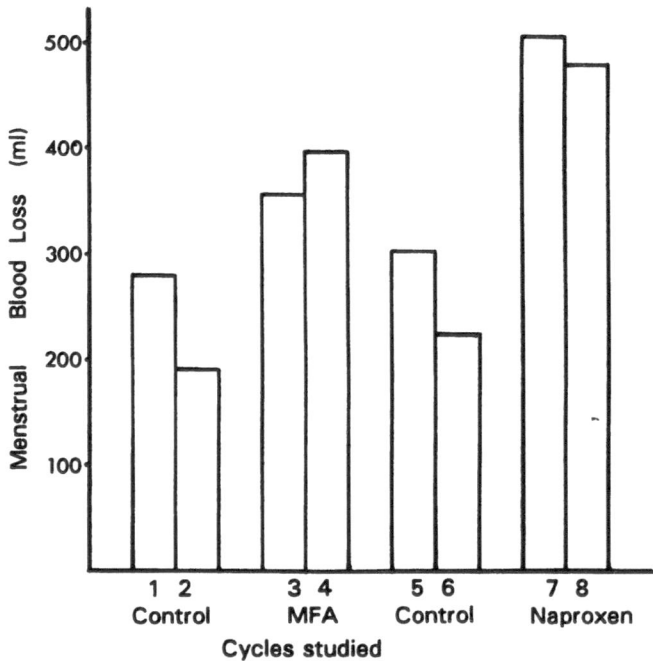

Fig. 5.3. Measured menstrual blood loss in a woman with menorrhagia followed through eight successive cycles, when she was untreated (control; four cycles), or treated with one of two prostaglandin inhibitors (mefenamic acid; MFA: two cycles; or naproxen: two cycles). Menstrual blood loss increased substantially during treatment with both prostaglandin inhibitors. Reproduced with permission from Fraser [30].

response is probably that patients become less meticulous about dosage as time goes by, although there is evidence from the field of rheumatology that some individuals do need to have their NSAIDs rotated in order to maintain an optimal response. This has never been tested for menorrhagia, but may apply in some individuals. We have tested a small group of individuals who participated in a clinical trial of mefenamic acid and have demonstrated maintained responses ten years after the initial trial.

It is important to note that other symptoms, such as dysmenorrhoea, menstrual headaches and menstrually related diarrhoea, nausea and depression also improve with mefenamic acid treatment and this improvement is maintained over more than one year [3,24]. Anecdotally, symptoms of premenstrual syndrome (PMS) will sometimes also improve, but this is the exception rather than the rule. However, there is good evidence that PMS symptoms will improve with mefenamic acid given throughout the luteal phase in a substantial proportion of cases [39].

There are few data in the literature about the effect of prostaglandin inhibitors on menorrhagia due to causes other than dysfunctional bleeding. The exception is menorrhagia associated with use of an IUD. Recent evidence indicates that there is a 74% increase in measured menstrual loss with insertion of most modern copper IUDs, and this can be prevented by use of a prostaglandin inhibitor [13]. Numerous reports confirm the efficacy of prostaglandin inhibitors for the treatment of menorrhagia due to IUDs [40–46], indeed the first major report on the use of a PG inhibitor for menorrhagia was on mefenamic acid and IUDs [20]. There is encouraging evidence that mefenamic acid may be helpful to a substantial proportion of women with adenomyosis, endometriosis and occasionally other conditions causing menorrhagia [3,10]. However, these drugs are not usually helpful with myomata [10,32] and some coagulation disorders [34].

Individual differences in response are an important aspect of PG inhibitor use, but only a few comparative trials have been carried out with different PG inhibitors or comparing a PG inhibitor against other agents in the same patient. The small number of randomised studies of this type show that mefenamic acid and naproxen are probably similar in effect, provided that sufficient dosages are used [26,30], although not all patients who respond well to one will respond to the other. Hence, there is a place for considering use of an alternative PG inhibitor if one does not work. Mefenamic acid has also been compared against danazol and oral contraception [27,30], with remarkably similar results in the first cycle of treatment, provided that tolerance and side effects are taken into account. Danazol produces a very much greater reduction with continued use than most other agents (see below). Comparative studies have also been carried out with prostaglandin inhibitors and tranexamic acid [35,36] and with progesterone-releasing IUDs [28,36], demonstrating that the PG inhibitors are less effective than these other treatments. There is currently no information about the possible use of prostaglandin inhibitors in combination with hormonal therapies.

Side effects are an important consideration with any form of long-term therapy, and medical treatment of menorrhagia may be necessary for many years. Numerous side effects have been reported with prostaglandin inhibitors, but in general the dosage regimen with intermittent use for only a few days out of each month is remarkably free of problems. In our initial trial of mefenamic acid over two cycles in 69 patients equal numbers of side effects were recorded in treatment and placebo groups [3], and in the one-year follow-up only two out of 36 women withdrew because of gastrointestinal side effects [24]. However, it is important to recognise that a range of gastrointestinal, central nervous system and other effects have been recorded with prolonged use, and there have even been cases of renal failure in older or systematically ill women using mefenamic acid. These serious effects have not been recorded with short-term or cyclical use of PG inhibitors.

In view of the variability of cycles and the difficulties of compliance with frequent dosage each day of every menstruation, there is a need to develop delivery systems for prostaglandin inhibitors. It would be ideal if systems could be developed which would deliver constant dosages over several days and could be controlled by the woman herself. Since dosages are in the gram range each day the most appropriate system would be a vaginal ring, provided that these drugs are absorbed effectively from this surface. Since indomethacin is well absorbed from rectal suppositories, a vagina device should be realistic.

Hormonal

Numerous hormonal regimens have been promoted in the literature but few have any good substantiation for the efficacy. The most popular therapy for ovulatory DUB in the United Kingdom is luteal phase norethisterone (NET), and the rationale for this is a paper by Bishop and de Almeida [47] which reports subjective improvement in women with both ovulatory and anovulatory DUB. It is now clear that women have great difficulty in determining both absolute amounts of menstrual loss and changes in loss from day to day and cycle to cycle [1–4], and therefore subjective reports cannot be relied on to give an accurate picture. The first reports of objective measurements of menstrual blood loss in women treated with progestogens have only just appeared in the last few years. A small reduction of around 16% has been reported in menstrual blood loss (MBL) with oral NET given during the luteal phase [28]. This degree of improvement is too small to be clinically useful. Luteal phase progestogen therapy is probably very useful in women with anovulatory DUB, where objective reductions of more than 50% have been reported [48]. In these women the pattern and duration of loss were also beneficially influenced. More prolonged therapy of durations up to three weeks out of every four is probably necessary to produce optimal reductions in MBL in women with ovulatory DUB. With these regimens objective mean reductions of 35% have been reported [48].

It is my view that luteal phase oral progestogens, such as NET 5 mg bd/tds or medroxyprogesterone acetate (MPA) 10 mg bd/tds, are good first-line therapy for anovulatory bleeding, but not for ovulatory bleeding where longer courses which will inhibit the unopposed oestrogen effect on the endometrium are needed [48]. Continuous oral progestogen therapy has also been recommended anecdotally, and may be highly satisfactory as long as breakthrough bleeding is not a problem. This produces an effect on the endometrium similar to that of depot-medroxyprogesterone acetate (DMPA) injections, following which amenorrhoea is the eventual rule, but a substantial proportion experience erratic and sometimes prolonged breakthrough bleeding. DMPA is probably not a good therapy for DUB unless amenorrhoea is first produced with oral MPA.

The best way of administering progestogens in order to obtain dramatic reductions in menstrual blood loss with ovulatory, and probably anovulatory, DUB is with an intrauterine device. Preliminary data from the progesterone-releasing IUD (Progestasert, Alza Corporation) suggested that reductions of the order of 70%–80% could be obtained [28,49]. Even better results have now been recorded from several centres with the new levonorgestrel-releasing IUDs. Andersson and Rybo [50] have reported reductions in menstrual blood loss of around 85% at 3 months, 90% at 6 months and 95% at 12 months after device insertion.

The mechanism of action of progestogens is not known, but it is fairly safe to assume that arachidonic acid metabolism is changed substantially with reduced exposure to unopposed oestrogen and increased exposure to high dose progestogens. Exposure of the endometrium to large amounts of progestogen leads to inhibition of proliferation followed by suppressed secretory change and eventually atrophy. These changes presumably reduce the capacity of the endometrium to mobilise arachidonic acid from membrane phospholipids, and may also affect synthesis of individual prostaglandins from any arachidonic acid and endoperoxides that may be formed. However, the main mechanisms of action may be by the inhibition of fibrinolytic activity and by reduction in endometrial vascularity. Much work needs to be done to elucidate these mechanisms.

Gestrinone is an antiprogesterone and antioestrogen with some androgenic activity, and has been shown to be beneficial for ovulatory menorrhagia when given in a dosage of one capsule twice weekly [51].

Combined oral contraceptives (COCs) have been an effective method of treatment of menorrhagia for many years, and overall appear to produce a 40%–50% reduction in MBL in ovulatory DUB [30,52]. A minority of individuals do not obtain satisfactory benefit or else experience troublesome side effects. There is also the consideration that long-term therapy may be inappropriate for women with contraindications like cigarette smoking. COCs may work for endometriosis and some of the coagulation disorders, but probably do not help adenomyosis and myomata. Objective data are lacking.

In some menstrual disorders, including dysmenorrhoea and premenstrual syndrome, there is a significant placebo response, but this does not appear to play any role in the reduction of MBL by active therapies in women with menorrhagia [53]. On the other hand, attention to psychosomatic aspects is probably very important in obtaining the best long-term results with any therapy in menorrhagia.

Danazol is a highly effective drug for producing amenorrhoea during treatment for endometriosis, and usually does the same for ovulatory and anovulatory DUB. Danazol is also effective at reducing menstrual blood loss dramatically at dosages as low as 200 mg or even 100 mg daily over several months [30,53]. Reduction of menstrual blood loss is limited during the first cycle of therapy but increases greatly with subsequent cycles of continued therapy. Short-term treatment with danazol may be limited by side effects such as weight gain, acne, mood changes and muscle cramps, and long-term therapy should not generally be used because of concerns about cardiovascular and liver effects. Therefore, this is a drug to be used for severe menorrhagia when profound reduction in menstrual blood loss is required to allow thinking time before more definitive treatment is instituted.

Gonadotrophin-releasing hormone analogues (GnRHa) have been used in very limited studies as treatments for menorrhagia. Shaw and Fraser have reported highly effective reductions in measured loss in four women with ovulatory DUB [54]. These are the only agents capable of producing a reasonably effective medical approach to the management of myomata [55], but unfortunately, their use is limited by side effects in the short term and metabolic concerns and costs in the long term. In principle, there are several ways in which they might be used for the short and long term management of DUB [56], and they could be highly effective especially when combined with low dose hormone replacement therapy. Unfortunately, the major stumbling block to their use will be the high cost of continuous therapy and at the present time it is not possible to see any hope of worthwhile reductions even with genetic engineering and bacterial synthesis techniques.

Fibrinolytic Inhibitors

Fibrinolytic inhibitors have been extensively evaluated for menorrhagia, especially in Scandinavia [35,36,52,57], and have been shown to be highly effective. Objective reductions in measured loss are dose related and reach a mean of 50% in most studies. The preferred drug is tranexamic acid since side effects are infrequent (mainly gastrointestinal) and complications are exceedingly rare. Epsi-aminocaproic acid has been associated with occasional spontaneous thromboses and should preferably not be used. The only disadvantage of this approach is the dosage which requires use of large tablets or sachets which many patients find difficult to ingest over the long term. Bioavailability may improve with modifications to the tablets. The way in which fibrinolytic inhibitors interrelate with prostaglandins is uncertain, and whether a combination of fibrinolytic inhibitor with a prostaglandin inhibitor would be better than either on its own is also unclear. However, it does seem that fibrinolytic and prostaglandin mechanisms are both highly important in the pathogenesis of most cases of ovulatory DUB, and a dual approach to therapy could have some merit.

Other Treatments

Other treatments include the use of ethamsylate, which has been reported to be of value with IUDs and DUB [58]; tamoxifen, which has been used for myomata and myometrial hypertrophy [59]; injections of long-acting vasopressin analogues such as glypressin [60]; and older treatments such as toluidine blue and protamine sulphate [61].

Choices

How does one decide which therapy is the most appropriate? Table 5.1 compares some of the different approaches. Individual use depends greatly on the doctor's familiarity with the different drugs and the information and encouragement which is given to the patient. This does not mean hoodwinking the patient with extravagant claims, but providing no-nonsense basic information on benefits, side effects, dosage regimens, the need for compliance and the availability of alternative treatments. This should include a long-term plan (which may involve surgery such as endometrial ablation or hysterectomy).

Table 5.1. Chart comparing some of the more important features of different therapies for menorrhagia due to ovulatory dysfunctional uterine bleeding

| | Prostaglandin inhibitors | Fibrinolytic inhibitors | Progestogens | | OCP | Danazol | Endometrial ablation[b] | Hyster-ectomy[b] |
			Short cycle[a]	Long cycle[a]				
Mean % reduction in blood loss	30	50	15	35	50	80	90	100
% showing substantial reduction	60	90	20	70	80	90	95	100
Convenience of regimen	+++	++	++	++	++	++	+	(+)
Cost	+	+	+	+	+	++	++	+++
Reversibility	+++	+++	+++	+++	+++	+++	0	0
Minor side effects	+	+	+	++	+	+++	+	++
Complications	(+)	(+)	(+)	(+)	(+)	+	+	++

+++, high; ++, moderate; +, low; (+), very low.
[a] Short cycle, luteal phase only; long cycle, follicular + luteal therapy. OCP, oral contraceptive pill.
[b] In skilled hands.

Surgical Therapy

Surgical therapy has a major role in the long-term management of menorrhagia due to DUB because there is no known medical cure for this condition in older women. Medical therapy is merely a palliative for as long as it is given.

Curettage

Dilatation and curettage (D&C) has long been recommended as an emergency treatment for menorrhagia, but without objective evidence of its effectiveness. It may be a helpful diagnostic measure in the acute case, but does not always help to stop excessive bleeding. In chronic menorrhagia there is good evidence that D&C will greatly reduce bleeding in the next cycle, but will then be followed by an increase in measured blood loss in the second cycle before finally reverting to the precurettage pattern [22,52].

Hysterectomy

The traditional and highly effective surgical approach to management of menorrhagia has been hysterectomy, and this has become so widely used that in several countries up to 40% of women will undergo this major surgery at some time during their lifetime [62,63]. A careful look at the figures suggests that about 25% of the women will have this operation before the menopause and, of these, in about 40% it will be for a diagnosis of DUB. Most others will be for myomata, endometriosis and neoplasia, of which a substantial number will have menorrhagia as a component of their symptomatology. Although this is major surgery, many surgeons consider that one major operation, with very low mortality when undertaken for benign disease and a reasonably low long-term morbidity in skilled hands, will be preferable to medical therapy prolonged over many years [5]. It is essential to consider whether the approach should be abdominal or vaginal, and whether removal should be total or subtotal. It seems that the approach used by a particular surgeon is generally dictated more by anecdote and familiarity than by thorough clinical and scientific evaluation.

Endometrial Ablation

Increasing criticism of the large numbers of hysterectomies and concern about possible psychological and medical sequelae of this major operation accompanied by advances in endoscopic technology have led to a rapid refinement of the procedures known by the term endometrial ablation. This is a logical surgical procedure which aims to remove that part of the uterus which bleeds abnormally and allow the uterine lumen to become lined by a thin layer of fibrous tissue. This can be accomplished by an operation which takes 30–60 min and is handled as a day case or with an overnight stay [64–66].

Several techniques are currently used with some success. These include the neodymium-YAG laser [64], the hysteroresectoscope with resection loop [65] or roller ball [66] element and the radiofrequency probe [67]. It needs to be remembered that these are relatively new techniques which require much more extensive evaluation before they can be routinely offered as alternatives to hysterectomy.

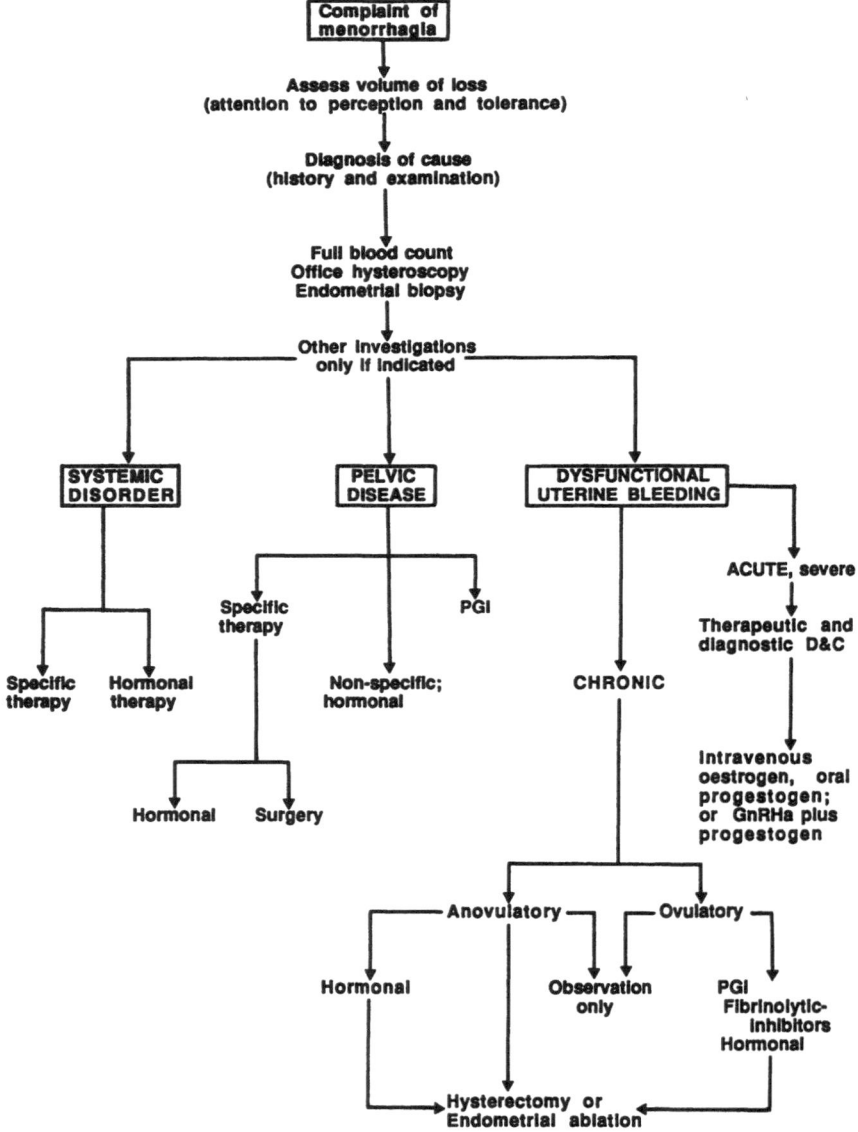

Fig. 5.4. Flow chart for the management of menorrhagia (modified from Fraser [5]). PGI, prostaglandin inhibitors; GnRHa, gonadotrophin-releasing hormone agonists.

Conclusions

Menorrhagia provides problems with assessment of blood loss; precision of diagnosis, lack of understanding of mechanisms and individualisation of management. Counselling is essential after appropriate investigations and before the careful selection of relevant medical or surgical therapy. Fig. 5.4 illustrates a flow chart summarising some of the main steps which need to be considered in an overall plan of management for the patient with menorrhagia.

References

1. Hallberg L, Hogdahl A-M, Nilsson L, Rybo G. Menstrual blood loss – a population study. Acta Obstet Gynecol Scand 1966; 45:320–51.
2. Chimbira T, Anderson ABM, Turnbull AC. Relation between measured menstrual blood loss and patients' subjective assessment of loss, duration of bleeding, number of sanitary towels used, uterine weight and endometrial surface area. Br J Obstet Gynaecol 1980; 87:603–9.
3. Fraser IS, Pearse C, Shearman RP, Elliott PM, McIlveen J, Markham R. Efficacy of mefenamic acid in patients with a complaint of menorrhagia. Obstet Gynecol 1981; 58:543–51.
4. Fraser IS, McCarron G, Markham R. A preliminary study of factors influencing perception of menstrual blood loss volume. Am J Obstet Gynecol 1984; 149: 788–93.
5. Fraser IS. Treatment of menorrhagia. In: Drife JO, ed. Dysfunctional uterine bleeding and menorrhagia. Bailliere's Clinical Obstetrics and Gynaecology 1989; 3:391–402.
6. Fraser IS, McCarron G, Markham R. Blood and total fluid content of menstrual discharge. Obstet Gynecol 1985; 65:194–8.
7. Rock JA, Hurst BS. Clinical significance of prostanoid concentration in women with endometriosis. In: Chadha DR, Buttram VC, eds. Current concepts in endometriosis. Progress in clinical and biological research, Vol. 323. New York: Alan R Liss, 1990; 61–80.
8. Smith SK. The endometrium and endometriosis. In: Thomas EJ, Rock JA, eds. Modern approaches to endometriosis. Dordrecht: Kluwer Academic Publishers, 1991; 57–77.
9. Fraser IS. Hysteroscopy and laparoscopy in women with menorrhagia. Am J Obstet Gynecol 1990; 162:1264–9.
10. Fraser IS, McCarron G, Markham R. Objective measurement of menstrual blood loss in women with a complaint of menorrhagia associated with pelvic disease or coagulation disorder. Obstet Gynecol 1986; 68:630–3.
11. Kauppila A, Puolakka J, Ylikorkala O. Prostaglandin biosynthesis inhibitors and endometriosis. Prostaglandins 1979; 18:655–61.
12. Baird DT, Abel MH, Kelly RW, Smith SK. Endocrinology of dysfunctional uterine bleeding: the role of endometrial prostaglandins. In: Crosignani PG, Rubin BL, eds. Endocrinology of human infertility; new aspects. New York: Academic Press, 1981; 399–417.
13. Pizarro E, Schoenstedt G, Mehech G, Hidalgo M, Romero C, Munoz G. Uterine cavity and the location of IUDs following administration of meclofenamic acid to menorrhagic women. Contraception 1989; 40:413–23.
14. Brooks PG, Serden SP. Hysteroscopic findings after unsuccessful dilatation and curettage for abnormal bleeding. Am J Obstet Gynecol 1888; 158:1354–7.
15. Loffer FD. Hysteroscopy with selective endometrial sampling compared with dilatation and curettage for abnormal uterine bleeding: the value of a negative hysteroscopic view. Obstet Gynecol 1989; 73:16–20.
16. Whitehouse HB. The physiology and pathology of uterine haemorrhage. Lancet 1914; i:951–7.
17. Boctor A, Eickholt M, Pugsley IA. Meclofenamate sodium is an inhibitor of both the 5-lipoxygenase and cyclo-oxygenase pathways of the arachidonic cascade in vitro. Prostaglandin Leukotrienes Med 1986; 23:229–38.
18. Flowers RJ, Vane JR. Inhibition of prostaglandin synthesis. Biochem Pharmacol 1974; 23:1439–50.

19. Rees MCP, Canete-Soler R, Bernal AL, Turnbull AC. Effect of fenamates on prostaglandin E receptor binding. Lancet 1988; i:541–2.
20. Anderson ABM, Haynes PJ, Guillebaud J, Turnbull AC. Reduction of menstrual blood loss by prostaglandin synthetase inhibitors. Lancet 1976; i:774–6.
21. Jacubowicz DL, Wood C. The use of the prostaglandin synthetase inhibitor mefenamic acid in the treatment of menorrhagia. Aust NZ J Obstet Gynaecol 1979; 18:135–42.
22. Haynes PJ, Flint AP, Hodgson H, Anderson ABM, Turnbull AC. Studies in menorrhagia: a) mefenamic acid; b) endometrial prostaglandin concentration. Int J Gynaecol Obstet 1980; 17:567–72.
23. Wood C, Jacubowicz DL. The use of mefenamic acid in the treatment of menorrhagia and other menstrual symptoms in specialist practice. Res Clin Forums 1982; 14:111–22.
24. Fraser IS, McCarron G, Markham R. Long-term treatment of menorrhagia with mefenamic acid. Obstet Gynecol 1983; 61:109–12.
25. Muggeridge J, Elder MG. Mefenamic acid in the treatment of menorrhagia. Res Clin Forums 1983; 5:83–8.
26. Hall P, Maclachlan N, Thorn N, Hudd MWE, Taylor CG, Garrioch DB. Control of menorrhagia by the cyclo-oxygenase inhibitors naproxen sodium and mefenamic acid. Br J Obstet Gynaecol 1987; 94:554–8.
27. Dockeray CJ. The use of prostaglandin synthetase inhibitors in dysfunctional uterine bleeding. In: Shaw RW, ed. Dysfunctional uterine bleeding. Carnforth: Parthenon Press, 1990; 117–25.
28. Cameron IT, Haining R, Lumsden MA, Thomas VR, Smith SK. The effects of mefenamic acid and norethisterone on measured menstrual blood loss. Obstet Gynecol 1990; 76:85–8.
29. Grover V, Usha R, Gupta U, Kaira S. Management of cyclical menorrhagia with a prostaglandin synthetase inhibitor. Asia Oceania J Obstet Gynaecol 1990; 16:255–9.
30. Fraser IS, McCarron G. Randomised trial of two hormonal and two prostaglandin inhibiting agents for the treatment of menorrhagia. Aust NZ J Obstet Gynaecol 1991; 31:66–70.
31. Rybo G, Nilsson S, Sikstrom B, Nygren KG. Naproxen in menorrhagia. Lancet 1981; i:608–9.
32. Ylikorkala O, Pekonen F. Naproxen reduces idiopathic but not fibromyoma-induced menorrhagia. Obstet Gynecol 1986; 68:10–16.
33. Vargyas JM, Campeau JD, Mishell DR, jr. Treatment of menorrhagia with meclofenamate sodium. Am J Obstet Gynecol 1987; 157:944–50.
34. Makarainen L, Ylikorkala O. Primary and myoma-associated menorrhagia: role of prostaglandins and effect of ibuprofen. Br J Obstet Gynaecol 1986; 93:974–83.
35. Ylikorkala O, Viinikka L. Comparison between antifibrinolytic and antiprostaglandin treatment in the reduction of increased menstrual blood loss in women with intrauterine contraceptive devices. Br J Obstet Gynaecol 1983; 90: 78–87.
36. Milsom I, Andersson K, Andersch B, Rybo G. A comparison of flurbiprofen, tranexamic acid and a levonorgestrel-releasing intrauterine contraceptive device in the treatment of idiopathic menorrhagia. Am J Obstet Gynecol 1991; 164:879–93.
37. Fraser IS. The treatment of menorrhagia with mefenamic acid. Res Clin Forums 1983; 5:93–9.
38. Meyboom RH, Bonsema K, Huisman-Klein Haneveld PM. Can naproxen impair menstruation? Ned Tijdschr Geneeskd 1989; 133:1326–7.
39. Mira M, Fraser IS, McNeil D, Vizzard J, Abraham S. The use of mefenamic acid in treatment of premenopausal tension sufferers. Obstet Gynecol 1986; 68:395–8.
40. Guillebaud J, Anderson ABM, Turnbull AC. Reduction by mefenamic acid of increased menstrual blood loss associated with intrauterine contraception. Br J Obstet Gynaecol 1978; 85:53–60.
41. Ylikorkala O, Kauppila A, Siljander M. Antiprostaglandin therapy in prevention of side-effects of intrauterine contraceptive devices. Lancet 1978; ii:393–5.
42. Davies AJ. Reduction of menstrual blood loss by naprooxen in intrauterine contraceptive device users. Int J Gynaecol Obstet 1980; 17:353–4.
43. Davies AJ, Anderson ABM, Turnbull AC. Reduction by naproxen of excessive menstrual bleeding in women using intrauterine devices. Obstet Gynecol 1981; 57:74–8.
44. Roy S, Shaw ST. Role of prostaglandins in IUD-associated uerine bleeding – effect of a prostaglandin synthetase inhibitor (ibuprofen). Obstet Gynecol 1981; 58:101–6.
45. Toppozada M, Anwar M, Abdel Rahman H, Gaweesh S. Control of IUD-induced bleeding by three non-steroidal anti-inflammatory drugs. Contracept Deliv Systems 1982; 3:117–25.
46. Makarainen L, Ylikorkala O. Ibuprofen prevents IUCD-induced increases in menstrual blood loss. Br J Obstet Gynaecol 1986; 93:285–8.
47. Bishop PMF, de Almeida JCC. Treatment of functional menstrual disorders with norethisterone. Br Med J 1960; 1:1103–6.

48. Fraser IS. Treatment of ovulatory and anovulatory dysfunctional uterine bleeding with oral progestogens. Aust NZ J Obstet Gynaecol 1990; 30:353–6.
49. Bergqvist A, Rybo G. Treatment of menorrhagia with intrauterine release of progesterone. Br J Obstet Gynaecol 1983; 90:255–8.
50. Andersson K, Rybo G. Levonorgestrel-releasing intrauterine device in the treatment of menorrhagia. Br J Obstet Gynaecol 1990; 97:690–4.
51. Turnbull AC, Rees MCP. Gestrinone in the treatment of menorrhagia. Br J Obstet Gynaecol 1990; 97:713–15.
52. Nilsson L, Rybo G. Treatment of menorrhagia. Am J Obstet Gynecol 1971; 110:713–20.
53. Chimbira T, Anderson ABM, Turnbull AC. Reduction of menstrual blood loss with danazol in unexplained menorrhagia; lack of effect of placebo. Br J Obstet Gynaecol 1980; 87:1152–7.
54. Shaw RW, Fraser HM. Use of a superactive luteinizing hormone-releasing hormone agonist in the treatment of menorrhagia. Br J Obstet Gynaecol 1984; 91:913–19.
55. McLachlan RI, Healy DL, Burger HG. Clinical aspects of LHRH analogues in gynaecology: a review. Br J Obstet Gynaecol 1986; 93:431–54.
56. Petrucco OM, Fraser IS. The potential for use of GnRH agonists for the treatment of dysfunctional uterine bleeding. In: Developments in the treatment of benign gynecological disorders. Am J Obstet Gynecol, (Suppl) 1992 (in press).
57. Nilsson L, Rybo G. Treatment of menorrhagia with an anti-fibrinolytic agent, tranexamic acid (AMCA): a double blind investigation. Acta Obstet Gynecol Scand 1967; 46:572–80.
58. Harrison R, Campbell S. A double-blind trial of ethamsylate in the treatment of primary and intrauterine device menorrhagia. Lancet 1976; ii:283–5.
59. Fraser IS. Menorrhagia due to myometrial hypertrophy and its successful treatment with the anti-estrogen, tamoxifen. Obstet Gynecol 1987; 27:244–7.
60. Pavlin V, Flynn MJ, Mulder JL, Cort JH. The treatment of uterine bleeding with vasopressin homonogen (Glypressin) – a pilot study. Br J Obstet Gynaecol 1978; 85:801–5.
61. Rumbolz WL, Moon CF, Norelli JC. Use of protamine sulphate and toluidine blue for abnormal uterine bleeding. Am J Obstet Gynecol 1952; 63:1029–36.
62. Selwood T, Wood C. Incidence of hysterectomy in Australia. Med J Aust 1978; 2:201–4.
63. McIntosh MCM. Incidence of hysterectomy in New Zealand. NZ Med J 1987; 100:345–7.
64. Goldrath MH, Fuller TA, Segal S. Laser photovaporization of endometrium for the treatment of menorrhagia. Am J Obstet Gynecol 1981; 140:14.
65. Magos AL, Baumann R, Lockwood GM, Turnbull AC. Experience with the first 250 endometrial resections for menorrhagia. Lancet 1991; 337:1074–8.
66. Townsend DE, Richart RM, Paskowitz RA, Woolfork RE. "Rollerball" coagulation of the endometrium. Obstet Gynecol 1990; 76:310–13.
67. Phipps JH, Lewis BV, Roberts T, Prior MV, Hand JW, Elder M, Field SB. Treatment of functional menorrhagia by radiofrequency-induced thermal ablation. Lancet 1990; 335:374–6.

Discussion

Calder: Would Professor Fraser care to speculate further about why some of these patients get worse on PGE synthetase inhibitors? Is it something to do with selective effects, which maybe are reducing the beneficial effects of $PGF_{2\alpha}$?

Fraser: I have no idea. There are so many possible mechanisms involved in the control of volume of bleeding at the time of menstruation that we could speculate on a number of possible mechanisms. But it would be interesting to study some of these women perhaps and see what their endometrium is doing.

Keirse: Could there be two mechanisms, one which has an influence on the prostaglandin system within the uterus, and the second, which we all know, is that they increase or decrease the coagulability of blood and prolong bleeding time? If they do not have an effect for one reason or another on the prostaglandin system within the uterus, or if for one reason or another the prostaglandin system is not involved in the whole process, then there is only the negative effect of more difficult haemostasis and prolonged bleeding times and therefore there is a likelihood of bleeding a little bit more.

Fraser: It is possible that a prolonged bleeding time or some other bleeding-related mechanism may well play a part in it, because in this particular woman we did see a substantially greater increase in the volume of bleeding with naproxen compared with mefenamic acid. I gather there is evidence that suggests that naproxen has a greater effect on bleeding time than mefenamic acid does, but I suspect it was probably through more than one mechanism.

Amy: Miss Rees and Professor Fraser have both alluded to the fact that fenamates are more effective in vitro than other PGSIs. As far as I understand the data mentioned in the literature on the control of dysmenorrhoea, it seems that except for salicylic acid, which is much less effective than other PGSIs, all of the PGSIs are equally effective in controlling dysmenorrhoea. Granted dysmenorrhoea is a subjective phenomenon, but are there similar data on control of the blood loss in vivo? Have there been controlled studies showing that fenamates are more effective than, for instance, naproxen sodium, which I use regularly for the control of blood loss?

Fraser: It is a very good question because few of these things have been systematically investigated. The clinical data are even less than those of the laboratory comparisons.

The biggest problem with this is that there is variability within individual women from one cycle to another and there is considerable variability from one woman to another, and therefore in order to compare different preparations very large studies need to be done under the same conditions by the same group, and one would need to do a comparative study with one prostaglandin inhibitor for a couple of cycles and then perhaps a washout with control cycles, and then compare the results against the other prostaglandin inhibitor. There are relatively few of those studies in the literature; there are five which have measured menstrual blood loss under those circumstances and they have not been able to show any significant difference, but the numbers have all been small. It is impossible to say that there is not some difference.

Rees: Many of the studies do not investigate their treatment failures. In a study of gestrinone those who did not respond to gestrinone had unsuspected uterine pathology such as polyps or submucous fibroids and fibroids produce prostacyclin. In the presence of pathology, medication tends not to work. Most of these studies have not defined their population and investigated them to find that they were normal to start off with, although now with outpatient hysteroscopy this is a possibility.

Fraser: That is a very good point, that many of those studies have not investigated their patients beforehand. Nowadays we try to do this always, but we had four patients with fibroids in our first study of 70 women and they were unsuspected at the beginning of the study.

Amy: Some less recent data in the literature suggested that the administration of the PGSI would be more effective when started extremely early during menstruation, meaning at the first sign or symptom that menstruation was about to start. I still insist with my patients that they should start as soon as they feel that menstruation is about to appear. Does this rest on any rational findings or is it purely a placebo effect?

Fraser: There are several questions in that. I think that this does not rest on good scientific basis. I do exactly the same and I advise my women to make sure that they carry their PGSI with them at all times in case menstruation starts early and that they do start at the very earliest time. I think there is a proportion of patients who do get optimum benefit if they start very early, and quite clearly there are some who do not get benefit if they start several hours after the onset of menstruation. But Anne Anderson showed in the late 1970s, that women with dysmenorrhoea as a group did not get increased benefit, subjective benefit, in the treatment of their dysmenorrhoea whether they started treatment the day before or at the onset of bleeding.

The majority of women probably get just as good benefit if they start it at the onset of bleeding as if they started previously, but there may be a small group who get more benefit by a very early start.

Calder: A distinction has been made between anovulatory and ovulatory menorrhagia. Does it really matter all that much in terms of success of treatment?

Fraser: I think it does. Again anecdotally, we have very little benefit for the treatment of anovulatory menorrhagia with prostaglandin inhibitors. We have not done a large study, we just have a small number of anecdotal cases, and it seems quite clear to me that those women do better by replacing the progesterone that they are not making themselves and that the majority will then get good benefit simply from that treatment. I believe that there is some scientific validity in trying to determine whether the woman is predominantly anovulatory or predominantly ovulatory. One can be a little more logical about the way in which one then uses the sequence of treatments until one gets a good result.

MacKenzie: How is the anovulatory woman defined? How is the diagnosis reached?

Fraser: In broad terms it can usually be done by asking two questions: her age, and whether her menstrual cycles are regular or irregular. The majority will be sorted out from those two questions. But there is a group of women who have anovulatory cycles who have moderately regular periods, and there is a group of women, particularly in the perimenopausal age group, who are often ovulating and who are sometimes irregular. So it is not a clear distinction.

In clinical terms one has to determine what lengths one wishes to go to to determine whether they are predominantly anovulatory or not. I use the word "predominantly" advisedly because we showed some 17 or 18 years ago in a group of women in the perimenopausal age group whom we thought were probably anovulatory that sometimes they were ovulating, sometimes they had a proliferative endometrium at the end of the cycle and were anovulatory, sometimes they had cystic glandular hyperplasia. And this was the same woman, if we investigated her over the year, she varied in what was happening at different times.

Calder: I was intrigued by the biopsy diagnosis of adenomyosis. Is that something that is done at hysteroscopy?

Fraser: Not as a routine. These were women who had bulky uterus, no evidence on ultrasound that they had discrete fibroids, and they were relatively young women in their 20s who wished to retain their fertility. One was done as a mini-laparotomy biopsy. She had a uterus that was about 10-week size and it did look as if she almost certainly had a major degree of adenomyosis producing an even enlargement of the uterus. The other was a hysteroscopic fundal biopsy.

Smith: A word of warning about the adenomyosis. Those of us who go to resection meetings should be aware that the French are able to diagnose adenomyosis by looking through the hysteroscope without a biopsy, and when these studies are published adenomyosis is present.

Fraser: I would caution that these are the severe degrees of adenomyosis. One certainly can sometimes see those apparent small holes in the endometrium which may be dilated glands. I do not think we have good correlation on biopsy data but we do sometimes. But quite often no matter how carefully one looks at the endometrium, one will not pick up a clue as to the presence of a moderate adenomyosis.

Husslein: If one talks about progestational agents and treatment, one differentiates between short cycle, i.e., only luteal phase, and long cycle meaning follicular and luteal phase. Why not give more consideration to continuous progesterone treatment because that will drive a large number of women into amenorrhoea and solve the problem almost as efficiently as endometrial ablation, but still be reversible?

Fraser: If we give the progestogens long term there are more problems with side effects and a significant proportion of women get breakthrough bleeding.

For the purposes of this meeting I limited my discussion to just those two regimens of treatment, but if one is individualising, one may vary them considerably.

Calder: And many women do not want, or like, to be amenorrhoeic.

Rees: I would suspect that women would prefer to have regular light predictable periods, taking a medication only when they need it. That explains why PGSIs and antifibrinolytic agents are so popular and why one should be striving at making a super agent working slightly higher up the pathway.

MacKenzie: I have seen data previously on progesterone-containing IUCDs, which have phenomenal results. It almost looks as though women with menstrual problems could throw away their PGSIs and have a coil put in until they wanted to get pregnant. Are they really as good as is suggested?

Fraser: They really are as good as on that first study, and a number of other centres have got good data now. The problem is that there is some erratic bleeding in the first three to six months after their insertion and some women do not like that and find it difficult to cope with. But the majority who have had them in for six months find them fantastic and they really do not want to have them taken out.

MacKenzie: And why are the results so much better than with orally administered progestogens?

Fraser: I suspect that it is purely a matter of concentration and they are producing a very atrophic, thin, or histologically atrophic endometrium. Whether it is a true atrophy or a high degree of suppression by progestogens I do not know, but certainly the same concentration of progestogen at the endometrium cannot be produced by giving it orally.

MacKenzie: But they continue to cycle.

Fraser: Some of the progestogen is absorbed systematically and we see a range of effects on ovarian function. Probably 50%–60% have normal cyclical ovarian function if it is assessed purely on oestradiol and progesterone secretion. Another 20% or 30% will have some degree of luteal deficit and a small proportion will not ovulate at all, and will have some follicular activity.

Calder: Do we know anything about the ectopic pregnancy rate?

Fraser: It is extremely low.

Calder: That is surprising in a way.

Fraser: No. There are quite good data on different concentrations of progesterone or progestogens released within the uterine cavity. At levels of around 2 μg/day release of norgestrel there is a significant increase in the ectopic pregnancy rate. However, at higher doses, 10μg or 20 μg/day, all released within the uterine cavity, the pregnancy rate is exceedingly low and very few of those have been ectopics. If a very low level of progestogen is released within the uterine cavity, there may well be an increase in ectopics, but at higher levels the rate drops dramatically.

Early Pregnancy

Chapter 6

Prostaglandins and Implantation

S. K. Smith

Introduction

The mechanism of implantation is perhaps the least well understood aspect of human reproduction, because hitherto there has been a lack of interest in endometrial function. Implantation is a complex process involving the cyclical preparation of a receptive endometrium, the development of a normal embryo, the attachment and penetration of trophoblast, decidualisation and the maternal recognition of pregnancy. Research is inevitably hindered by the physical and ethical difficulty of obtaining suitable human material.

It is difficult to know how many pregnancies fail to thrive because of failed or impaired implantation, but Wilcox et al. [1] estimate that 30% of spontaneous pregnancies fail and this figure is higher in pregnancies arising from assisted conception cycles [2,3], in which failed implantation of replaced embryos is the principal cause of failure.

Animal studies, principally in rodents, demonstrated an absolute requirement for prostaglandins (PGs) in the process of implantation but it is now clear that their function is even more extensive than originally thought, largely due to the role of eicosanoids as intracellular second messengers. In this chapter consideration will initially be given to the synthesis of PGs by endometrium and the factors which regulate this synthesis. In the second half of the chapter, the putative roles of PGs will be considered in an attempt to determine their specific functions in the process of human implantation.

Prostaglandin Synthesis and Metabolism

Prostaglandins are the product of PG synthase metabolism of free arachidonic acid (AA), this being the rate-limiting step in the release of PGs from cell membrane phospholipids. The release of AA from the cell membrane is mediated by a group of phosphodiesterases which are central to the regulation of PG synthesis.

Phospholipases A_2

Phospholipases A_2 (PLA$_2$) hydrolyse the sn-2 fatty acyl ester bond of 3-sn-membrane phospholipids like phosphatidylethanolamine (PE) and phosphatidylcholine (PC) to release free AA. Two families of PLA$_2$ exist: type I found in elapid snakes and characterised by human pancreatic PLA$_2$ also found in lung [4], and type II PLA$_2$s present in viperid and crotalid snake venom. The non-pancreatic type II PLA$_2$ is a 124 amino acid peptide found in human rheumatoid arthritic fluid [5], platelets [6] and placental membranes [7]. Different forms of this enzyme are present suggesting differential splicing from a single gene [8]. Human endometrium has PLA$_2$-type activity [9] but it is not known which PLA$_2$ is active. These PLA$_2$s are Ca^{2+} sensitive and contain a Ca^{2+} binding domain.

Phospholipase C

The heterogeneity of PLA$_2$ expression appears simple when compared to phospholipase C (PLC) expression. This group of enzymes is recognised as a large family of bacterial and mammalian enzymes which mediate receptor-coupled activation initiating a whole host of cellular events ranging from proliferation and differentiation to secretion [10]. The principal substrates are phosphatidylinositol (PI) and PC. Little is known of the expression or activity of PC–PLC in human endometrium but PI–PLCs are expressed in this tissue (D. S. C. Jones, personal communication). Three isozymes, PLC γ, β and δ, have been isolated from bovine and rat brain [11]. These peptides contain two conserved regions each extending for 150 and 120 amino acids, and their molecular weights range from 150 and 140 to 85 kDa. A fourth PLC, not similar in structure to these other PLCs, has been identified in guinea-pig uterus and rat basophilic leukaemia cells (RBL-1) with a molecular weight of 62 kDa [12]. This PLC is expressed by human endometrium and endometrial carcinoma cell lines.

The substrates for PLC are phosphatidylinositol 4,5-bisphosphate (PIP$_2$), PI 4-phosphate or PI. The byproducts of the hydrolysis of PIP$_2$ are diacylglycerol (DG) and inositol phosphates, notably inositol 1,4,5-trisphosphate (IP$_3$) [13]. DG may be further degraded to AA by the actions of di- and monoglycerol lipases but, in combination with Ca^{2+} and phosphatidylserine (PS), DG activates protein kinases C [14]. This latter action is associated with a host of intracellular phosphorylations which may activate or inactivate a large number of intracellular peptides. IP$_3$ binds to specific IP$_3$ receptors on the endoplasmic reticulum and releases intracellular pools of Ca^{2+}, raising cytosolic Ca^{2+} levels. PI$_3$-kinase converts IP$_3$ into IP$_4$, which may facilitate transport of Ca^{2+} into the cell [15].

Phospholipase D

The actions of PLA$_2$ and PI–PLC might be expected to produce a rapid rise of DG, IP and PG levels but this would not explain chronic activation of this signalling system. Hydrolysis of phosphatidylcholine has been suggested to be the source of chronic elevation of DG activity [16]. The degradation of PC to yield phosphatidic acid (PA) and choline is induced by phospholipase D. Phosphatidic acid is further degraded to DG by the action of phosphatidic acid phosphohydrolase. The secondary source of DG is responsible for the biphasic rise of DG levels following PIP_2 hydrolysis [17].

Prostaglandin Synthase

Arachidonic acid is converted into PGs by the action of PG cyclo-oxygenase (COX) whose ovine and human sequence has been determined and which is present in human endometrium principally in the glandular cells [18] and at the site of implantation in the rat [19]. Several species of PG–COX exist but it is not yet clear which of them is the biologically active isozyme. Regulation of COX expression and activity clearly will influence PG and, via the lypoxygenase pathway, leukotriene synthesis.

Prostaglandin Synthesis in Human Endometrium

Initial studies measured endogenous levels of PG in tissue by radioimmunoassay. These levels were thought to reflect the response of the tissue to the trauma of tissue collection. PGs are not stored in tissues. These early studies found higher levels of PGF in tissue removed in the luteal phase of the cycle compared to that removed in the proliferative phase [20,21]. Decidua of early pregnancy has very low levels of PG [22], irrespective of whether the embryo was in the uterine cavity or not [23].

This picture became more complicated with the introduction of in vitro studies. Abel and Bird [24], using whole tissue explants, found that secretory endometrium released more PGs than proliferative endometrium but this was contradicted by Tsang and Ooi [25], and Schatz et al. [26], who found the converse to be true. Separation of the endometrium into predominantly glandular and stromal compartments by partial digestion [27] further confused the issue. Schatz et al. [26] and Smith and Kelly [28] found that glandular cells were the principal source of PGs whereas Gal et al. [29] found the converse to be the case. However, in the latter case, the cells were maintained for over seven days in culture compared to the first two studies in which cells were not kept for more than four days in culture. Further evidence for the glands being the main source of PGs is the presence of COX immunoreactivity in the glands [18], and the observation that decidualisation in rodents (known to require PG synthesis) is abolished by removal of epithelial cells [30].

More recent studies suggest a more sophisticated release of PGs. Using culture systems with an established extracellular matrix in which epithelial cells obtain a structure similar to that found in vivo, Glasser et al. [31] and Cherny and Findlay [32] found polarity in PG synthesis, most being secreted from the basal aspect of the cells. Separated cells of human endometrium release more PGs in the proliferative phase of the cycle with the lowest amounts of PGs being released from decidual epithelial cells [28].

Prostaglandins and Implantation

Initial interest in the role of PGs in implantation centred on their increased release at the site of implantation in rodents. Their role was thought to involve their action on vascular permeability and tone. It is now evident that PGs are the product of polyphosphoinositide hydrolysis (PPI) and that they play a crucial role in many aspects of cellular function ranging from proliferation to differentiation yet still possibly playing a part in the local mechanism of implantation itself.

Prostaglandins and Preparation of the Endometrium

Implantation in women occurs on an oestradiol-primed endometrium exposed to progesterone. This relationship between a discrete steroid pattern and implantation is most clearly seen in rodents, where an implantation window occurs. Though not as obvious in women, there is still a broad requirement for steroids. However, more recently, attention has turned to the paracrine and autocrine factors mediating steroid reponses. Nelson et al. [33] have shown in ovariectomised mice, that development of the reproductive tract is mediated by epidermal growth factor (EGF) quite independently from oestrogens. Human endometrium expresses EGF and transforming growth factor (TGFa), both of which are ligands for the EGF receptor [34,35]. The angiogenic growth factors, acidic and basic fibroblast growth factor (a and b FGF), are also present in human endometrium and promote growth of both endothelial cells and vascular smooth muscle cell. In mice and humans, EGF stimulates proliferation of epithelial cells [35–37].

In addition to growth factors, PGs are required to induce endometrial proliferation. Inhibitors of PG synthesis prevent the DNA synthesis induced by oestradiol, an action which is attenuated by the addition of PGF [37]. These two puzzling observations are now being seen to be related. Both EGF and FGF bind to transmembrane receptors with intrinsic tyrosine kinase activity. Binding of the ligand results in dimerisation of the receptor in the case of EGF and phosphorylation of PI–PLCγ1. PIP_2, the substrate of PI–PLCγ1 will not bind to unphosphorylated PLC because it is bound to profilin. Phosphorylation of the enzyme permits it to bind to PIP_2 and cause the release of DG and IP_3. The precise mechanisms whereby these metabolites cause proliferation are unclear but three pathways are becoming clear. First, DG activates protein kinase C, whose overexpression has long been associated with proliferation. Second, GTPase activating protein (GAP) exerts a negative modulatory role on cell growth [21, 38,39]. Tyrosine phosphorylation of this peptide inactivates it, suggesting for example, that binding of EGF to its receptor would result in the phosphorylation of GAP and promote the growth of the cell. DG can bind to GAP and exerts a similar inactivation of the peptide [30]. Third, a new 60 kDa protein has recently been described which is activated by DG and which functionally opposes GAP activity. Finally, the early release of Ca^{2+}, induced by IP_3, derived from PIP_2 is maintained by chronic hydrolysis of PC. Elevation of intracellular Ca^{2+} persists due to Ca^{2+} influx and this is maintained whilst the growth factor is in contact with the cell [40,41].

These observations put into perspective the findings of elevated PGF release from epithelial cells in the proliferative phase of the cycle and begin to provide a more coherent picture as to the local events involved in the preparation of endometrium for implantation.

Prostaglandins and the Local Response to Implantation

Animal Studies

The clearest evidence for a role of PGs in the mechanism of implantation has been obtained in rodents, most notably through the work of Kennedy [42,43], and reviewed recently [44]. Increased vascular permeability and oedema characterise the implantation site and raised levels of PGs are found there compared to non-implantation sites. Inhibitors of PG synthesis reduce PG release in endometrium, reduce the local oedema associated with implantation sites, and impair implantation. In addition, the decidual changes seen in stromal cells beneath the implantation site arise by the action of eicosanoids.

A suggestion as to whether in mice the PAF derived from embryo or stroma is reponsible for the increased vascular permeability at the site of implantation is provided by Spinks et al. [45]. They showed that treatment of donor and recipient mice on day 3 of pregnancy with PAF antagonists reduced implantation of transferred embryos, whereas treatment of only the donor mouse on day 4 prevented implantation, suggesting that it is the embryo-derived PAF that provides the initial recognition signal to the mother. What is the response that this embryo-derived PAF induces in endometrium?

PAF, PGs and Human Endometrium

Pharmacological doses of PAF induce a dose-dependent rise of PGE_2 synthesis from epithelial cells of human endometrium obtained from women in the secretory phase of the menstrual cycle [46]. This response is not elicited from stromal cells taken from this tissue, nor from epithelial cells obtained in the proliferative phase of the cycle. PAF did not stimulate $PGF_{2\alpha}$ synthesis. PGE_2 is most consistently elevated in rodents at the site of implantation and induces vasodilation and oedema in many experimental systems.

PGs could be derived from the action of PLA_2 or PLC-like activity. In order to investigate the mechanism of action of PAF, its ability to elevate IP_3 levels in human endometrium was studied. Pharmacological doses of PAF induced a rapid

(30 s) rise in IP_3 levels after prelabelling of cells with *myo*-inositol [47]. Addition of lithium chloride to the explant incubates, which prevents re-accumulation of inositol into lipid stores, caused a significant elevation of IP_1 levels at 30 min. This effect of PAF was demonstrated only in secretory endometrium, it being absent in proliferative endometrium and decidua of early pregnancy. Specific PAF receptor antagonists attenuated this response in a dose-dependent manner. As labelled *myo*-inositol was the precursor for these studies, the conclusion is that PAF binds to a specific receptor, only expressed in luteal-phase endometrium, which activates PI–PLC activity. This would elevate IP_3, intracellular Ca^{2+} and DG, resulting in potentially significant events in the cell but specifically a rise of PG levels.

This would promote only a rapid short-lived response but substantial release of DG arises from the degradation of phosphatidylcholine [48,49]. PAF causes a rapid rise of choline in human secretory endometrium suggesting PLD-like activity which is confirmed by trans-phosphatidylation studies, a reaction catalysed only by PLD [50]. From the same studies, it is clear that PAF stimulates a whole range of phospholipases including PI–PLC, PC–PLC, PLA_2 and PLD.

These studies were conducted with pharmacological doses of PAF but as the experiments were conducted on whole tissue and as PAF in vitro not only binds to albumin but is also metabolically unstable, it is still likely that these events in vitro may be arising in vivo. The precise role of PAF in human endometrium still needs to be determined but it is now clear that the ability of human endometrium to respond to PAF involves a series of pathways known to be important in proliferation, differentiation and secretion, and that this response is a key aspect of the cyclical development of the endometrium.

Maintenance of Pregnancy

The key to successful implantation in women, as far as the role of eicosanoids is concerned, is to induce a local rise of PG synthesis whilst not stimulating a more widespread elevation of PG release, which would lead to myometrial contractility, spiral arteriolar construction, and menstruation. In other species, uterine PGs induce luteolysis [51]. This does not occur in women, but raised levels of PG are found at menstruation and exogenous PGs induce bleeding and abortion in early pregnancy [52].

It is now clear that in sheep conceptus secretory proteins inhibit PG synthesis [53,54]. These proteins are similar to interferon, and human α-interferon suppresses PG release from ovine endometrium [55]. This mechanism does not operate in humans, demonstrating a significant difference in the establishment of pregnancy between epitheliochorial and haemochorial placentation. Interferon has little effect on PG synthesis by human endometrium, whereas progesterone reduces both PGF and PGE release [56]. Thus far, there is no evidence for any other agent, over and above progesterone as the suppressor of uterine PG synthesis and the mediator of the myometrial relaxation that occurs throughout pregnancy.

Conclusion

Animal studies have long demonstrated the crucial role that PGs play in implantation. Inevitably restrictions on experimentation have hampered progress in understanding their role in human implantation. However, some aspects of their function are becoming clearer, though still often by inference. First, there is an important change in PG synthesis, from a local stimulation at the site of implantation to a generalised suppression of their synthesis to prevent menstruation. Local elevation of PG synthesis could be mediated by PAF, released either by the embryo or from the stromal cells of the endometrium. PAF acts on the epithelial cells of secretory endometrium to release PGs and together PG and PAF induce the local oedema, vasodilation and vascular permeability associated with implantation sites. This presumably facilitates the nurture of the very early embryo before the development of trophoblastic lacunae and the more formal interrelationship between the vascular system of the mother and fetus. It is not known if disorders of this mechanism result in infertility or failed pregnancy after embryo transfer. Nor is it known if non-steroidal anti-inflammatory drugs (NSAIDs) which inhibit synthesis of PG increase the risks of failed pregnancy if taken at the time of implantation.

It is not known if the increased PG release at the implantation site is required to facilitate the correct development of the embryo, or to promote the successful invasion of the trophoblast into the decidual blood vessels and the decidua itself. Quite apart from these direct effects of PGs on implantation, their role as mediators or even by-products of the signal of transduction mechanisms of growth factors, raises crucial questions about the role of growth factors in the preparation and differentiation of endometrium and the subsequent regulation of embryo–endometrial interactions. These are fundamental questions concerning human reproduction and there is an increasing need for these questions to be addressed. Further studies will need to determine in which respect PGs function – whether as discrete paracrine regulators of cell to cell dialogue, or as intracellular second messengers for other cell signalling molecules.

References

1. Wilcox AJ, Weinberg CR, O'Connor JF et al. Incidence of early pregnancy loss. N Engl J Med 1988; 319:189–94.
2. Yovich JL, Matson PL. Early pregnancy wastage after gamete manipulation. Br J Obstet Gynaecol 1988; 95:1120–7.
3. Weinberg CR, Wilcox AJ. Incidence rate of implantation in "non-pregnant" patients. Fertil Steril 1988; 50:993.
4. Seilhammer JJ, Randall TL, Yamanaka M, Johnson LK. Pancreatic phospholipase A2; isolation of the human gene and cDNAs from porcine pancreas and human lung. DNA 1986; 5:519–27.
5. Seilhammer JJ, Pruzanski W, Vadas P, Plant S, Miller JA, Kloss J, Johnson LK. Cloning and recombinant expression of phospholipase A2 present in rheumatoid arthritic synovial fluid. J Biol Chem 1989; 264:5335–8.
6. Kramer RM, Hession C, Johansen B et al. Structure and properties of a human non-pancreatic phospholipase A2. J Biol Chem 1989; 264:5738–75.

7. Lai CY, Wada K. Phospholipase A2 from human synovial fluid: purification and structural homology to the placental enzyme. Biochem Biophys Res Comm 1988; 157:488–93.
8. Seilhammer JJ, Randall TL, Johnson LK, Heinzmann C, Klisak I, Sparkes RS, Lusis AJ. Novel gene exon homologous to panacreatic phospholipase A$_2$: sequence and chromosomal mapping of both human genes. J Cell Biochem 1989; 39:327–37.
9. Bonney RC, Franks S. Phospholipase C activity in human endometrium: its significance in endometrial pathology. J Endocrinol 1987; 27: 307–20.
10. Little C. Phospholipase C. Biochem Soc Trans 1989; 17:271–3.
11. Rhee SG, Suh PG, Ryu SH, Lee SY. Studies of inositol phospholipid-specific phospholipase C. Science 1989; 244:546–50.
12. Bennett CF, Crooke ST. Purification and characterisation of a phosphoinositide-specific phospholipase C from guinea pig uterus. J Biol Chem 1987; 262:13789–97.
13. Berridge MJ, Irvine RF. Inositol triphosphate, a novel second messenger in cellular signal transduction. Nature 1984; 312:315–21.
14. Nishizuka Y. The molecular heterogeneity of protein kinase C and its implications for cellular regulation. Nature 1988; 344:661–5.
15. Morris AP, Gallacher DV, Irvine RF, Peterson OH. Synergism of inositol trisphosphate and tetrakisphosphate in activating Ca^{2+}-dependent K$^+$ channels. Nature 1987; 330:653–5.
16. Billah MM, Lapetina EG, Cuatrecasas P. Phospholipase A2 and phospholipase C activities of platelets. Differential substrate specificity, Ca^{2+} requirement, pH dependence, and cellular localization. J Biol Chem 1980; 255:10227–31
17. Loffeeholz K. Receptor regulation of choline phospholipid hydrolysis. Biochem Pharmacol 1989; 38:1543–9.
18. Rees MCP, Parry DM, Anderson ABM, Turnbull AC. Immunohistochemical localisation of cyclooxygenase in the human uterus. Prostaglandins 1982; 23:207–14.
19. Parr MB, Parr EL, Munaretto K, Clark MR, Dey SK. Immunohistochemical localisation of prostaglandin synthase in the rat uterus and embryo during the peri-implantation period. Biol Reprod 1988; 38:333–43.
20. Downie J, Poyser N, Wunderlich M. Levels of prostaglandins in human endometrium during the normal menstrual cycle. J Physiol 1974; 236:465–72.
21. Singh EJ, Baccarini IM, Zuspan FP. Levels of prostaglandins F$_{2\alpha}$ and E$_2$ in human endometrium during the menstrual cycle. Am J Obstet Gynecol 1975; 121:1003–6.
22. Maathuis JB, Kelly RW. Concentration of prostaglandins F$_{2\alpha}$ and E$_2$ in endometrium throughout the menstrual cycle after the administration of clomiphene or an oestrogen–progesterone pill and in early pregnancy. J Endocrinol 1978; 77:361–71.
23. Abel MH, Smith SK, Baird DT. Suppression of concentration of endometrial prostaglandin in early intra-uterine and ectopic pregnancy in women. J Endocrinol 1981; 85:379–86.
24. Abel MH, Baird DT. The effect of 17β-estradiol and progesterone on prostaglandin production by human endometrium maintained in organ culture. Endocrinology 1980; 106:1599–606.
25. Tsang BK, Ooi TC. Prostaglandin secretion by human endometrium. Am J Obstet Gynecol 1982; 142:626–33.
26. Schatz F, Markiewicz L, Barg P, Gurpide E. In vitro effects of ovarian steroids on prostaglandin F$_{2\alpha}$ output by human endometrium and endometrial epithelial cells. J Clin Endocrinol Metab 1985; 61:361–7.
27. Satyaswaroop PG, Bressler RS, de la Pena MM, Gurpide E. Isolation and culture of human endometrial glands. J Clin Endocrinol Metab 1979; 48:639–41.
28. Smith SK, Kelly RW. The release of PGF$_{2\alpha}$ and PGE$_2$ from separated cells of human endometrium and decidua. Prostaglandins Leukotrienes Essential Fatty Acids 1988; 33:91–6.
29. Gal D, Casey ML, Johnston JM, Macdonald PC. Mesenchyme–epithelial interactions in human endometrium. Prostaglandin synthesis in separated cell types. J Clin Invest 1982; 70:798–805.
30. Lejeune B, van Hoeck J, Leroy F. Transmitter role of the luminal uterine epithelium in the induction of decidualisation in rats. J Reprod Fertil 1981; 61:235–40.
31. Glasser SR, Julian J, Decker GL, Tang JP, Carson DD. Development of morphological and functional polarity in primary cultures of immature rat uterine epithelial cells. J Cell Biol 1988; 107:2409–23.
32. Cherny RA, Findlay JK. Separation and culture of ovine endometrial epithelial and stromal cells: evidence of morphological and functional polarity. Biol Reprod 1990; 43:241–50.
33. Nelson KG, Takahashi T, Bossert NL, Walmer DK, McLachlan JA. Epidermal growth factor replaces estrogen in the stimulation of female genital-tract growth and differentiation. Proc Natl Acad Sci USA 1991; 88:21–5.
34. Haining REB, Schofield JP, Jones DSC, Rajput-Williams J, Smith SK. The identification of

mRNA for EGF and TFGα present in low copy number in human endometrium and decidua using RT-PCR. J Mol Endocrinol 1991; 6:207–14.

35. Haining REB, Cameron IT, van Papendorp C, Davenport AP, Prentice A, Thomas EJ, Smith SK. Epidermal growth factor in human endometrium: proliferative effect in culture and immunocytochemical localisation in normal and edometriotic tissues. Human Reprod 1991; 6:1200–5.

36. Tomooka Y, DiAugustine RP, McLachlan JA. Proliferation of mouse uterine epithelial cells in vitro. Endocrinology 1986; 118:1011–18.

37. Orlicky DJ, Lieberman R, Williams C, Gerschenson LE. Requirements for prostaglandin $F_{2\alpha}$ in 17β-estradiol stimulation of DNA synthesis in rabbit endometrial cultures. J Cell Physiol 1987; 130:292–300.

38. Zhang K, DeClue JE, Vass WC, Papageorge AG, McCormick F, Lowy DR. Suppression of c-ras transformation by GTPase-activating protein. Nature 1990; 346:754–6.

39. Tsai M-H, Yu C-L, Stacey DW. A cytoplasmic protein inhibits the GTPase activity of h-ras in a phospholipid-dependent manner. Science 1990; 250:982–5.

40. Magni M, Meldolesi J, Pandiella A. Ionic events induced by epidermal growth factor. B J Biol Chem 1991; 266:6329–35.

41. Huang C-L, Takenawa T, Ives HE. Platelet-derived growth factor-mediated Ca^{2+} entry is blocked by antibodies to phosphatidylinositol 4,5-biphosphate but does not involve heparin-sensitive inositol 1,4,5-triphosphate receptors. J Biol Chem 1991; 266:4045–8.

42. Kennedy TG. Embryonic signals and the initiation of blastocyst implantation. Aust J Biol Sci 1983; 36:531–43.

43. Kennedy TG. Prostaglandins and blastocyst implantation. Prost Perspec 1985; 1:1–3.

44. Smith SK. The role of prostaglandins in implantation. In: Seppala M, ed. Factors of importance for implantation. Clinical Obstetrics and Gynaecology, Bailliere Tindall, London, 1991; 5:95–115.

45. Spinks NR, Ryan JP, O'Neill CO. Antagonists of embryo-derived platelet-activating factor act by inhibiting the ability of the mouse embryo to implant. J Reprod Fertil 1990; 88:241–8.

46. Smith SK, Kelly RW. Effect of platelet-activating factor on the release of PGF-2a and PGE-2 by separated cells of human endometrium. J. Reprod Fertil 1988; 82:271–6.

47. Ahmed A, Smith SK. Platelet activating factor stimulates phospholipase C activity in human endometrium. J Cell Physiol 1992; in press.

48. Kennedy TG. Prostaglandins and blastocyst implantation. Prost Perspec 1987; 1:1–3.

49. Billah MM, Anthes JC. The regulation and cellular functions of phosphatidylcholine hydrolysis. Biochem J 1990; 269:281–91.

50. Ahmed A, Ferriani RA, Smith SK. Activation of multiple phospholipases – catalysed phosphatidylcholine hydrolysis is by platelet activating factor in human endometrium. Biochim Biophys Acta 1992; in press.

51. Bazer FS, Vallett JL, Roberts RM, Sharp DC, Thatcher WW. Role of conceptus secretory products in establishment of pregnancy. J Reprod Fertil 1986; 76: 841–50.

52. Smith SK, Baird DT. The use of 16-16-dimethyl-trans 2 PGE_1 methyl ester (ONO 802) vaginal suppositories for the termination of early pregnancy. A comparative study. Br J Obstet Gynaecol 1980; 87: 712–17.

53. Vallet JL, Bazer FW. Effect of ovine trophoblast protein-1, oestrogen and progesterone on oxytocin-induced phosphatidylinositol turnover in endometrium of sheep. J Reprod Fertil 1989; 87:755–61.

54. Helmer SD, Gross TS, Newton GR, Hansen PJ, Thatcher WW. Bovine trophoblast protein-1 complex alters endometrial protein and prostaglandin secretion and induces an intracellular inhibitor of prostaglandin synthesis in vitro. J Reprod Fertil 1989; 87:421–30.

55. Salamonsen SA, Stuchbery SJ, O'Grady CM, Godkin JD, Findlay JK. Interferon-α mimics effects of ovine trophoblast protein 1 on prostaglandin and protein secretion by ovine endometrial cells in vitro. J Endocrinol 1988; 117:R1–R4.

56. Mitchell SN, Smith SK. Progesterone and human interferon α-2 have a different effect on the release of prostaglandin $F_{2\alpha}$ from human endometrium. Recent Adv Prost Thombox Leuk Res 1991; 21:823–6.

Chapter 7

Menstrual Induction

J. E. Norman

Introduction

"Menstrual induction" describes the use of medical agents to induce menses in women in whom menstruation is delayed – traditionally before pregnancy could always be confirmed, though assays for serum human chorionic gonadotrophin (hCG) are now so sensitive that pregnancy can be diagnosed confidently at the time of the first missed menses. In this chapter, the term menstrual induction is taken to include medical termination of early pregnancy at up to eight weeks of amenorrhoea. The use of prostaglandins for menstrual induction and the advantages of menstrual induction compared to "menstrual regulation" (a surgical procedure) will be reviewed. Menstrual induction using a prostaglandin/ antiprogestin combination will also be described, and the role of menstrual induction in the 1990s will be discussed.

Abortion and Menstrual Regulation

It has been estimated that 40–60 million abortions are performed world wide each year [1]. In some countries, where abortion is used as a method of contraception, the abortion rate (the number of abortions per 1000 women of reproductive age per year) may be as high as 180 [2]. In England, despite the ready availability of contraceptive services, 184 000 abortions were performed in 1989, giving an abortion rate of 13.4 [3]. Surgical termination of pregnancy in the first trimester requires skilled personnel. It may involve a general anaesthetic and there is a risk of damage to the uterine cervix [4] or body. The complication rate of surgical termination of pregnancy increases by 15%–30% for every week of delay after eight weeks gestation [5]. In early pregnancy, within a few weeks of the missed menses, abortion can be performed without cervical dilation, using a flexible plastic cannula attached to a suction device, under local anaesthesia [6,7]. This method of uterine evacuation shortly after the first missed period became known as menstrual regulation, and in a wish to use the method as early as possible, it was often used before a pregnancy test became positive [8]. Uterine evacuation before pregnancy can be confidently diagnosed, is ethically more acceptable to some, and this is felt to outweigh the disadvantages of undergoing an unnecessary procedure, should the patient not actually be pregnant [9]. In some countries where abortion itself is illegal, menstrual regulation is not a crime, and allows women to avail themselves of medical help [10]. With time, however, it became obvious that menstrual regulation had more side effects than was initially thought; even when local anaesthesia was used, the incidence of syncope during the procedure was as high as 20% in one study, and the incidence of incomplete abortion and/or endometritis was 4% [11]. Follow-up was felt to be necessary, to ensure complete abortion, and histological examination of the products of conception recommended to exclude ectopic pregnancy [12].

Menstrual Induction

Use of Prostaglandins in Abortion

As methods of menstrual regulation were being developed, interest was increasing in the use of prostaglandins to terminate pregnancy. Ravenholt had described the ideal method of fertility control as a "non-toxic and completely effective substance which when self administered by the woman on a single occasion will ensure non-pregnancy at the completion of one monthly cycle" [13], and initially it was hoped that prostaglandins would provide this ideal method. The uterotonic effects of prostaglandins had been apparent since an active substance in the seminal plasma [14], later termed "prostaglandin" [15], was first described but it was not until after the prostaglandins were isolated and their structure described that this effect could be exploited for fertility control. The use of natural $PGF_{2\alpha}$ as an abortifacient was first described in the early 1970s in women in the late first trimester and second trimester; complete abortion was achieved in 13 of 15 women following intravenous administration of $PGF_{2\alpha}$ (50 μg min^{-1}) [16], and in 3 of 11 women following intravenous PGE_2 (1–10 μg min^{-1}) or $PGF_{2\alpha}$ (10–50 μg min^{-1}), or subcutaneous $PGF_{2\alpha}$ (5 mg 3 hourly) [17].

Properties of the Ideal Menstrual Induction Agent

Menstrual induction within a few weeks of the missed menses has some potential advantages over medical termination of pregnancy at a later gestation. First, spontaneous abortions before the eighth week of pregnancy are often complete, probably due to a lack of anchoring villi which develop later in pregnancy, suggesting that menstrual induction at this early stage of pregnancy is unlikely to be complicated by incomplete abortion. Second, blood loss after medical termination is proportional to gestation [18]. Menstrual induction could feasibly be performed at home (in countries where this is legal), and because it is done at an early gestation would be ethically more acceptable than suction termination of pregnancy. However, since the corpus luteum is the main source of progesterone in very early pregnancy, the ideal medical abortifacient should provoke not only uterine activity and abortion but also luteolysis, otherwise asynchrony between the ovarian and endometrial cycles would occur [19]. This would cause confusion, especially in women who may rely on menstrual induction as a method of contraception, and would reduce patient acceptability of the method [20]. A luteolytic agent would also increase the uterine activity and uterine sensitivity to oxytocic agents [21]. Prostaglandins were thought to have some of the properties required of the ideal menstrual induction agent; not only do they induce uterine activity, but they also induce luteolysis in animals [22].

The Use of Natural Prostaglandins for Menstrual Induction

The first description of prostaglandins for menstrual induction involved the use of $PGF_{2\alpha}$ as a continuous intravenous infusion (up to 3 mg min^{-1}) for 7 h to twelve women at up to 17 weeks' gestation. Abortion occurred in all seven women at up to nine weeks' gestation within 24 h, and in three of the other five women after a second course of treatment the following day. The apparent increased effectiveness in the earlier stage of pregnancy was attributed to decreased cervical resistance and a more vulnerable vascular connection between the conceptus and the uterus at this early stage of pregnancy [23]. The 100% rate of complete abortion in early pregnancy was not achieved by other workers. In another study, 13 women reporting a menses delay of between 6 and 18 days (34–47 days of amenorrhoea) were given $PGF_{2\alpha}$ intravenously (50 μg min^{-1}) for 8 h 20 min [24]. Nine of the 13 women were subsequently found to have been pregnant (by measurement of hCG by radioimmunoassay, with a sensitivity to 5 miu ml^{-1}). Five patients aborted completely; four continued to have a positive immunological pregnancy test following treatment. Histological evaluation of products of conception obtained at uterine evacuation from these latter four women showed severe trophoblastic damage. The authors concluded that caution should be exercised in the use of $PGF_{2\alpha}$ as a post-conceptive agent for fertility control, because of lack of reliability of the method and because of concern about adverse effects on the pregnancy should the pregnancy continue. In addition, abortion was not an inevitable consequence of vaginal bleeding, so that follow-up was necessary to determine outcome.

Vaginal Administration of Prostaglandins for Menstrual Induction

One of the advantages of menstrual induction over menstrual regulation is the potential for self-medication. The fact that this is not possible with intravenous prostaglandins encouraged exploration of other routes of administration of prostaglandins. Vaginal $PGF_{2\alpha}$ in THAM solution was administered to nine women at between 34 and 40 days amenorrhoea every 2–4 h for 24 h, up to a total dose of 1100 mg $PGF_{2\alpha}$ [25]. Three of the nine women aborted completely. Evidence of adequate absorption into the systemic circulation was confirmed by finding serum prostaglandin levels 2.5–8 times higher after treatment than before. Although there was a decrease in concentrations of luteal hormones (17-hydroxyprogesterone) after treatment, this occurred only after a fall in serum hCG, suggesting that prostaglandins did not induce luteolysis directly. Variable rates of success of between 50% and 80% have been achieved by other groups, using vaginal prostaglandins within a few weeks of the first missed period [26–29], although gastrointestinal side effects were found to be a problem in most of these studies. Again, the lack of efficacy and poor correlation between vaginal bleeding and eventual abortion meant that follow-up was necessary.

The "Prostaglandin Impact"

A modification of the use of prostaglandins for early pregnancy termination was suggested by Csapo and Pulkkinen who proposed that the mechanism of action of prostaglandins in inducing abortion was biphasic. The initial effect was to promote uterine activity; this resulted in suppression of the endocrine function of the fetoplacental unit and subsequent withdrawal of progesterone, which in turn increased spontaneous uterine activity [30]. The success of prostaglandin in abortion depended therefore on the initial "prostaglandin impact" [31]. Although this was initially described in women at nine weeks' gestation (i.e. after the luteoplacental shift), it also appeared to operate in early pregnancy, with the insult to the endocrine function of the fetoplacental unit leading to luteolysis. From these observations, it seemed sensible to administer prostaglandins as a bolus, thereafter the above mechanism would ensure the development of uterine activity without further doses of prostaglandin being given. Clinical studies used intrauterine administration of prostaglandins, so that a large dose of the drug could be given directly to the target organ. Complete abortion rates of 91% (in 22 women at a mean of 11 days after the missed menses following a single intrauterine injection of 5 mg $PGF_{2\alpha}$ [32], and 100% (65 women with a mean of eleven days after the missed menses given either 5 mg $PGF_{2\alpha}$ ($n=50$) or 1 mg PGE_2 ($n=15$) [33] were achieved. Similar success rates were found after intrauterine prostaglandin therapy by other workers [34,35]. An American study had a lower complete abortion rate of 65%, using a similar protocol at a slightly later gestation of 38–47 days amenorrhoea and the authors felt that the incidence of side effects (up to 35%), including hypertension and haemorrhage, and septic abortion in those who failed to abort completely [36] made the method unsuitable for routine use. Despite the apparent success of extraovular prostaglandin for menstrual induction, some disadvantages of the regime were becoming obvious. In all the above studies – with the exception of one [34] – premedication was required, and the route of administration precluded self-administration. Side effects were greater than experienced with vacuum aspiration; in a comparison between intrauterine $PGF_{2\alpha}$ (5 mg) and vacuum aspiration under intramuscular analgesia alone, in 200 women of up to 56 days amenorrhoea [37] the incidence of vomiting in the prostaglandin-treated group was 30%, significantly greater than in the group undergoing vacuum aspiration (9%), although the rate of complete abortion was high in each group, and only one patient (in the vacuum aspiration group) failed to abort completely.

Second Generation Prostaglandins for Menstrual Induction

When prostaglandins are administered by a route which involves systemic absorption, repeated high doses have to be given because of the short half-life of the natural prostaglandins in the circulation. The development of a synthetic prostaglandin with an alkyl group at C-15 so that oxidation at C-15 does not occur, and activity is increased [38] offered a prostaglandin which could be given once only. The effects of 15-methyl $PGF_{2\alpha}$ on uterine contractility were found to be 100–400 times greater than that of the natural compound, depending on the route of administration [39]. The abortifacient effects of 15-methyl $PGF_{2\alpha}$ and PGE were initially demonstrated in the late first trimester and second trimesters, with 91% rate of complete abortion [40,41]. When 15-methyl $PGF_{2\alpha}$ was used for menstrual induction, complete abortion was achieved in 8 of 9 women [42] and 32 of 34 women [43], at up to 60 days' gestation following multiple or single intramuscular injections, respectively. The latter study also investigated the effects of vaginal therapy with the synthetic prostaglandin, which has the advantage that it could be given at home. Thirty women were given the first dose of prostaglandin in hospital, and subsequently self-administered further doses at home; all aborted completely. Many investigators subsequently reported their results with vaginal 15-methyl $PGF_{2\alpha}$ therapy, and initially promising success rates were achieved with complete abortion without further therapy of 70%–94% in women up to 61 days from the last menstrual period [44–48]. However, 15-methyl $PGF_{2\alpha}$ is not an ideal abortion method, since repeated doses are necessary, making non-compliance a problem, gastrointestinal side effects are still a significant feature, occurring in up to 50% of patients, and premedication was still required in all but two [46,48] of the above studies. A long-acting suppository of 15-methyl $PGF_{2\alpha}$ has been developed which gives a sustained release of prostaglandins [49]. In women with less than 50 days amenorrhoea, the rate of complete abortion after a single vaginal pessary was dose-dependent; 120 of 128 women aborted following a single 3 mg dose [50]. Although compliance is not a problem with this regime, gastrointestinal side effects are still excessive. The development of a regime giving consistent results remains elusive. In addition, objective measurement of blood loss shows a mean blood loss during abortion of 131 ml, and a mean blood loss during menstruation 2–4 months later at the upper limit of normal, perhaps reflecting continued presence of trophoblast [47]. Notwithstanding these problems, vaginal 15-methyl $PGF_{2\alpha}$ has become the method of choice of early abortion in some countries [51].

Use of the Third Generation of Prostaglandins for Menstrual Induction

Introduction of methyl groups at C-16 has generated prostaglandins which are more resistant to oxidation of the 15-hydroxy group, thus increasing activity in vivo. These compounds are called the third generation of prostaglandins. Four have been extensively investigated for their use in pregnancy termination: 16-phenoxy-tetranor PGE_2 methyl sulphonylamide (sulprostone); 16,16-dimethyl

PGE$_2$; 16,16-dimethyl PGE$_1$ methyl ester (gemeprost); and 9-deoxo 16,16-dimethyl 9-methylene PGE$_2$ (9-methylene PGE$_2$).

These compounds were first administered as extraovular injections; a complete abortion rate of 95% was achieved in a study of 240 women with up to 6–14 days menstrual delay following a single 50 μg dose of sulprostone into the uterine cavity [52]. Intramuscular administration of sulprostone gives success rates of 94%–100% in women with less than 49 days' amenorrhoea [30, 53–55]. In the largest of these studies, 90 women with a mean menstrual delay of 17 days were given intramuscular injections of 500 μg sulprostone 4 hourly to a maximum of 2 mg; the complete-abortion rate was 96% and the incidences of vomiting and diarrhoea were 26% and 10%, respectively [53]. Following treatment, women who had previously also undergone surgical termination of pregnancy were asked which method they preferred; 89% preferred menstrual induction with prostaglandins.

16,16-Dimethyl PGE$_2$ has been administered as a vaginal suppository; abortion rates of 87%–100% have been achieved by using up to 4 mg in divided doses in women with less than 56 days' amenorrhoea. Gastrointestinal side effects were seen in up to 50% of patients [56,57]. The advantages of the newer prostaglandins are indicated by the greater effectiveness and lower incidence of gastrointestinal side effects in women at a similar gestation treated with vaginal 16,16-demethyl PGE$_2$ compared to vaginal 15-methyl PGF$_{2\alpha}$, although a randomised comparison was not performed [57].

Vaginal administration of 16,16-dimethyl PGE$_1$ (1 mg every 1–3 h; up to 5 mg) induces abortion in 87% of patients with up to 49 days of amenorrhoea [58]. We have recently used a 6-hourly regime in 151 women with up to 56 days amenorrhoea (to a total of 3 mg) and achieved an abortion rate of 87%. Despite a lower total amount of prostaglandins administered, the incidence of side effects was similar to that previously reported, with 38% of women vomiting, and 40% having diarrhoea after prostaglandin treatment.

Finally, 9-methylene PGE$_2$ has also been administered vaginally; abortion occurs in 92%–98% of women, depending on the dose [55].

Menstrual Induction Compared to Vacuum Aspiration

Several trials have compared menstrual induction, using one of the third generation prostaglandins, to vacuum aspiration under local or general anaesthesia. Menstrual induction using vaginal administration of up to 3.6 mg of 16,16-dimethyl PGE$_2$ [56], up to 5 mg of 16,16-dimethyl PGE$_1$ [58], up to 120 mg 9-methylene PGE$_2$ [59] or up to 1.5 mg intramuscular sulprostone [60], is as effective as vacuum aspiration, either under local anaesthesia or under premedication only. Premedication was not given routinely in any of these studies, but between 12% and 30% of women required an injection of opiate analgesia, and most investigators highlight the greater incidence of gastrointestinal side effects in women undergoing menstrual induction, compared with vacuum aspiration. In a study of 473 women, mean duration of bleeding was 9 days in the prostaglandin-treated group compared with 4 days in the vacuum aspiration group ($P<0.001$) [60]; similar trends were observed in the other three studies. Objective measurement of total blood loss shows a mean loss of 70–85 ml in women treated with prostaglandin, vacuum aspiration under local anaesthesia or vacuum aspiration under general anaesthesia, with no significant differences between the groups [58].

In two of the above studies, menstrual induction was undertaken wholly or partially at home. When women at up to 49 days' gestation were asked which of three methods of abortion they would prefer, 35 of 51 patients opted for menstrual induction (using prostaglandins) at home, 8 opted for menstrual induction in hospital and only 8 wished to undergo vacuum aspiration, despite an awareness that menstrual induction would be more painful [59]. Women were subsequently randomised to one of the three treatment groups. Both the analgesic requirements and the incidence of gastrointestinal side effects were lower in the group undergoing menstrual induction at home rather than in hospital. Those who underwent menstrual induction at home were very positive about the method at the end of the study, confirming previous work by the same group [55,61].

Few studies have compared the long-term effects of menstrual induction and vacuum aspiration. In an analysis of 132 women in their second pregnancy who had previously undergone menstrual induction with intrauterine prostaglandin, the prematurity rate was 8% [62]. The authors compare this to Hungarian data showing a greater prematurity rate (of 13%–20%) in women who had previously undergone therapeutic abortion, largely by dilation and curettage [63]. However, a randomised comparison was not performed, and accepted data fail to demonstrate an increased prematurity rate following vacuum aspiration [64].

Antiprogestins

The prostaglandin impact postulated by Csapo for menstrual induction achieves its effects first with a large dose of prostaglandins to stimulate uterine activity and second through disruption of the endocrine function of the fetoplacental unit, luteolysis and generation of spontaneous uterine activity. If the hormonal output of the fetoplacental unit can be reduced directly, the use of a large initial dose of prostaglandins (with its attendant side effects) could be avoided. No agent has been produced which consistently induces luteolysis in the human in the presence of hCG [65], so attention has turned to inhibition of synthesis, or antagonism, of the luteal hormones. There is good evidence that progesterone is responsible for the inhibition of uterine activity in early pregnancy [21,66], and both the progesterone synthetase inhibitor epostane and the antiprogesterone mifepristone have been investigated for menstrual induction [67–70]. Although the use of these compounds resulted in a lower requirement for opiate analgesia than the use of the third generation of prostaglandins, the complete abortion rate compared poorly with that of the prostaglandins. In addition, nausea and vomiting are a problem with doses of epostane sufficient to induce abortion. A higher complete abortion rate can be achieved if treatment is confined to women at an early gestation, but even in women within 14 days of the missed menses, the efficacy of mifepristone alone reaches only 85% [71].

Antiprogestins and Prostaglandins

Mifepristone not only increases spontaneous uterine activity, but also increases uterine sensitivity to exogenous prostaglandins [72]. In a study of 34 women with up to 49 days' amenorrhoea, 94% aborted completely using mifepristone 25 mg twice daily for 4 days, followed by 0.25 mg sulprostone intramuscularly on day 4. This high rate of success is similar to that seen using sulprostone alone for menstrual induction, but pretreatment with mifepristone allows one-sixth of the dose of sulprostone to be used. The improved abortion rate when mifepristone is used in combination with prostaglandins, compared to the use of mifepristone alone, has been confirmed in other studies using a combination of mifepristone and sulprostone, with abortion rates of 89%–95% achieved in women with less than 50 days' amenorrhoea [73,74]. Pretreatment with mifepristone for 3 days before treatment with sulprostone appears to be as effective as pretreatment with mifepristone for 4–6 days.

Other prostaglandins have also been used in combination with mifepristone. Abortion rates of 94%–100% [75–78] can be achieved in women given 0.5–1 mg gemeprost 48–72 h after mifepristone. There was no significant difference in abortion rates between the smaller and larger dose of gemeprost used (0.5 mg or 1.0 mg) [79].

The use of oral prostaglandins has potential advantages. First, the oral route of administration is more acceptable than vaginal or intramuscular routes. Second, it allows self-administration. However, the combination of oral PGE_2 (1–2 mg) and mifepristone (25 mg twice daily for four days) was initially no more successful than that of mifepristone and placebo [80], with an overall complete abortion rate of 59%. One of the newer prostaglandins, 9-methylene PGE_2 seems to be more active orally. An abortion rate of 95% can be achieved using 600 mg mifepristone followed 3 and 4 days later by 10 mg 9-methylene PGE_2 [81]. Recently, we have investigated the combination of other oral prostaglandins with mifepristone, as although 9-methylene PGE_2 is effective it has to be given in solution, a formulation which is unsuitable for routine use. Misoprostol (Cytotec) is an oral prostaglandin which is marketed for the treatment of peptic ulcer disease. Manipulation of its chemical structure has generated a compound which has fewer gastrointestinal side effects than natural prostaglandins. Doses of 200–600 μg misoprostol effect an increase in uterine tone; and an increase in uterine activity is seen in women pretreated with mifepristone (Figs. 7.1 and 7.2). Clinically, the combination of 200–600 mg mifepristone followed 48 h later by 200–1000 μg misoprostol appears to be effective, with complete abortion rates of 95% in women with up to 49 days' amenorrhoea [82] and 86% in women with up to 56 days' amenorrhoea [83]. However, further work is required to determine whether this combination has fewer side effects than the combination of mifepristone and sulprostone or gemeprost.

The combination of mifepristone and prostaglandin allows a smaller total dose of prostaglandin to be used, compared to the use of prostaglandin alone for menstrual induction. Mifepristone alone appears to cause few side effects (other than vaginal bleeding). However, in a study of over 500 women given mifepristone and gemeprost, 26% and 13% of patients reported vomiting and diarrhoea respectively as a new symptom in the 4 h following prostaglandin treatment, and 28% required opiate analgesia [78]. In a large French trial of over 2000 women, the reported incidence of vomiting and diarrhoea was 15% and 7% respectively,

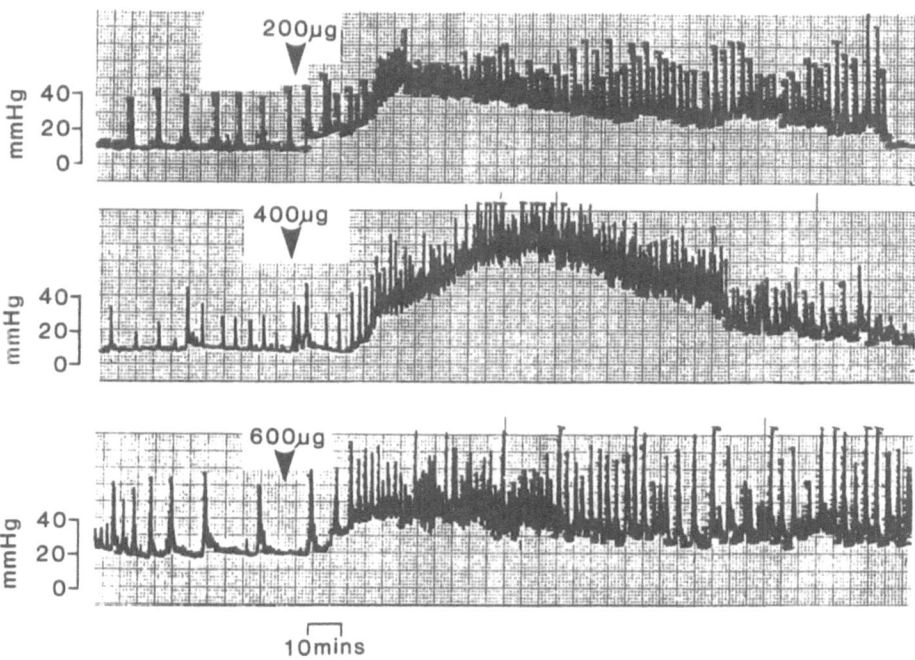

Fig. 7.1. Intrauterine pressure tracings (mmHg) from three women in early pregnancy who received 200, 400, or 600 μg misoprostol orally at ➡, 48 h after administration of 200 mg mifepristone.

and the overall requirement for opiate analgesia was 1%. However, some of these women were given premedication [84]. The degree of abdominal pain experienced is related to prostaglandin dosage [84], and since smaller doses of prostaglandins are as effective as the larger doses used in these studies [79,84], this offers a method of reducing side effects without any reduction in efficacy. Median blood loss during abortion using mifepristone and gemeprost has been found to be 81 ml in a series of 13 women (range 32–222 ml) [75] and 71 ml in a series of 206 women (range 14–512 ml) [18]. Duration of amenorrhoea has a major influence on blood loss, and the median blood loss in seven women with 56–63 days' amenorrhoea was 154 ml (range 84–341 ml) [18]. The requirement for blood transfusion was 0.1% in the first 10 000 women treated in France from October 1988 [85].

We have recently performed a comparative study of gemeprost alone (1 mg 6 hourly to a maximum of 3 mg) or mifepristone (200–600 mg) followed 48 h later by 1 mg gemeprost to induce abortion [86]. Of the 301 women studied, 150 were given mifepristone and gemeprost and 151 were given gemeprost alone. The complete abortion rate in the mifepristone and gemeprost group was 95%, significantly greater than that (87%) in the gemeprost alone group (P=0.004). The requirement for analgesia was significantly greater in the group treated with gemeprost alone (P=0.0001). In addition, over half the women in the gemeprost-alone group required three pessaries, and most of these stayed in hospital overnight; this was not a feature of the women treated with mifepristone and gemeprost.

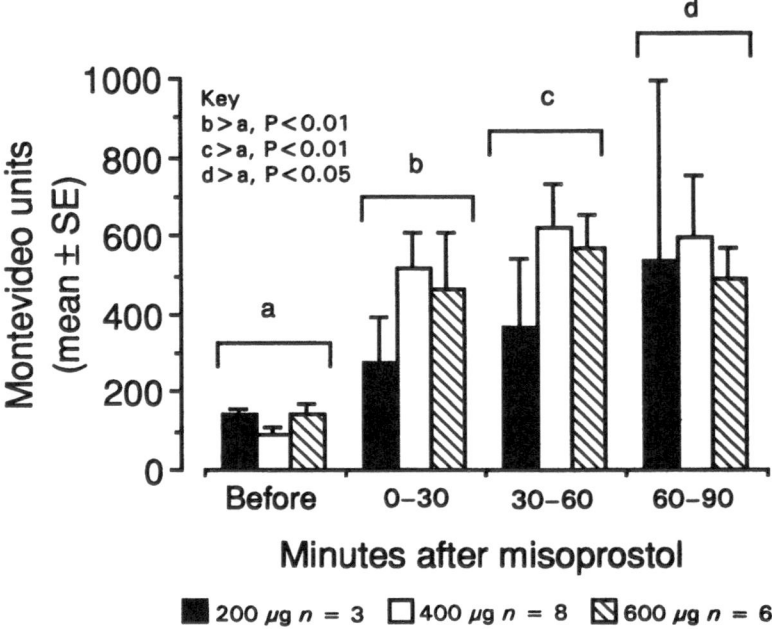

Fig. 7.2. Mean (SEM) uterine activity before and at varying times after misoprostol at three doses following pretreatment with mifepristone.

Menstrual Induction

Since Ravenholt [13] described the properties of the ideal menstrual induction agent in 1968, the realisation of this is much nearer. Whereas prostaglandins alone seem unlikely to provide the optimal method of menstrual induction, the combination of mifepristone and prostaglandins may provide the best method. The combination of mifepristone and prostaglandin appears to be safe in early pregnancy, mean blood loss in women with up to 56 days' amenorrhoea is similar to the upper limit of normal for menstruation, and the requirement for blood transfusion is low. Women at an early gestation (within 1–2 weeks of the missed menses) could feasibly be treated at home. Since 1968, advances in assays for serum human chorionic gonadotrophin have ensured that women (at least in the Western world) are able to purchase a pregnancy test which is sensitive enough to confirm pregnancy within a few days of the missed menstrual period, so that only women who have conceived following a cycle of unprotected intercourse will require treatment. The side effects induced by the mifepristone–prostaglandin combination are not inconsiderable, but are mainly related to the dose of prostaglandin used. The lowest effective dose of mifepristone and of prostaglandin has not yet been established. Newer prostaglandin analogues, such as the oral prostaglandin misoprostol, offer hope of a more easily administered prostaglandin with reduced side effects. Since the rate of complete abortion induced by mifepristone and prostaglandin compares with that of surgical termination of pregnancy, a similar protocol for follow-up can be employed in each case to determine whether abortion is complete.

In the UK it seems unlikely that menstrual induction will become popular as a method of contraception. Not only is the method unacceptable in principle to a proportion of women (43% of women questioned) [20], but, because of variability of length of the succeeding cycle, many women will become confused as to when it is appropriate to perform a pregnancy test. In addition, the legal position of menstrual induction is likely to be similar to that of termination of pregnancy. Under current legislation, it is the intention to procure an abortion (whether or not the woman is actually pregnant) which is illegal in England under the Offences Against the Person Act (1861); both menstrual induction and abortion can be performed only under the conditions laid down under the 1967 Abortion Act. In Scotland, the situation is different, and the legal position of menstrual induction is unclear. However, no method of contraception is 100% effective, and despite the ready availability of contraception in the UK the abortion rate is still rising. The requirement for abortion is therefore likely to continue for the forseeable future. In the 1990s, menstrual induction offers a safe, straightforward method of early abortion with minimal side effects. The ideal method is probably a combination of an antiprogestin and a prostaglandin. The onus is on all those concerned with women's health to encourage women with an unwanted pregnancy to present early for consideration of abortion, and on those who provide abortion services to respond early to her request, so that menstrual induction rather than surgical termination of pregnancy can be performed.

References

1. Tietze C, Henshaw SK. Induced abortion: a world review. London: Alan Guttmacher, 1986.
2. Segal SJ, LaGuardia KD. Termination of pregnancy – a global view. Ballieres Clin Obstet Gynaecol 1990; 4:235–47.
3. Office of Population Censuses and Surveys. OPCS Monitor 1990; AB 90:3.
4. Johnstone FD, Beard RJ, Boyd IE, McCarthy TG. Cervical diameter after suction termination of pregnancy. Br Med J 1976; i:68–9.
5. Cates W Jr, Shulz KF, Grimes DA, Tyler CW Jr. Short-term complications of uterine evacuation techniques for abortion at 12 weeks' gestation or earlier. In: Zatunchni G, Sciarra JJ, Speidel JJ, eds. Pregnancy termination: procedures, safety and new developments. Hagerstown: Harper and Row, 1979; 127–35.
6. Goldsmith S, Margolis AJ. Aspiration abortion without cervical dilation. Am J Obstet Gynecol 1971; 110:580–2.
7. Karman H, Potts M. Very early abortion using syringe as vacuum source. Lancet 1972; i:1051–2.
8. Anonymous. Menstrual regulation. Lancet 1974; i:84.
9. Potts M, Diggory P, Peel J. Abortion. Cambridge: Cambridge University Press, 1977.
10. Anonymous. Menstrual regulation. Lancet 1976; i:947.
11. Landesman R, Kaye RE, Wilson KH. Menstrual extraction: review of 400 procedures at Women's Services, New York, NY. Contraception 1973; 8:527–39.
12. Atienza MF, Burkman RT, King TM, Burnett LS, Lau HL, Parmley TH, Woodruff JD. Menstrual extraction. Am J Obstet Gynecol 1975; 121:490–5.
13. Ravenholt RT. In: Hall RE, ed. Abortion in a changing world, vol 2, New York: Columbia University Press, 1968; 49–52.
14. Kurzrok R, Lieb C. Biochemical studies of human semen: II. The action of semen on the human uterus. Proc Soc Exp Biol Med 1930; 28:268–72.

15. Von Euler US. Uber die spezifische blutdrucksenkende Substanz des menschlichen Prostata- und Samenblasensekretes. Klin Wochenschr 1935; 14:1182–3.
16. Karim SMM, Filshie GM. Therapeutic abortion using prostaglandin $F_{2\alpha}$. Lancet 1970; i:157–9.
17. Roth-Brandel U, Bygdeman M, Wiqvist N, Bergstrom S. Prostaglandins for induction of a therapeutic abortion. Lancet 1970; i:190–1.
18. Rodger MW, Baird DT. Blood loss following induction of early abortion using mifepristone (RU 486) and a prostaglandin analogue (gemeprost). Contraception 1989; 40:439–47.
19. Baird DT, Cameron IT. Menstrual induction: surgery versus prostaglandins. In: Abortion: medical progress and social implications. Ciba Foundation Symposium 115. London: Pitman, 1985; 178–91.
20. Louden N, quoted in Baird DT, Cameron IT. Menstrual induction: surgery versus prostaglandins. In: Abortion: medical progress and social implications. Ciba Foundation Symposium 115. London: Pitman, 1985; 178–91.
21. Csapo AI, Pulkkinen MO, Wiest WG. Effects of luteectomy and progesterone replacement therapy in early pregnant patients. Am J Obstet Gynecol 1973; 115:759–65.
22. Horton EW, Poyser NL. Uterine luteolytic hormone: a physiological role for prostaglandin $F_{2\alpha}$. Physiol Rev 1976; 56:913–9.
23. Wiqvist N, Bygdeman M. Induction of therapeutic abortion with intravenous prostaglandin $F_{2\alpha}$. Lancet 1970; i:889.
24. Wentz AC, Jones GS. Intravenous prostaglandin $F_{2\alpha}$ for induction of menses. Fertil Steril 1973; 24:569–77.
25. Corlett RC, Sribyatta B, Mishell DR, Ballard C, Nakamura RM, Thorneycroft IH. Termination of early gestation with vaginal prostaglandin $F_{2\alpha}$ tablets. Prostaglandins 1972; 2:453–64.
26. Sato T, Ami K, Matsumoto S. The induction of abortion and menstruation by the intravaginal administration of prostaglandin $F_{2\alpha}$. Am J Obstet Gynecol 1973; 116:287–9.
27. Bolognese RJ, Corson SL. Abortion of early pregnancy by the intravaginal administration of prostaglandin F2α. Am J Obstet Gynecol 1973; 117:246–50.
28. Tredway DR, Mishell DR. Therapeutic abortion of early human gestation with vaginal suppositories of prostaglandin $F_{2\alpha}$. Am J Obstet Gynecol 1973; 116:795–8.
29. Jones JR, Perez RJ, Bienart W. Intravaginal PGE$_2$ in early abortion. Prostaglandins 1974; 7:149–63.
30. Csapo AI, Pulkkinen MO. The mechanism of prostaglandin action on the early pregnant human uterus. Prostaglandins 1979; 18:479–90.
31. Csapo AI, Ruttner B, Wiest WG. First trimester abortions induced by a single extraovular injection of PGF$_{2\alpha}$. Prostaglandins 1972; 1:365–71.
32. Csapo AI, Moscary P, Nagy T, Kaihola HC. The efficacy and acceptability of the "prostaglandin impact" in inducing complete abortion during the second week after the missed menstrual period. Prostaglandins 1973; 3:125–39.
33. Moscary P, Csapo AI. "Delayed menstruation" induced by prostaglandin in pregnant patients. Lancet 1973; ii:683.
34. Karim SMM. Intrauterine prostaglandins for outpatient termination of very early pregnancy. Lancet 1973; ii:794.
35. Ylikorkala O, Jouppila P, Ylostalo P, Jarvinen PA. Intrauterine injection of PGF$_{2\alpha}$ for termination of early pregnancy in out-patient. Prostaglandins 1974; 7:57–70.
36. Lichtman AS, Brenner P, Mishell DR. Intrauterine administration of PGF$_{2\alpha}$ as an outpatient procedure for termination of early pregnancy. Contraception 1974; 9:403–8.
37. Ragab I, Edelman DA. Early termination of pregnancy: comparative study of intrauterine prostaglandin $F_{2\alpha}$ and vacuum aspiration. Prostaglandins 1976; 11:275–83.
38. Bundy G, Lincoln F, Nelson N, Pike J, Schneider W. Novel prostaglandin syntheses. Ann NY Acid Sci 1971; 180:76–90.
39. Karim SMM, Sharma SD. Termination of second trimester pregnancy with 15-methyl analogues of prostaglandin E$_2$ and F$_{2\alpha}$. J Obstet Gynaecol Br Commonw 1972; 79:737–43.
40. Lauersen NH, Wilson KH. Serial intramuscular injection of 15(S)-15-methyl prostaglandin $F_{2\alpha}$ in the induction of abortion. Prostaglandins 1975; 10:1029–36.
41. Lauersen NH, Wilson KH. Midtrimester abortion induced by serial intramuscular injections of 15(S)-15-methyl-prostaglandin $F_{2\alpha}$. Am J Obstet Gynecol 1975; 121:273–6.
42. Lauersen NH, Wilson KH. Luteolytic and abortifacient effects of serial intramuscular injections of 15(S)-15-methyl prostaglandin F_{2a} in early pregnancy. Am J Obstet Gynecol 1976; 124:425–9.
43. Fylling P, Jerve F. 15(S)15-methyl prostaglandin F_{2a} for termination of very early human pregnancy. A comparative study of a single intramuscular injection and vaginal suppositories. Prostaglandins 1977; 14:785–90.

44. Bygdeman M, Martin JN Jr, Leader A, Lundstrom V, Ramadan M, Eneroth P, Green K. Early pregnancy interruption by 15(S) 15 methyl prostaglandin $F_{2\alpha}$ methyl ester. Obstet Gynecol 1976; 48:221–4.
45. Ylikorkala O, Jarvinen PA, Puukka M, Viinikka L. Abortifacient efficiency of 15(S) 15-methyl prostaglandin F_{2a} methyl ester administered vaginally during early pregnancy. Prostaglandins 1976; 12:609–24.
46. Zoremthangi B, Agarwal N, Puri CP, Laumas KR, Hingorani V. Evaluation of 15(S) 15-methyl-$PGF_{2\alpha}$ methyl ester suppositories with a two dose schedule for termination of early pregnancy. Contraception 1976; 14:519–27.
47. Hamberger L, Nilsson L, Bjorn-Rasmussen E, Atterfelt P, Wiqvist N. Early abortion by vaginal prostaglandin suppositories; blood loss in relation to elimination of serum chorionic gonadotrophin, progesterone and estradiol 17-β. Contraception 1978; 17:183–94.
48. Lauersen NH, Wilson KH. Early pregnancy interruption with two 15-ME-$PGF_{2\alpha}$ suppositories. Contraception 1980; 21:273–82.
49. Spilman CH, Beuving DC, Forbes AD. Evaluation of vaginal delivery systems containing 15(S) 15-methyl $PGF_{2\alpha}$ methyl ester. Prostaglandins 1976; 12 (suppl): 1–16.
50. Green K, Bygdeman M, Bremme K. Interruption of early first trimester pregnancy by single vaginal administration of 15-methyl-$PGF_{2\alpha}$-methyl ester. Contraception 1978; 18:551–60.
51. Population information program. Prostaglandins: the use of PGs in human reproduction. Popul Rep [G]; 8:79–119.
52. Karim SMM, Rao B, Ratnam SS, Prasad RNV, Wong YM, Ilancheran A. Termination of early pregnancy (menstrual induction) with 16-phenoxy-ω-tetranor PGE_2 methyl sulfonylamide. Contraception 1977; 6:377–81.
53. Csapo AI, Peskin EG, Sauvage JP et al. Menstrual induction in preference to abortion. Lancet 1980; i:90–1.
54. Fleischer A, Schulman H, Blattner P, Jagani N, Fayemi A. Early pregnancy – abortion model using sulprostone. Prostaglandins 1982; 23:643–55.
55. Bygdeman M, Christensen NJ, Green K, Zheng S, Lundstrom V. Termination of early pregnancy: future development. Acta Obstet Gynecol Scand Suppl 1983; 113:125–9.
56. Lundstrom V, Bygdeman M, Fotiou S, Green K, Kinoshita K. Abortion in early pregnancy by vaginal administration of 16,16-dimethyl-PGE_2 in comparison with vacuum aspiration. Contraception 1977; 16:167–73.
57. MacKenzie IZ, Embrey MP, Davies AJ, Guillebaud J. Very early abortion by prostaglandins. Lancet 1978; i:1223–6.
58. Smith SK, Baird DT. The use of 16,16-dimethyl trans $\Delta2$ PGE_1 methyl ester (ONO 802) vaginal suppositories for the termination of early pregnancy. A comparative study. Br J Obstet Gynaecol 1980; 87:712–17.
59. Rosen A-S, von Knorring K, Bygdeman M, Christensen NJ. Randomised comparison of prostaglandin treatment in hospital or at home with vacuum aspiration for termination of early pregnancy. Contraception 1984; 29:423–35.
60. WHO Task Force on post-ovulatory methods for fertility regulation. Menstrual regulation by intramuscular injections of 16-phenoxy-tetranor PGE_2 methyl sulfonylamide or vacuum aspiration. A randomised multicentre study. Br J Obstet Gynaecol 1987; 94:949–56.
61. Bygdeman M, Christensen NJ, Green K, Zheng S. Self administration of prostaglandin for termination of early pregnancy. Contraception 1981; 24:45–52.
62. Moscary P, Csapo AI. Effect of menstrual induction on prematurity rate. Lancet 1978; i:1159–60.
63. Csapo AI. The prospects of PGs in postconceptional therapy. Prostaglandins 1973; 3:245–89.
64. WHO Task Force on Sequelae of Abortion. Gestation, birth weight, and spontaneous abortion in pregnancy after induced abortion. Lancet 1979; i:142–5.
65. Baird DT. Control of luteolysis. In: Jeffcoate SL, ed. The luteal phase. Chichester: John Wiley. 1985; 25–42.
66. Csapo AI, Pulkkinen MO, Kaihola HL. The effect of estradiol replacement therapy on early pregnant luteectomized patients. Am J Obstet Gynecol 1973; 117:987–90.
67. Birgerson L, Olund A, Odlind V, Somell C. Termination of early human pregnancy with epostane. Contraception 1987; 35:111–20.
68. Crooj MJ, de Nooyer CCA, Rao BR, Berends GT, Gooren LJG, Janssens J. Termination of early pregnancy by the 3β-hydroxysteroid dehydrogenase inhibitor epostane. N Engl J Med 1988; 319:813–17.
69. Herrmann W, Wyss R, Riondal A, Philibert D. Teutsch G, Sakiz E, Baulieu EE. Effect d'un steroide anti-progesterone chez la femme: interruption du cycle menstruel et de la grossesse au debut. C R Acad Sci [III] 1982; 294:933–8.

70. Kovacs L, Sas M, Resch BA, Ugocsai G, Swahn ML, Bygdeman M, Rowe RJ. Termination of very early pregnancy by RU 486 – an antiprogestational compound. Contraception 1984; 29:399–410.
71. Couzinet B, Le Strat N, Ulman A, Baulieu EE, Schaison G. Termination of early pregnancy by the progesterone antagonist RU 486 (mifepristone). N Engl J Med 1986; 315:1565–70.
72. Bygdeman M, Swahn ML. Progesterone receptor blockade. Effect on uterine contractility and early pregnancy. Contraception 1985; 32:45–51.
73. Swahn ML, Bygdeman M. Termination of early pregnancy with RU486 (mifepristone) in combination with a prostaglandin analogue (sulprostone). Acta Obstet Gynecol Scand 1989; 68:293–300.
74. WHO Task Force on post-ovulatory methods for fertility regulation. Termination of early human pregnancy with RU 486 (mifepristone) and the prostaglandin analogue sulprostone: a multi-centre, randomised comparison between two treatment regimens. Hum Reprod 1989; 4:718–25.
75. Cameron IT, Michie AF, Baird DT. Therapeutic abortion in early pregnancy with antiprogesto-gen RU 486 alone or in combination with prostaglandin analogue (Gemeprost). Contraception 1986; 34:459–68.
76. Rodger MW, Baird DT. Induction of therapeutic abortion in early pregnancy with mifepristone in combination with prostaglandin pessary. Lancet 1987; ii:1415–18.
77. Dubois C, Ulman A, Aubeny E et al. Contragestation par le RU-486: interet de l'association a un derive prostaglandine. C R Acad Sci [III] 1988; 306:57–61.
78. UK Multicentre Trial. The efficacy and tolerance of mifepristone and prostaglandin in first trimester termination of pregnancy. Br J Obstet Gynaecol 1990; 97:480–6.
79. Rodger MW, Logan AF, Baird DT. Induction of early abortion with mifepristone (RU 486) and two different doses of prostaglandin pessary (gemeprost). Contraception 1989; 39:497–502.
80. Swahn ML, Ugocasi G, Bygdeman M, Kovacs L, Belsey EM, Van Look PFA. Effect of oral prostaglandin E_2 on uterine contractility and outcome of treatment in women receiving RU 486 (mifepristone) for termination of early pregnancy. Hum Reprod 1989; 4:21–8.
81. Swahn ML, Gottlieb C, Green K, Bygdeman M. Oral administration of RU 486 and 9-methylene PGE_2 for termination of early pregnancy. Contraception 1990; 41:461–73.
82. Aubeny E, Baulieu EE. Contragestation with RU 486 and an orally active prostaglandin. CR Acad Sci [III] 1991; 312:539–46.
83. Norman JE, Thong JT, Baird DT. Uterine contractility and induction of abortion in early pregnancy by misoprostol and mifepristone. Lancet 1991; 338:1233–6.
84. Silvestre L, Dubois C, Renault M, Rezvani Y, Baulieu EE, Ulman A. Voluntary interruption of pregnancy with mifepristone (RU 486) and a prostaglandin analogue. A large scale French experience. N Engl J Med 1990; 322:645–8.
85. Aubeny E. First congress of European Society of Contraception, Paris 1990.
86. Norman JE, Thong KJ, Rodger MW, Baird DT. Medical abortion in women of 56 days amenorrhoea: comparison between gemeprost (a PGE_1 analogue) alone and mifepristone and gemeprost. Br J Obstet Gynaecol in press.

Discussion

Lumsden: It is obvious that progesterone is important during the period of implantation. Do we have any information about what progesterone does to, for example, EGF?

Smith: No. We do have data in terms of the effect of oestradiol on EGF but I know of no direct evidence on progesterone and EGF. It would be very disappointing if it switched it off. The evidence would suggest it was the opposite.

There are other growth factors, e.g., CSF, whose expression is significantly switched on by progesterone.

López Bernal: Would Professor Smith clarify the point about PAF effects being mediated by either PLC or PLB? He said that rapid effects would be mediated by the PLC pathway whereas long-term effects would be mediated by the phospholipase. I can understand that IP_3 would have a very rapid effect, but protein kinase C would be activated through the pathway, and would have long-term effects on growth.

Smith: There are several experiments that have shown that the principal substrate for chronic activation of cells, certainly in terms of proliferation, is PC not PI. The PI response produces the early trigger of calcium, which I know is relevant in labour, but that is only a transient response. If we look at diacylglyceride (DAG) release, for example, there is almost always a biphasic response of DAG and there are many other studies which have shown that that is arising principally from PC hydrolysis. There are PC PLCs and PLDs; what we were trying to describe was how PAF might be all very well in a culture dish in 5 seconds but it did not seem to have great physiological significance.

There are two mechanisms, but there are extra data to show that it is the PC hydrolysis which is the most important for chronic activation of a whole host of cellular events from proliferation, differentiation and secretion.

Olson: What are the second messengers with the phospholipase D phosphatidylcholine mechanism to generate phosphatidic acid and choline? Is choline a second messenger, or is phosphatidic acid?

Smith: Phosphatidic acid is definitely a second messenger in that it enhances expression of GAP. We are discussing how the second messengers affect genomic events and it is a huge area. Specifically the question was whether choline or phosphatidic acid, which are the products of PLD activity, have any demonstrable effects in the cell and I was saying that phosphatidic acid has been shown to activate GTPase activating protein, which is part of the *ras* oncogene product and GAP and GTPase inhibiting protein (GIP) mechanisms involved in cell proliferation, probably the third most important pathway in terms of inducing proliferation.

Furthermore arachidonic acid is able to antagonise that by enhancing expression of GIP, and therefore there is a direct effect.

The crucial issue is whether phosphatidic acid and arachidonic acid bind to the genome and activate promoters. That is the crucial issue and nobody, to the best of my knowledge, has as yet demonstrated that specific action.

There are other issues like the cyclic AMP, in that again cyclic AMP has response elements or similar structures to response elements in the genome, so it may be that they are acting through yet another system or another integrated system.

But the answer is that yes they do have direct effects.

Greer: We have heard about the effects of prostaglandins and menstrual induction and we have probably all largely assumed that this is purely a uterine contractility effect. Is there any evidence that PGF, or PGE, or one of the analogues, could have a direct embyropathic effect, perhaps through the growth factors that Professor Smith has described?

Smith: I do not know of any data. I cannot think of any data.

Greer: We have heard of ectopic pregnancies being injected with $PGF_{2\alpha}$ but I am not clear whether that is an embryopathic phenomenon or whether it is contractility in the tube which causes a tube abortion.

Smith: There is some evidence that some interleukins can be toxic, but I do not know of any data.

Kelly: There is some evidence that antiprotestins can cause arterial constriction, and therefore energy deprivation of the fetus. It is one of the early events, which suggests that it could again be a toxin.

Calder: Dr Husslein might comment on management of ectopic pregnancy with prostaglandins.

Husslein: From our experience with the use of prostaglandins for the treatment of ectopic pregnancy, we believe that efficacy is explained by the vasoconstrictive and the tuboconstrictive effect, but not necessarily by an effect that is directly embryotoxic.

Nathanielsz: That is a very interesting question. There is some information, particularly in the pig, that there is a change in the profiles of PGs in the uterine secretions, and this may have direct effects on the embryo.

Smith: This is the exocrine release of PGs into the cavity.

Nathanielsz: Right. This is a very different situation. The pig embryo does not implant until it is 33 days old and very long. It is a very different type of implantation process.

Smith: There is evidence in humans; I think Dr Finlay has some original data showing basal release of PGs.

Kelly: Can Professor Smith explain why these elongating blastocysts need to produce such huge amounts of PGE?

Smith: The obvious answer is no. The point is that in rodents the elevation of PGE is associated with the site of implantation and if that mechanism should be inhibited, then presumably it is either something to do with the embryo or something to do with the implantation site.

Human embryos produce PG; we did that pilot work in Edinburgh, and other workers have similarly shown PG production from embryos. The production of prostaglandins in the embryo itself which probably induces elongation or is involved in the elongation mechanism in the pigs is clearly involved in the proliferation of human blastocyst, but exactly how, I do not know.

Amy: I was asked last year to contribute to an encyclopaedia of bioethics that is being written in French and so I was obliged to think about the subjects I was to write on. One of the subjects was the interruption of pregnancy and after thinking about it I have developed objections to the use of expressions such as interruption of pregnancy, contra gestation, and menstrual induction, and I would plead for the use of the term very early abortion instead of menstrual induction. It is not the induction of menstruation; it is the induction of very early abortion.

Husslein: I wanted to make the same comment. I do not want to discuss the ethics of abortion but I believe that we have to realise it is a sensitive issue and I believe that we owe it to ourselves and the lay public, who perhaps do not know about all the details of the methodology, to speak in clear terms. There is a difference between menstrual induction, to induce menstruation, at least from the point of view of the lay public, and an early termination of pregnancy. The problem does not disappear if we say what we are doing: we are terminating an early pregnancy and we should state what we are doing.

MacKenzie: It would be acceptable, would it not, when referring to what Dr Norman said about giving it in the luteal phase, when indeed it is inducing abortion if conception does occur? It is perfectly reasonable to call that an induced menstruation. But I am sure that to talk about giving prostaglandins or antiprogestins at 56 days of amenorrhoea is not quite menstrual induction.

Norman: Was the phrase not coined originally because the technique was used in women whose pregnancy had not been confirmed because there was no access to sensitive pregnancy tests?

MacKenzie: That was in the first six weeks or so of amenorrhoea, beyond which physiological pregnancy tests are reasonably reliable.

Nathanielsz: I was very interested in the data on RU486 and the conclusion that its effects on myometrial activity were not prostaglandin dependent. There are interesting data from Miles Novy's group where giving RU486 in late pregnancy in the monkey gives rise to a very different pattern of myometrial activity from labour and delivery, although it goes into labour if the monkey is examined clinically. I thought the pattern after giving a PGSI was really rather different. The basal tone was much higher, the frequency of the individual contractile epochs was much less, and one has to keep an open mind about ruling out the role of prostaglandins in the effects of RU486.

Greer: Dr Norman showed a bell-shaped time course with regard to PG production in response to RU486 in the decidua experiments, and yet those same individuals had a straightforward, almost time-dependent increase in uterine activity. How is the lack of correlation to be explained, and also the fact of the bell-shaped time course?

Norman: The bell-shaped time course may be because the decidua by this stage is so necrotic that it is not synthesising PGs in the same way, or it may be that the arachidonic acid sources are exhausted so that it will not have the same synthetic capacity. I do not know why uterine activity carries on increasing. It does not seem to be related to PG production so it is not surprising that as PGs decline, uterine activity does not decline.

Greer: I have a second point about analgesic requirements in these studies. We accept that there is quite a high analgesic requirement with gemeprost, but I am not really sure when we compare it with the RU486 pretreatment whether we are genuinely comparing like with like. The dose of gemeprost we give is probably a very high dose and probably higher than is necessary to induce abortion. Are there any data where much smaller doses of gemeprost are compared with RU486 plus gemeprost to see if it is purely the fact that we have given too much prostaglandin that dictates the analgesic requirements as opposed to a difference in the methodologies?

Norman: No. And the time course is completely different. If PGs are used alone to induce abortion it can take till the third PG pessary, which is given 12 h after the first, whereas if RU486 plus a prostaglandin is used, the majority of women have aborted by 4 h.

The time course is also different and it is very difficult to compare doses.

Chapter 8

Prostaglandins and Midtrimester Abortion

I. Z. MacKenzie

For a method of pregnancy termination to become widely adopted, it must have a high degree of efficacy, it must be acceptable to patients and staff, and it must be safe at the time of abortion, during the early recovery period and in the long term. In addition, for terminations performed as a consequence of a positive prenatal diagnostic test, the method should allow the diagnosis to be confirmed and the woman given appropriate advice for future conceptions. In many respects, the methods involving the administration of prostaglandins have been found to fulfil these objectives.

Prostaglandins were first used for midtrimester abortion in the early 1970s [1,2], and by 1973 they were being used increasingly in gynaecological departments in the UK. By 1975, abortions performed with prostaglandins were being recorded specifically in the abortion statistics for England and Wales collected by the Office of Population Censuses and Surveys [3]. Fig. 8.1 shows that the number of second trimester abortions each year in England and Wales has remained relatively constant although representing a declining proportion of the total. There has, however, been a gradual increase in the number and proportion of abortions performed with prostaglandins. In 1989, a total of 183 974 terminations was performed, of which 26 550 were during the second trimester and 8091 were performed with prostaglandins [4]. It is possible that developments during the past decade may lead to an even greater use of this medical approach to midtrimester termination using some of the newer strategies described below.

Administration Routes and Drug Regimens

Since the introduction of the prostaglandins for pregnancy termination, there have evolved four main routes of administration. Intravenous infusions were

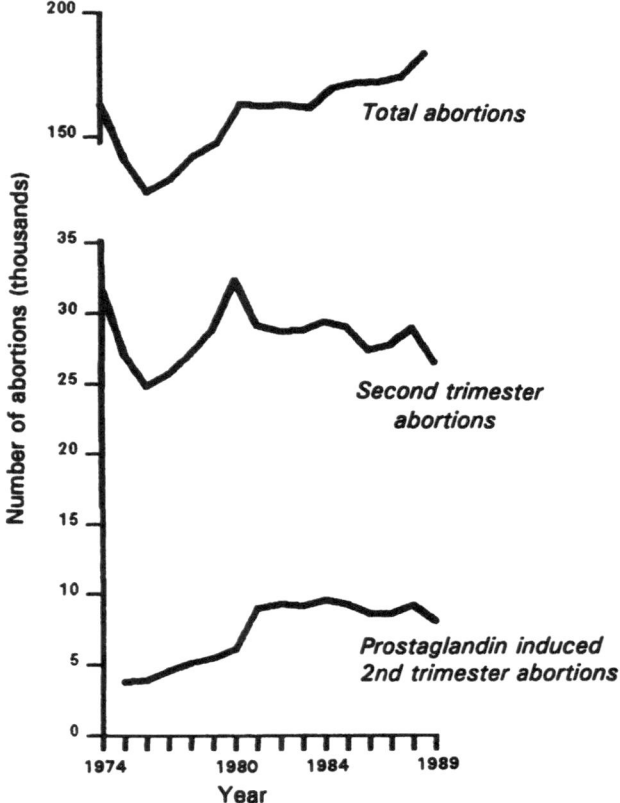

Fig. 8.1. Trends in total abortions, second trimester abortions, and prostaglandin-induced abortions in England and Wales, 1974–1989.

initially used, but the required dosages resulted in unacceptable side effects and the route is no longer used to any extent. The decision over which of the four established routes to use is determined largely by personal preference, but pregnancy gestation and availability of the various prostaglandin analogues influence the choice.

Extra-amniotic Administration

This route has been widely used for 20 years with great success. It is appropriate throughout the whole of the second trimester, but if used beyond 18 weeks' gestation it has the disadvantage of inducing abortion with the fetus expelled showing signs of life. The natural prostaglandins PGE_2 and $PGF_{2\alpha}$ and a variety of analogues have been used and regimens have varied, involving intermittent hourly or two hourly injections, continuous infusions, or single bolus injections in a viscous gel. Schedules of extra-amniotic treatment have included the use of prostaglandins alone or in combination with other substances such as ethacridine lactate [5] or an intravenous infusion of oxytocin. As shown in Table 8.1, which shows some examples of different protocols, the results obtained are broadly similar with the different schedules, except that some are less demanding of nursing and medical staff time. Intravenous oxytocin augmentation shortens the induction to abortion intervals, and some protocols reduce the incidence of associated side effects. Gestation has little effect on abortion times over the period of pregnancy when the extra-amniotic route is used; there thus seems little justification for delaying admission for abortion until 16 weeks' gestation as is practised by some. However, as with other routes of administration, shorter abortion times are achieved for multiparae compared with nulliparae [7,8,17].

Intra-amniotic Administration

This route of administration has generally been reserved for pregnancies terminated at 16 weeks' gestation and over. With the widespread availability and use of ultrasound scanning, the intra-amniotic route can be used at earlier gestations, but there appears to be no advantage over the extra-amniotic approach. Either single injection schedules, often combined with an intravenous infusion of oxytocin, or repeated injections at 6-, 12- or 24-h intervals using an indwelling intra-amniotic catheter have been used. Table 8.1 illustrates some examples of intra-amniotic protocols that have been developed, and the results obtained.

As with the extra-amniotic route, an intact fetal circulation is likely to be encountered at delivery at gestations over 18 weeks and to avoid this, either air embolism of the fetus can be performed, or 100–200 ml of amniotic fluid can be withdrawn and replaced with some hypertonic solution. Apart from ensuring that the fetus is dead at abortion, induction to abortion intervals can be significantly reduced using the addition of a hypertonic solution and it almost guarantees success in achieving abortion with a single instillation. Serious complications are associated with the use of hypertonic solutions, notably a consumptive coagu-lopathy with all the hypertonic solutions used, and hypernatraemia with hyper-tonic saline – problems which do not occur when prostaglandins are used alone [18–21]. In consequence, it seems appropriate to reserve these combination methods for the few cases performed when the risk is justified.

With the intra-amniotic route, it is particularly important to ensure that the tip of the injecting needle or self-retaining cannula is correctly sited within the amniotic sac either by continuous ultrasound screening, or by repeated aspiration of aliquots of amniotic fluid during the injection of the prostaglandins. The dosages used with this route are relatively large and if injected directly into the systemic circulation by inadvertent dislodgement of the needle-tip or cannula into a myometrial vessel, sudden collapse will occur which requires supportive management for the next 15–30 min. Maternal deaths have occurred during prostaglandin-induced abortion, and some almost certainly have been due to acute massive overdosage into the circulation (see below).

Intramuscular Injections

A variety of synthetic analogues of both the E and F prostaglandins have been explored for repeated intramuscular injections. This approach represents the

Table 8.1. Results of prostaglandin-induced midtrimester abortion using different administration methods and protocols

Protocol	n	Induction–abortion interval			Side effects		Reference
		Mean (h)	<24 h	<36 h	Vomiting	Diarrhoea	
Extra-amniotic							
15MePGF$_{2\alpha}$ 0.92 mg gel single injection	660	16.2/13.1[a]	NR	80%	38%	32%	[6]
15MePGF$_{2\alpha}$ 1 mg gel single injection	1569	15.4/13.6[a]	71%	78%	36%	34%	[7]
PGE$_2$ 1.5–2.5 mg gel single inj. +i.v. oxytocin at 6 h	1608	14.8	83%	96%	45%	17%	[8]
Intra-amniotic							
15MePGF$_{2\alpha}$ 2.5 mg single inj.	430	20.6/17.7[a]	69%	88%[b]	42%	24%	[7]
PGF$_{2\alpha}$ 25+25 mg at 6 h	717	19.7	61%	80%[b]	53%	15%	[9]
PGE$_2$ 5–10 mg single inj. +i.v. oxytocin at 6 h	700	14.8	89%	98%	39%	5%	[8]
PGF$_{2\alpha}$ 10 mg + urea	180	16.3	78%	95%	70%	1%	[10]
Intramuscular							
16-phenPGE$_2$ 1 mg 8 hourly	145	14.8	NR	88%[d]	50%	25%	[11]
15MePGF$_{2\alpha}$ 250 µg 2 hourly laminaria for 12 h pre-PG	294	23.2[c]	NR	94%[c]	64%	65%	[12]
16-phenPGE$_2$ 500 µg 2 hourly laminaria for 12 h pre-PG	298	22.8[c]	NR	96%[c]	41%	17%	[12]
Vaginal							
15MePGF$_{2\alpha}$ 3 mg 3 hourly	310	14.2	88%	92%[b]	67%	70%	[13]
15MePGF$_{2\alpha}$ 3 mg	288	14.7	NR	78%[b]	72%	77%	[14]
16,16diMePGE$_1$ 1 mg 3 hourly ×5	113	19.3	82%	NR	14%	20%	[15]
16,16diMePGE$_1$ 1 mg 3 hourly ×3 + i.v. oxytocin at 6 h	349	18.3	78%	92%	28%	23%	[16]

n = number of subjects
[a] nulliparous/multiparous.
[b] in 48 h.
[c] includes 12 h with laminaria in situ.
[d] in 30 h.

least invasive midtrimester termination method and is appropriate up to 18 weeks' gestation. A number of studies published in the 1970s examined these analogues using different dosages and injection frequencies from 2 hourly to 8 hourly; virtually all protocols result in acceptable induction to abortion intervals but at the expense of very high rates of vomiting and diarrhoea (Table 8.1). In many, these high rates of gastrointestinal side effects occur despite 2–6 hourly administration of antiemetics and antidiarrhoeal agents.

To try to improve the results, laminaria tents have been inserted into the cervix for 12–18 h before prostaglandin administration. Although prostaglandin to abortion intervals are reduced, the overall treatment to abortion times frequently approach 24 h and in consequence the method has little to commend it.

Vaginal Administration

Initial studies of vaginal administration of the natural prostaglandins indicated that the dosage required caused very high rates of vomiting and diarrhoea and the approach was abandoned. With the introduction of some of the synthetic anologues, the route was explored further. Large multicentre studies using 15Me-$PGF_{2\alpha}$ were conducted by the World Health Organization, but side effects were still a significant drawback, although abortion times were acceptable. During the past ten years, gemeprost, the PGE_1 analogue 16,16-dimethyl-trans 2-PGE_1, has been increasingly used and much more acceptable results have been achieved. Table 8.1 gives the results of some of the reported series. Those obtained with gemeprost, whether given as five doses at 3-hourly intervals or three doses at the same intervals with intravenous oxytocin augmentation at 6 h, are essentially similar, though surprisingly, the side effect rates appear to be higher with the lower total dose of prostaglandin.

We recently reported the results of 450 patients in a randomised study comparing the three dose protocol with extra-amniotic PGE_2 2.5 mg as a single injection and intra-amniotic PGE_2 10 mg as a single injection; all groups received oxytocin augmentation at 6 h [22]. The cumulative abortion times are illustrated in Fig. 8.2. The mean±SD induction to abortion interval with the pessaries was 19.5±8.4 h which was significantly ($P<0.001$) longer than the 14.4±9.3 for extra-amniotic treatment and 16.1±6.8 h for intra-amniotic treatment; the incidence of vomiting for the respective groups was 31%, 37%, and 13% and diarrhoea was 27%, 14% and 2%. The vaginal route, however, is less invasive and simpler but it requires more prostaglandins and abortion takes longer and is thus more expensive. In addition it has the very important potential to provide a safer option than the two intra-uterine administration routes.

Prostaglandins and the Antiprogestins

In the 1980s, the antiprogestins were introduced into clinical practice for assessment. Two forms of antiprogestin have been studied: the 3β-hydroxy-steroid dehydrogenase inhibitor, "epostane", which prevents the essential con-

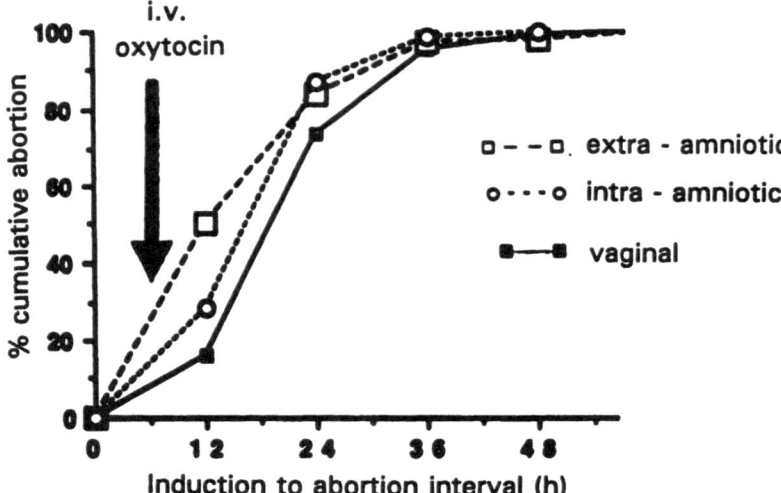

Fig. 8.2. Cumulative abortion rates of a randomised trial comparing gemeprost 1 mg 3 hourly for three doses with a single injection of PGE$_2$ 2.5 mg extra-amniotically or PGE$_2$ 10 mg intra-amniotically: all regimes included intravenous oxytocin titration 6 h after the start of prostaglandin treatment.

version of pregnenolone into progesterone, and the progesterone receptor blocker, "mifepristone", which deforms the receptor–agonist complex, and prevents the stimulation of RNA synthesis. Both have been shown to be powerful antagonists to the myometrial suppressant properties of progesterone but neither has been found to be sufficiently reliable in inducing abortion when used alone.

The impact of a combination treatment using prostaglandin preceded by an antiprogestin was first demonstrated by Webster et al. [23], using a combination of oral epostane and vaginal PGE$_2$ for terminating early first trimester pregnancy. The potential value of antiprogestins for second trimester prostaglandin induced abortion was subsequently demonstrated also using epostane [24]. Double-blind placebo-controlled trials were then conducted, which indicated that if epostane is given orally for 24–72 h prior to the administration of PGE$_2$, it reduces the induction-to-abortion intervals by 50%–70% [25]; the longer the duration of epostane treatment, the shorter the abortion interval. Measurements of intra-uterine pressure in these studies demonstrated the enhanced myometrial contractility in response to prostaglandins, but not oxytocin. These studies also illustrated that the fall in circulating progesterone resulting from epostane treatment was associated with increased myometrial sensitivity when compared with placebo [26].

Similar effects on myometrial contractility have been demonstrated using mifepristone in the first trimester of pregnancy in uncontrolled studies [27], and in the second trimester [28]. As with epostane, the prior exposure of the patient to mifepristone has been shown to reduce abortion times by up to 50% if it is given at least 24 h before prostaglandin treatment with extra-amniotic administration using historical controls [29] or placebo controls [28], and vaginal treatment using placebo controls [30].

Table 8.2 illustrates the impact of antiprogestin treatment on abortion times in published studies. All demonstrate a reduction in abortion times, two show

Table 8.2. Published results of controlled studies using an antiprogestin and prostaglandins for second trimester abortion

Reference	Protocol	Total studied	Total PGs given	Induction–abortion-interval (min)	
				Treated	Control
				(mean±SD)	
[25,26,31]	Epostane 72 h±EA PGE$_2$	10	1.5 mg	490±271	1432±640
	Epostane 72 h±IA PGE$_2$	10	5.0 mg	553±70	944±503
	Epostane 72 h±EA PGE$_2$	25	1.5 mg	406±223 ⎫	1343±560
	Epostane 24 h±EA PGE$_2$		1.5 mg	662±388 ⎭	
[30]	RU486 36 h±PGE$_1$	100	3.0 mg (trt)[a]	408	948
			5.0 mg (con)[a]		
[29]	RU486 24 h±EA PGE$_2$[c]	40	11.0 mg (trt)[b]	550	730
			18.0 mg (con)[b]		
[28]	RU486 48 h±EA PGE$_2$	20	1.5 mg	512±321	1128±606
	RU486 48 h±IA PGE$_2$			630±360 ⎫	
	RU486 24 h±IA PGE$_2$	24	5.0 mg	678±366 ⎬	966±462
	RU486 4 h±IA PGE$_2$			1032±516 ⎭	

[a] Median values.
[b] Mean values.
[c] Study used historical controls; the others were placebo controlled.
trt, treated; con, controls.

reduced prostaglandin requirements [29,30] and one found an increased analgesia requirement [29] and one a decrease [30].

The ideal protocol for antiprogestin administration has yet to be identified, but to date it appears that a 24 h interval is probably necessary between antiprogestin and prostaglandin treatment [27]. Whether varied doses of the antiprogestin and prostaglandin can maintain or enhance the improved abortion times and reduce side effects and analgesic requirements, remains to be investigated [32].

Prostaglandins and Cervical Preparation for Surgical Termination in the Second Trimester

There has been very little work undertaken to explore the role of prostaglandins prior to cervical dilatation and uterine evacuation (D&E) during the second trimester. Choo et al. [33] reported reasonably good results up to 16 weeks' gestation with a prostaglandin-to-surgery interval of 12–14 h, but the results were accompanied by gastrointestinal side effects in 30% of patients. More recent work indicates that cervical changes can be demonstrated within 3 h in most cases with much reduced side effect rates, and since the preoperative administration of prostaglandins also produces a significant reduction in operative blood loss there would seem to be good reason to examine their role further in this situation.

Safety of Prostaglandin-Induced Midtrimester Abortion

When assessing the complications associated with abortion,. morbidity encountered during the abortion procedure as well as that occurring shortly after
abortion and at a much later date all need to be considered.

Immediate and Short-term Morbidity

Complications encountered during the abortion vary marginally between the
different prostaglandin protocols described. Excess blood loss appears to be the
commonest problem occurring in 1.7% cases with transfusion being given to
0.6% [8]. Cervical trauma, especially cervicovaginal fistulae, were reported in a
number of series in the early 1970s. They appear to be largely related to the intra-
amniotic approach, and in particular those employing the augmenting effect of
intra-amniotic hypertonic solutions which produce short induction-to-abortion
intervals by provoking strong uterine contractions against an unyielding cervix.
The extra-amniotic route appears less likely to cause cervical damage, and the
relatively small numbers of cases managed to date in the United Kingdom with
vaginal pessaries have not yet led to any relationships being detected. The
incidence of ruptured uterus during midtrimester prostaglandin-induced abortion
is unknown. There have been the occasional anecdotal reports from which no
specific aetiological factors can be discerned [34–36]. It would thus seem that this
is an infrequent complication, but one which should be borne in mind when acute
pelvic symptoms present or the patient collapses during or shortly after the
abortion process.

Postabortal sepsis rates are always difficult to assess, but experience suggests
from the few large series reported that this occurs in 1%–2% cases. There is no
good prospective evidence from randomised trials to support the need for routine
antibiotic prophylaxis during midtrimester prostaglandin-induced abortion. We
do not use routine antibiotic prophylaxis in the management of midtrimester
prostaglandin abortions in Oxford: in an analysis of 2308 cases, managed with
intra-amniotic (700 cases), or extra-amniotic (1608) PGE_2, only 1.9% received
antibiotics when any concern arose about possible sepsis, and only two patients
developed any evidence of pelvic sepsis during the early postabortive period [8].

Incomplete abortion is a function of gestation as illustrated in Fig. 8.3.
Although some advocate routine surgical uterine evacuation following abortion
[37], this would seem inappropriate, provided that skilled experienced personnel
are caring for the patients, examining the expelled placenta and performing a
bimanual examination following abortion to determine whether complete
expulsion has occurred. Hospital readmission rates for re-evacuation are around
1%–2%, similar to those following first trimester aspiration termination, and
from personal experience, readmission occurs whether immediate postabortal
evacuation and curettage had been performed or omitted [38]. The immediate
postabortion management will influence the duration of hospitalisation: with the
selective approach to postabortion curettage in Oxford, only 23% patients are in
hospital for more than one night [8] compared with the national figure of 79% [4].

When comparing morbidity rates with dilatation and uterine evacuation

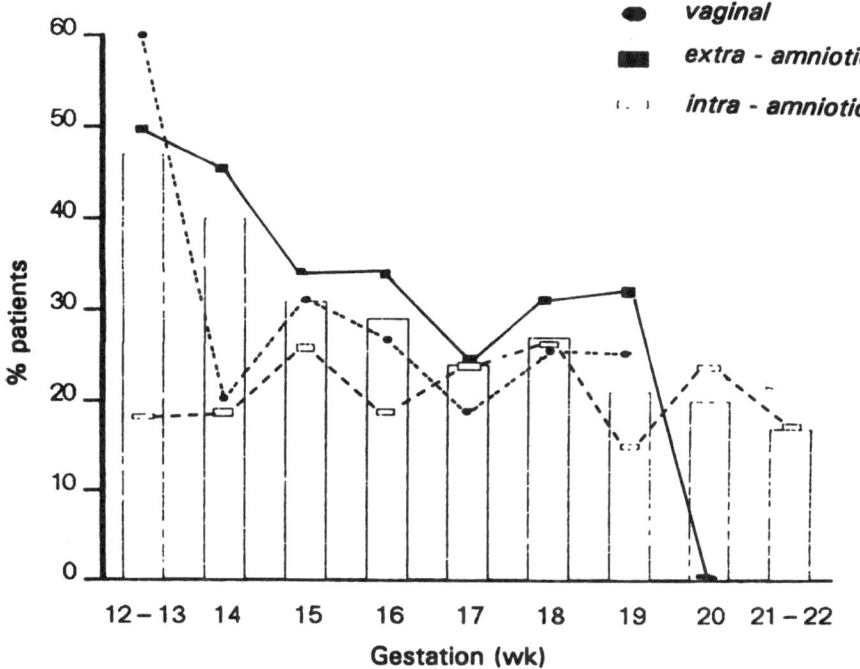

Fig. 8.3. Influence of gestation on rate of incomplete abortion during prostaglandin-induced midtrimester termination using extra-amniotic, intra-amniotic and vaginal administration. (Derived from references [8] and [9].)

(D&E), as the alternative approach to second trimester abortion, the results we have obtained in the 2308 cases of prostaglandin-induced abortion in Oxford [8] are similar to those reported from individual series of D&E [30–44] as far as blood loss, sepsis and lower genital tract trauma are concerned. To use data derived from nationally collected statistics [4,45,46] involving very large numbers to determine morbidity rates for induced abortion, almost certainly yields misleading figures when compared to the large individual published series, especially if collected prospectively. It is hard to believe that there was a rate of excess haemorrhage of only 0.2% and sepsis of 0.01% among 141 558 therapeutic abortions performed in England and Wales in 1978 [46], compared with 3.5% and 1.3% respectively obtained in a prospective study of 6104 abortions in England and Wales performed at the same time [47].

Abortion Mortality

Improved abortion methods and greater experience have contributed to the improved morbidity figures for first and second trimester terminations; these factors have almost certainly led to the marked decline in the maternal death rate associated with the use of prostaglandins. Between 1973 and 1989, more than 100 000 prostaglandin-induced midtrimester abortions were performed in England and Wales. During this time, there were ten fatalities, eight during the period 1973–1981, at a rate of 11.1 per 100 000 operations, and two during 1982–1989, a rate of 3.1 per 100 000 operations. These mortality figures compare well with those for the USA during the 1970s of 9.9 per 100 000 D&E operations and 13.1 per 100 000 prostaglandin terminations [48].

Table 8.3 lists the stated cause of death for these maternal deaths during 1973 and 1989; four followed intra-amniotic infusion, and six followed extra-amniotic infusion. The number of patients in England and Wales managed by the two prostaglandin administration routes is not known, but the RCOG survey of 1982 [37] suggested that at that time approximately half the prostaglandin abortions were conducted with extra-amniotic injections and half with intra-amniotic injections. If vaginal administration becomes widely adopted as seems likely, especially if used in combination with an antiprogestational agent, deaths from prostaglandin overdosage should be virtually eliminated. A case of cardiac arrhythmia has been reported with the use of gemeprost vaginal pessaries [49], indicating that risks still exist and vigilance for this hazard is advised.

Table 8.3. Maternal deaths associated with the use of prostaglandins for induction of second trimester abortion in England and Wales: 1973–1989

Gestation	Method	Cause of death
18 weeks	Extra-amniotic	? overdosage (2 mg)
14 weeks	Extra-amniotic	ruptured uterus
15 weeks	Extra-amniotic	clostridial infection
15 weeks	Extra-amniotic	clostridial infection
18 weeks	Extra-amniotic	pulmonary embolism
14 weeks	Extra-amniotic	pulmonary embolism
17 weeks	Intra-amniotic	pulm oedema ? overdosage
14 weeks	Intra-amniotic	? overdosage
18 weeks	Intra-amniotic with urea	? air embolism
18 weeks	Intra-amniotic	? overdosage

Delayed Sequelae

There has been relatively few data about the long-term consequences of late abortion including those performed with prostaglandins. The data available suggest that there is probably minimal risk to subsequent fertility following a prostaglandin-induced abortion [50], and little if any risk to subsequent pregnancies or neonatal outcome [51]. It is not possible to comment on psychological sequelae specifically following a prostaglandin-induced midtrimester abortion compared with surgical abortion by D&E, although Kaltreider et al. [52] reported 24% of 30 women with guilt feelings studied after a medical abortion compared with none among 30 whose pregnancy was terminated surgically. This very important observation should be repeated.

Prostaglandins and Missed Abortions

The prostaglandins have been used for the past 20 years for evacuating pregnancies complicated by fetal death, both early missed abortions and late intra-uterine fetal deaths. All the routes described previously have been used, and a recent survey of consultant obstetric units in the United Kingdom indicated that of the 85% responding units, 87% used prostaglandins to evacuate missed abortions and 98% for later fetal deaths [53]. Table 8.4 gives some protocols and results of larger studies using intramuscular and vaginal administration.

Table 8.4. Selected large series of intramuscular or vaginal prostaglandins for the evacuation of missed abortion and late fetal death

Reference	Protocol	n	Induction–Abortion interval		Side effects	
			Mean (h)	<30 h	Vomiting	Diarrhoea
[54]	2α,2β-dihomo 15meF2α ME 0.5 mg/8 hourly i.m.	631	11.3	95%[a]	48%	
[55]	PGE₂ 20 mg 3–5 hourly vaginally	709	10.7[b]	95%	56%	43%
[56]	15-meF2α 125–250 μg 12 hourly i.m.	97	8.6	99%	52%	59%

[a] in 32 h.
[b] for 687 successfully treated.

In Oxford since 1976, we have used prostaglandins administered vaginally for the management of missed abortions. Table 8.5 gives an analysis of 209 cases with uterine sizes at 15–28 weeks inclusive; for smaller sizes, we prefer uterine aspiration under inhalational anaesthesia, and those larger than 28 weeks' gestational size are generally managed with lower prostaglandin doses. Patients have been treated with prostaglandins during the afternoon of admission and if pregnancy expulsion had not occurred by the following morning, an intravenous infusion of oxytocin at 100 mU/min is commenced and maintained till the fetus is expelled. There appears to be little difference in efficacy between the largest PGE₂ dose and the three gemeprost pessary protocol and, since there are restrictions on hospital pharmacies producing their own prostaglandin preparations for vaginal administration, it seems appropriate to advocate the use of the gemeprost protocol despite the higher rate of oxytocin augmentation; it is of note that with the lowest PGE₂ dose (10 mg), 73% cases required oxytocin augmentation the following morning. In consequence the PGE₂ 25 mg protocol was used from preference.

The advantage of using vaginal prostaglandins in these cases rather than extra-amniotic instillation is obvious, with the reduced interference for an already distressed patient. The place of the antiprogestins in this situation is unclear. Ulmann and Dubois [57] reported that following exposure to mifepristone 200 mg 8 hourly for 48 h in a double-blind prospective trial involving 92 patients, 63% of pregnancies were expelled within 72 h compared with only 17% receiving placebo: the majority in the trial were in the third trimester. However, Selinger [31], examining progesterone levels before and 24 h after treatment with epostane

Table 8.5. Oxford experience in 209 patients using prostaglandin vaginally for evacuation of missed abortions at 15–28 weeks gestational size

	Prostaglandin Protocol			
	PGE$_2$ 10 mg	PGE$_2$ 15 mg	PGE$_2$ 25 mg	Gemeprost 3 mg
Number treated	26	62	103	18
Gestation size (weeks) (mean)	20.0	20.4	20.5	18.1
Oxytocin at 18–20 h	73%	55%	29%	46%
IEI (h)				
Mean	14.7	17.8	13.2	13.7
<24 h	92%	72%	89%	89%
<36 h	100%	92%	96%	100%
Side effects				
Vomiting	15%	26%	29%	17%
Diarrhoea	0%	3%	9%	11%
Analgesia				
Analgesia given	92%	68%	81%	72%
Mean no. injections	2.5	0.9	1.3	1.1

IEI, inductin–expulsion interval.

in a small series of cases of fetal death, demonstrated that the existing low circulating progesterone levels could be reduced still further, but this did not significantly influence the clinical outcome when compared with controls not given antiprogestin. More work in this area is required, which should help to further knowledge of the mechanisms of parturition and the influence of progesterone on myometrial contractility.

Conclusions and Future Developments

In the United Kingdom, the prostaglandins have an established place in the management of midtrimester abortion. The evidence indicates that their use in experienced units results in morbidity rates that are as good as or better than those reported for D&E, and little worse than those for first trimester aspiration. The increasing popularity of vaginal administration protocols and reduced use of intra-amniotic administration could lead to even safer results, eliminating the risk of inadvertent intravascular overdosage. However, this will be at the expense of marginally prolonged abortion times and increased drug costs. The place of the intra-amniotic protocols, however, will remain for the management of the later gestation terminations.

With the licensing of the antiprogestin mifepristone, it is expected that in due course it will be used to facilitate second trimester prostaglandin-induced abortions with a consequent reduction in abortion times. Day-care medically induced midtrimester abortion has thus become a possibility for up to 50% of patients treated. Before this could become standard practice, however, more work is required to determine the optimum drug regimens and large studies will be necessary to assess the overall safety. It seems highly probable that this approach will be acceptable to NHS managers, providing it reduces costs. It is therefore essential to ensure that safety is not sacrificed for financial benefit.

References

1. Karim SMM, Filshie GM. Therapeutic abortion using prostaglandin $F_{2\alpha}$. Lancet 1970; i:157–9.
2. Embrey MP. Induction of abortion by prostaglandin E_1 and E_2. Br Med J 1970; 2:258–60.
3. Office of Population Censuses and Surveys. Abortion statistics 1975. London: HMSO, 1975.
4. Office of Population Censuses and Surveys. Abortion statistics 1989. London: HMSO, 1990.
5. Martin JN, Bygdeman M, Leader A, Wiquist N. Early second trimester abortion by the extraamniotic instillation of rivanol solution and a single $PGF_{2\alpha}$ dose. Contraception 1975; 11:523–31.
6. World Health Organisation Task Force. Single extra-amniotic administration of 0.92 mg of 15-methyl-prostaglandin $F_{2\alpha}$ in Hyskon for termination of pregnancies in weeks 10–20 of gestation; an international multicentre study. Am J Obstet Gynecol 1977; 129:597–600.
7. Tejuja SS, Choudhury SD, Manchanda PK. Use of intra- and extra-amniotic prostaglandins for the termination of pregnancies: report of multicentric trials in India. Contraception 1978; 18:641–52.
8. Hill NCW, MacKenzie IZ. 2308 second trimester terminations using extraamniotic or intraamniotic prostaglandin E_2: an analysis of efficacy and complications. Br J Obstet Gynaecol 1989; 96:1424–31.
9. World Health Organisation Task Force. Comparison of intra-amniotic prostaglandin $F_{2\alpha}$ and hypertonic saline for second trimester abortion. Br Med J 1976; i:1373–6.
10. Burkman RT, Atienza MF, King TM, Burnett LS. Intra-amniotic urea and prostaglandin $F_{2\alpha}$ for midtrimester abortion: a modified regimen. Am J Obstet Gynecol 1976; 126:328–33.
11. World Health Organisation Task Force. Termination of second trimester pregnancy by intramuscular injection of 16-phenoxy-ω-17,18,19,20-tetranor PGE_2 methyl sulfonylamide. Int J Gynaecol Obstet 1982; 20:383–6.
12. World Health Organisation Task Force. Termination of second trimester pregnancy with laminaria and intramuscular 15-methyl $PGF_{2\alpha}$ or 16-phenoxy-ω-17,18,19,20-tetranor PGE_2 methyl sulfonylamide. A randomised multicentre study. Int J Gynaecol Obstet 1988; 26:129–35.
13. World Health Organisation Task Force. Repeated vaginal administration of 15-methyl $PGF_{2\alpha}$ for termination of pregnancy in the 13th to 20th week of gestation. Contraception 1977; 16:175–81.
14. Tejuja SS, Choudhury SD, Manchanda PK, Malhotra U. Indian experience with a single long-acting vaginal suppository for the termination of pregnancies. Contraception 1979; 19:191–6.
15. Cameron IT, Michie AF, Baird DT. Prostaglandin induced pregnancy termination: further studies using gemeprost (16,16dimethyl-trans- 2-PGE_1 methyl ester) vaginal pessaries in the early second trimester. Prostaglandins 1987; 34:111–17.
16. MacKenzie IZ, Ferguson J, Selinger M. Gemeprost 1 mg pessaries for midtrimester induction of abortion: a reduced dose protocol. Unpublished data. 1991.
17. Karim SMM, Choo HT, Lim AL, Yeo KC, Ratnam SS. Termination of second trimester pregnancy with intramuscular administration of 16-phenoxy-ω-17,18,19,20-tetranor-PGE_2 methylsulfonylamide. Prostaglandins 1978; 15:1063–8.
18. Badraoui MHH, Bonnar J, Hillier K, Embrey MP. Coagulation changes during termination of pregnancy by prostaglandins and by vacuum aspiration. Br Med J 1973; i:19–21.
19. Burkman RT, Bell WR, Atienza MF, King TM. Coagulopathy with mid-trimester induced abortion. Association with hyperosmolar urea administration. Am J Obstet Gynecol 1977; 127:533–6.
20. MacKenzie IZ, Sayers L, Bonnar J, Hillier K. Coagulation changes during midtrimester abortion induced with intra-amniotic prostaglandin E_2 and hypertonic solutions. Lancet 1975; ii:1066–9.
21. Stander RW, Flessa HC, Gueck HI, Kisker CT. Changes in maternal coagulation factors after intraamniotic injection of hypertonic saline. Obstet Gynecol 1971; 37:660–5.

22. Hill NCW, Selinger M, Fergusson J, MacKenzie IZ. Mid-trimester termination of pregnancy with 16,16-dimethyl-trans- 2PGE$_1$ vaginal pessaries: a comparison with intra- and extra-amniotic prostaglandin E$_2$ administration. Int J Gynecol Obstet 1991; 35:337–40.
23. Webster MA, Phipps SL, Gillmer MDG. Interruption of first trimester human pregnancy following epostane therapy. Effect of prostaglandin E$_2$ pessaries. Br J Obstet Gynaecol 1985; 92:963–8.
24. Selinger M, Gillmer MD, MacKenzie IZ, Phipps S. Midtrimester myometrial sensitisation following antiprogesterone therapy. Abstracts of the 24th British Congress of Obstetrics and Gynaecology, London 1986; 273.
25. Selinger M, MacKenzie IZ, Gillmer MDG, Phipps SL, Ferguson J. Progesterone inhibition in midtrimester termination of pregnancy: physiological and clinical effects. Br J Obstet Gynaecol 1987; 94:1218–22.
26. Selinger M, MacKenzie IZ, Gillmer MD, Phipps SL, Ferguson J. The effect of epostane, a 3-beta-hydroxy steroid dehydrogenase inhibitor, on maternal and fetal steroid levels during mid-gestation. Br J Obstet Gynaecol 1988; 95:596–601.
27. Swahn ML, Bygdeman M. The effect of the antiprogestin RU 486 on uterine contractility and sensitivity to prostaglandin and oxytocin. Br J Obstet Gynaecol 1988; 95:126–34.
28. Hill NCW, Selinger M, Ferguson J, Lopez Bernal A, MacKenzie IZ. The physiological and clinical effects of progesterone inhibition with RU 38,486 (mifepristone) in the second trimester. Br J Obstet Gynaecol 1990; 97:487–92.
29. Urquhart DR, Bahzad C, Templeton AA. Efficacy of the antiprogestin mifepristone (RU 486) prior to prostaglandin termination of pregnancy. Hum Reprod 1989; 4:202–3.
30. Rodger MW, Baird DT. Pretreatment with mifepristone (RU 486) reduces interval between prostaglandin administration and expulsion in second trimester abortion. Br J Obstet Gynaecol 1990; 97:41–5.
31. Selinger M. Progesterone inhibition in mid-pregnancy with epostane. Contemp Rev Obstet Gynaecol 1988; 1:67–79.
32. Hill NCW, Selinger M, Ferguson J, MacKenzie IZ. Transplacental passage of mifepristone and its influence on maternal and fetal steroid concentrations in the second trimester of pregnancy. Hum Reprod 1991; 6:458–62.
33. Choo HT, Karim SMM, Cheng P. Extra-amniotic administration of single dose of 15(s)-15methyl-prostaglandin E$_2$ methyl ester for pre-operative cervical dilatation. J Asian Fed Obstet Gynaecol 1973; 4:71–3.
34. Emery S, Jarvis GJ, Johnson DNA. Uterine rupture after intraamniotic injection of prostaglandin E$_2$. Br Med J 1979; ii:51.
35. Propping D, Stubblefield PG, Golub J, Zuckerman J. Uterine rupture following midtrimester abortion by laminaria, prostaglandin F$_{2\alpha}$, and oxytocin. Am J Obstet Gynecol 1977; 128:689–99.
36. Sandler RZ, Knutzen VK, Milano CM, Gleicher N. Uterine rupture with the use of vaginal prostaglandin E$_2$ suppositories. Am J Obstet Gynecol 1979; 134:348–9.
37. Stanwell-Smith R. Procedures used for legal abortion. In: Alberman E, Dennis KJ, eds. Late abortions of England and Wales – report of a national confidential study. London: Royal College of Obstetricians and Gynaecologists, 1984; 45–67.
38. MacKenzie IZ, Hillier K, Embrey MP. Prostaglandin induced abortion: an assessment of operative complications and early morbidity. Br Med J 1974; iv:683–6.
39. Hodari AA, Peralta J, Quiroga PJ, Gerbi EB. Dilatation and curettage for second-trimester abortions. Am J Obstet Gynecol 1977; 127:850–4.
40. Edelman DA, Brenner WE, Berger GS. The effectiveness and complications of abortion by dilatation and vacuum aspiration versus dilatation and rigid metal curettage. Am J Obstet Gynecol 1974; 119:473–80.
41. Barr MM. Mid-trimester abortions – 12 to 20 weeks by dilatation and evacuation method under local anaesthetic. Adv Planned Parenthood 1978; 13:16–20.
42. Berger GS, Keith LG. Complications of second trimester abortion. In: Keirse MJNC, Gravenhorst JB, Va Lith DAF, Embrey MP, eds. Second trimester pregnancy termination. The Hague: Leiden University Press, 1982; 52–64.
43. Cates W, Schultz KF, Grimes DA, Horowitz AJ, Lyon FA, Kravitz FH, Frisch MJ. Dilatation and evacuation procedures and second trimester abortions. JAMA 1982; 248:559–63.
44. Peterson WF, Berry FN, Grace MR, Gulbranson CL. Second trimester abortion by dilatation and evacuation: an analysis of 11 747 cases. Obstet Gynecol 1983; 62:185–90.
45. Grimes DA, Cates W. Complications from legally induced abortion: a review. Obstet Gynecol Surv 1979; 34:177–91.

46. Office of Population Censuses and Surveys. Abortion Statistics 1978. London: HMSO, 1980; 29–33.
47. Frank PI, Kay CR, Wingrave SJ, Lewis TLT, Osborne J, Newell C. Induced abortion operations and their early sequelae: joint study of the Royal College of General Practitioners and the Royal College of Obstetricians and Gynaecology. J R Coll Gen Pract 1985; 35:175–80.
48. Speroff L. Is there a best way to do mid-trimester abortion? Contemp Obstet Gynecol 1979; 13:106–41.
49. Kalra PA, Litherland D, Sallomi DF, Critchley HOD, Falconer GF, Holmes AM. Cardiac standstill induced by prostaglandin pessaries. Lancet 1989; i:1460.
50. MacKenzie IZ, Fry A. A prospective self-controlled study of fertility after second-trimester prostaglandin-induced abortion. Am J Obstet Gynecol 1988; 158:1137–40.
51. MacKenzie IZ, Hillier K. Prostaglandin induced abortion and the outcome of subsequent pregnancies: a prospective controlled study. Br Med J 1977; ii:114–17.
52. Kaltreider NB, Goldsmith S, Margolis AJ. The impact of midtrimester abortion techniques on patients and staff. Am J Obstet Gynecol 1979; 135:235–8.
53. MacKenzie IZ, Boland J. The current uses of prostaglandins in obstetrics: a national survey. Singapore: Proceedings of the XIIIth Congr of Gynaecology and Obstetrics, 1991; 241.
54. Karim SMM, Ratnam SS, Hutabarat H et al. Termination of pregnancy in cases of intrauterine fetal death, missed abortion, molar and anencephalic pregnancy with intramuscular administration of 2a,2b-dihomo 15(s)-15methyl $PGF_{2\alpha}$ methyl ester – a multicentre study. Ann Acad Med Singapore 1982; 11:508–12.
55. Southern EM, Gutknecht GD, Mohberg NR, Edelman DA. Vaginal prostaglandin E_2 in the management of fetal intra-uterine death. Br J Obstet Gynaecol 1978; 85:437–41.
56. Wallenburg HCS, Keirse MJNC, Freie HMP, Blacquiere JF. Intramuscular administration of 15(s)-15methyl prostaglandin $F_{2\alpha}$ for induction of labour in patients with fetal death. Br J Obstet Gynaecol 1980; 87:203–9.
57. Ulmann A, Dubois C. Antiprogesterones in obstetrics, ectopic pregnancies and gynaecological malignancy. Baillière's Clin Obstet Gynaecol 1988; 2:631–8.

Chapter 9

Cervical Softening in Early Pregnancy

A. Rådestad

The concept of cervical "maturation", "ripening" or "priming" refers to the events leading to a soft, effaced and dilated uterine cervix in the third trimester of pregnancy, whereas cervical "preparation" or "softening" often refers to methods used to change the cervix from a stiff to a soft structure in the first and second trimesters.

In first and second trimester terminations of pregnancy, a soft cervix facilitates dilatation of the cervical canal. This leads to fewer short- and long-term complications, especially in young nulliparae [1,2].

At or near term, an unripe cervix is associated with an increased risk of complications if labour induction is indicated. Knowledge of the biochemical and physiological processes in cervical softening has resulted in a number of methods, mainly based on prostaglandin treatment, of ripening the cervix and dilating the cervical canal [3,4].

Women at risk of premature labour due to cervical incompetence may also benefit from research into the regulation of cervical ripening.

Structure of the Cervix

The uterine cervix is composed predominantly of fibroblasts, smooth muscle cells, and an extracellular matrix consisting of large bundles of collagen fibrils, elastic fibres and proteoglycans. The stroma is dominated by collagen, but a minor smooth muscle layer is located near the isthmus in the proximal part of the cervix. Compared to the uterus the contractility of the cervical tissue is negligible.

These findings were established by Danforth [5–7] as recently as 1947. Although these results were questioned by others who claimed that the human cervix possessed significant muscular contractility [8], his and his group's work should be acknowledged for the basic understanding of cervical morphology and function.

The cervix is stiffer in an area surrounding the cervical canal and progressively less stiff towards the periphery [9].

It is well known by all gynaecologists that the stiffness of the uterine cervix decreases during pregnancy. Morphologically, this corresponds to increased vascularity, migration of leukocytes (neutrophils and monocytes) from the blood, and a marked decrease in the overall collagen content of the tissue and in the size of the collagen fibril bundles [10,11]. Together with fibroblasts the inflammatory cells secrete proteinases which are capable of degrading collagen.

The ground substance, which consists of large molecules, can interact with the collagen, and is able to retain water. A loss of fluid leads to a loss of turgor which softens and dilates the cervix [12]. This is what happens when a stiff and dry Lamicel tent is inserted in the cervical canal and absorbs the tissue fluid, but does not, in contrast to the laminaria tent, apply any major pressure on the cervical canal [13].

The amount and composition of the ground substance may change during pregnancy. An increase in glycoproteins has been reported [14,15].

The cervical tissue can be influenced by a variety of endogenous and exogenous factors which alter its composition. These changes can occur within hours or days and can already be measured in the early stages of pregnancy.

The densely packed collaged fibres split up and dissolve in a characteristic way, which has been frequently observed in electron microscopic examinations of the cervix in term pregnancies [16,17]. A similar histological change in the cervix has been demonstrated in prostaglandin-induced cervical softening in the first and second trimesters [18,19].

The biomechanical properties of the cervical tissue may not be explained entirely by the connective tissue component. The presence of several biologically active neuropeptides has been demonstrated in the early pregnant uterine cervix, including neuropeptide Y (NPY), vasoactive intestinal polypeptide (VIP), peptide histidine–methionine (PHM), calcitonin gene-related peptide (CGRP), substance P (SP), enkephalin (ENK), gastrin-releasing peptide (GRP) and galanin (GAL) [20,21]. These findings indicate a role of the smooth muscle cells in the regulation of cervical softening. Smooth muscle cells may help maintain basal muscular tonus in the proximal part of the cervix [22].

Methods for Studying the Biomechanics of Cervical Softening in Early Pregnancy

Mechanical models have been used to describe the way collagen fibres in the uterine cervix behave under strain [23,24]. Strain-rate tests have shown that cervical tissue has the non-linear stress/strain curve typical of biological visco-elastic tissues, and that there is a large variation between individual cervices.

The deformation of the cervix depends primarily on two factors; the applied force per area and the rate at which the load is applied at the tissue [25]. Less force is required if the dilatation is more protracted.

In several studies of cervical softening in early pregnancy, the degree of cervical dilatation has been estimated subjectively as the diameter of the largest cervical dilator which can be passed through the internal os without resistance. The softness has been assessed in three or more categories during a series of dilatation steps using dilators of increasing diameter. These methods are too subjective and inaccurate for comparing the effect of different drugs on the cervix or for studying a small biomechanical change in the cervix. Instruments have therefore been designed to measure cervical resistance and dilatation objectively [26–31]. A consistent peak resistance has been found at a dilatation of 9 mm, from which it was concluded that this represented the first sign of tissue fracturing and that cervical dilatation beyond this limit should be avoided to minimise cervical damage [32]. However, in a more recent study no indications of tears were found and it was concluded that the resistance at 9 mm was an instrumentation artefact caused by the type of dilator used in the previous study [33].

Rath et al. [29] used a cervical tonometer of modified Hegar dilators in combination with a spring balance to study cervical softening. Compliant balloons inserted in the cervical canal have also been used to describe the characteristic pressure–volume curve reflecting the elasticity of the cervix [34].

In the search for pharmacological means of cervical softening, it is necessary to use methods which accurately reflect cervical stiffness. The ideal instrument should give a controlled rate of cervical dilatation and a continuous record of the load to allow a proper comparison between individuals in terms of stiffness. It should be noted that the force required to dilate the cervix decreases with parity and with gestational age [35].

We used a dilatation instrument with strain-gauged load cells which was specially developed to test cervical stiffness in situ, and measured the load acting on the tip of a Hegar dilator at serial dilatation steps from 4 to 11 mm. To standardise the procedure and minimise methodological error, one investigator carried out all dilatations and measurements. The values were divided by the increment of the cross-sectional area of the dilator used, which corresponded to the tissue deformation. These values expressed cervical stiffness and are presented as stress/strain curves (Fig. 9.1).

Agents Used for Cervical Softening in Early Pregnancy

A variety of agents and techniques have been used to soften the cervix and to dilate the cervical canal [36]. Both intracervical tents [37] and prostaglandins are used extensively and the possibility of using progesterone antagonists for this purpose has been suggested.

Intracervical Tents

The classical laminaria tent is an osmotic dilator made of seaweed sticks which absorb fluid, expand and exert pressure on the cervical canal. It dilates the canal within hours and seems to induce a soft cervix.

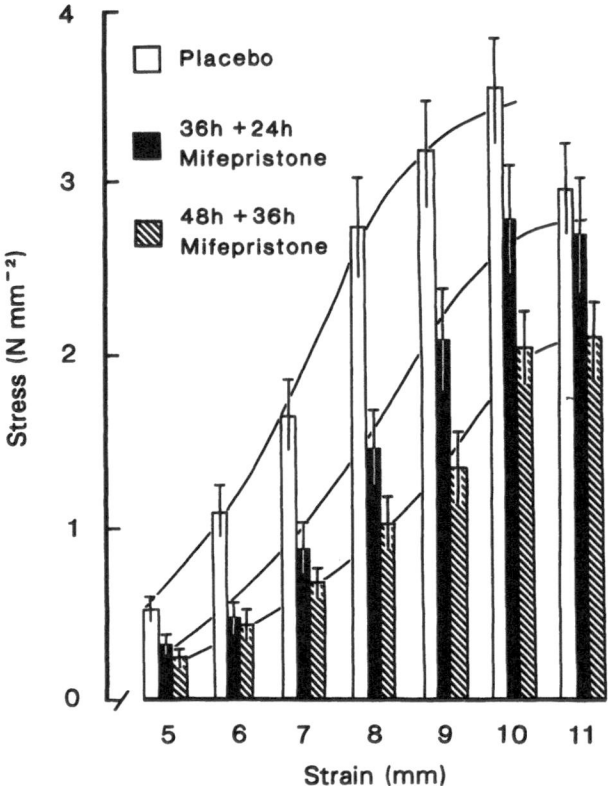

Fig. 9.1. The load acting on the tip of the dilators expressed as N mm^{-2} increment in cross-sectional area of the corresponding dilator plotted against tissue deformation expressed as the diameter (mm) of the dilated canal, reflecting the relation between applied loads and tissue deformation. The slope of the idealised curve reflects the stiffness of the cervical tissue.

Dilaphan is a synthetic tent with an action similar to that of the natural laminaria tent, but it seems to produce a more rapid cervical dilatation.

Lamicel is a polyvinyl alcohol polymer sponge impregnated with magnesium sulphate and compressed to a tent. It expands to form a soft sponge but is not capable of exerting mechanical pressure on the cervical canal.

All three tents are widely used to achieve cervical softening and dilatation [38–40]. Their insertion requires some skill and can sometimes be painful and associated with vasovagal symptoms and uterine cramps. It is probable that the laminaria and dilaphan tents exert their major effect on the cervix by applying a significant force per area for a relatively long time, whereas the lamicel tent works mainly by taking up fluid from the cervix. However, due to their mechanical effect on the cervix, all tents may increase the tissue production of prostanoids, and this may add to their clinical effect [41]. It has also been shown that lamicel treatment increases the collagenolytic activity and the sensitivity of the cervical smooth muscle to prostaglandin E_2 (PGE$_2$) [42].

Prostaglandins

Prostaglandin receptors have been demonstrated in the human uterine cervix [43]. The local production of prostaglandin increases in response to cervical softening. PGE_2 or $PGF_{2\alpha}$ or their analogues administered by various routes induce cervical softening. Several studies have shown that pretreatment with prostaglandin analogues prior to vacuum aspiration also results in significant dilatation of the cervical canal and a reduction of both operative and postoperative complications. In general, E-analogues are preferable to F-analogues with regard both to frequency of gastrointestinal side effects and to efficacy [44]. This is probably a direct effect on cervical tissue, but stimulation of endogenous prostanoid synthesis may also be important [45]. PGE_2 seems to have a greater effect on the cervix than $PGF_{2\alpha}$. The morphological changes in the tissue are similar to those observed in term pregnancies [16,18,46]. Intracervical application of a PGE_2 gel in nulliparae admitted for a first trimester abortion led to high collagenase activity in the cervical biopsies, suggesting that the tissue has a high capacity to degrade collagen [47]. However, these results contradict those of Rath et al. [18], who found no significant increase in enzyme activities and no evidence for the presence of collagen degradation products in cervical biopsies from patients having a first trimester abortion after intracervical pretreatment with the prostaglandin analogue sulprostone.

Progesterone Antagonists

Progesterone hormone receptor antagonists are compounds which bind to the progesterone receptor, thus inhibiting the hormone. Mifepristone (RU 486, Roussel-Uclaf) is a drug with strong antiprogesterone activity [48] as well as antiglucocorticoid activity and weak–moderate antiandrogen activity [49]. Its absorption after oral administration is high, with peak concentrations reached at 1–3 h. The half-life of mifepristone is in the range 26–48 h [50]. Other, more specific antigestagens are under investigation [51].

Mifepristone induces preterm delivery in several species (rat, guinea pig, monkey) and is effective as an abortifacient in early human pregnancy [52–55]. An increased uterine sensitivity to prostaglandins [56], and very few side effects after mifepristone treatment, have led to its clinical use in some countries together with prostaglandins for interruption of very early pregnancy [57,58].

Oral, single or multiple dose administration of 25–600 mg mifepristone is sufficient to decrease cervical stiffness in early pregnancy [59–65]. The clinical effect seems to be dose-related within the range 25–100 mg, whereas doses above 100 mg do not seem to improve the effect. The softening effect is, however, greater in multiparae or if the treatment is started 48 h instead of 24 h before vacuum aspiration [66] (Fig. 9.1). A disadvantage of the longer treatment is that more patients suffer preoperative vaginal bleeding. Mifepristone produces a smaller cervical dilatation than PGs. However, the absence of uncomfortable side effects makes the antigestagens more acceptable.

The exact mechanism of the softening effect of mifepristone on the cervix is not clear. Experiments in vitro have shown that progesterone decreases prostanoid synthesis in human endometrium, suggesting an inhibition of phospholipase A_2 [67] and that progesterone antagonists, by removing this inhibition, stimulate prostanoid [68,69]. This has led to the hypothesis that mifepristone acts via increased prostanoid synthesis [70]. However, this hypothesis must be questioned since it may not apply to the cervix. Cabrol et al. [71] recently showed that mifepristone-induced preterm delivery in the rat was antagonised by the cyclo-oxygenase inhibitor diclofenac, whereas cervical softening was not, as would have been expected if this effect of mifepristone on the cervix was mediated through increased prostanoid synthesis. These results agree with our data for humans (Rådestad et al., unpublished observations), in which no reduction of the softening effect of mifepristone was found on the early pregnant uterine cervix in patients who received the cyclo-oxygenase inhibitor naproxen.

It has also been suggested that mifepristone may exert its softening effect on the cervix via lipoxygenase. However, no qualitative or quantitative relationship was observed between mifepristone treatment and the capacity of human cervical tissue to produce lipoxygenase products (Heidvall et al., unpublished observations).

Studies in the rat of $PGF_{2\alpha}$ castration, oestradiol and mifepristone, showed that the latter was the most effective in causing cervical softening [72]. Light and scanning electron microscopy also showed an increase of collagen and a possible loosening of collagen fibres after mifepristone treatment. These observations agree with morphological findings in the uterine cervix of the guinea pig after treatment with the progesterone antagonist onapristone (ZK 98,299) [73].

Two electron microscope studies of human cervical softening after mifepristone treatment in the first trimester have been performed using a triple-blind randomised protocol. Rådestad et al. (unpublished observations) compared the interindividual change of cervical tissue morphology and found that 12 of the 18 patients had been correctly classified as representing the controls or the mifepristone treatment group. In the mifepristone group the morphology of the tissue was changed, with accumulation of mast cells, dissolution of collagen fibrils and outgrowth of blood capillaries. In the second study, Rådestad et al. (unpublished observations) compared the intraindividual change of tissue morphology in two cervical biopsies from the same patient. The first biopsy was taken before treatment and the second one week later, prior to vacuum aspiration but after oral administration of placebo or mifepristone 100 mg, 48 h and 36 h earlier. No significant change in cervical tissue morphology was observed when studying the same parameters as in the first study. These conflicting results show that re-evaluations and further investigations are necessary before any conclusions can be drawn from morphological studies after mifepristone treatment.

Summary and Future Aspects

It is of clinical importance to prepare the cervix before surgical evacuation of the uterus, particularly in more-advanced first trimester pregnancies in nulliparae as well as during the second trimester, before stimulating uterine contractility.

Treatment with intracervical tents, prostaglandins and the progesterone antagonist mifepristone induces cervical softening and dilatation.

It has often been suggested that endogenous prostaglandins are mediators of these changes [74] although other substances such as relaxin, cytokines and leukotrienes have also been proposed as possible mediators.

Although there are comparatively few studies [44], it seems that PGE analogues are more effective than the laminaria tent if the pretreatment period is limited to 3–4 h. Prostaglandins have additional advantages in simplicity of administration and the fact that the uterus will be contracted at surgery. Antiprogesterones may be found equally useful but comparative studies are, so far, lacking. The softening effect of antiprogesterone on the cervix, and the increased sensitivity of the myometrium to prostaglandins seem especially useful in second trimester abortion.

Intracervical tents may in the future be used as a vehicle for drugs, e.g. prostaglandin, which produce a soft cervix, for a direct and more specific effect on the cervix. This would probably make it easier to cope with the classical side effects of prostaglandins, e.g. uterine cramps and gastrointestinal symptoms.

It might be possible to extract specific cytokines, similar to those derived from inflammatory cells, which play a role in the degradation of collagen, and use them as cervical agents.

Relaxin, a protein produced by corpus luteum, the uterus and the placenta, seems to have a ripening effect on the cervix at term but whether the same applies to the cervix in early pregnancy remains to be shown.

References

1. Cates W, Schulz KF, Grimes DA, Tyler CW. Short-term complications of uterine evacuation techniques for abortion at 12 weeks' gestation or earlier. In: Zatuchni GI, Speidel SJJ, eds, Pregnancy termination procedures, safety and new developments. Hagerstown: Harper and Row, 1979; 127–35.
2. Merik O. Preterm birth and low birth weight related to complications in previous vacuum aspiration abortion. A case-control study within a cohort. Thesis, Acta Universitas Uppsala no. 422, 1982.
3. Wiqvist N, Beguin F, Bygdeman M, Fernström I, Toppozada M. Induction of abortion by extra-amniotic prostaglandin administration. Prostaglandins 1972; 1:34–53.
4. Calder AA, Embrey MP, Tait T. Ripening of the cervix with extra-amniotic prostaglandin E$_2$ in viscous gel before induction of labor. Br J Obstet Gynaecol 1977; 84:264–8.
5. Danforth DN. The fibrous nature of the human cervix, and its relation to the isthmic segment in gravid and nongravid uteri. Am J Obstet Gynecol 1947; 53:541–60.
6. Danforth DN. The distribution and functional activity of the cervical musculature. Am J Obstet Gynecol 1954; 68:1261–71.
7. Danforth DN. Early studies of the anatomy and physiology of the human cervix – implications for the future. In: Naftolin F, Stubblefield PG, eds, Dilatation of the uterine cervix – connective tissue biology and clinical management. New York: Raven Press, 1980; 3–15.
8. Schild HO, Fitzpatric RJ, Nixon WCW. Activity of the human cervix and corpus uteri. Lancet 1951; i:250–3.
9. Conrad JT, Ueland K. Physical characteristics of the cervix. Clin Obstet Gynecol 1983; 26:27–36.
10. Junqueira LCU, Zugaib M, Montes GS, Toledo OMS, Krisztán RM, Shigihara KM. Morphologic and histochemical evidence for the occurrence of collagenolysis and the role of neutrophilic polymorphonuclear leukocytes during cervical dilation. Am J Obstet Gynecol 1980; 138:273–81.
11. Uldbjerg N, Ekman G, Malmström A, Olsson K, Ulmsten U. Ripening of the human uterine cervix related to changes in collagen, glycosaminoglycans and collagenolytic activity. Am J Obstet Gynecol 1983; 147:662–6.
12. Tokarz RD, Williford JF, Söderström RM. Mobility of fluid as a factor in acute therapeutic dilation of the human cervix. Adv Planned Parenthood 1981; 16:22–9.

13. Rådestad A, Christensen NJ. Magnesium sulphate and cervical ripening. A biomechanical double-blind, randomized comparison between a synthetic polyvinyl sponge with and without magnesium sulphate. Contraception 1989; 39:253–63.
14. Karube H, Kanke Y, Mori Y. Increase of structural glycoprotein during dilatation of human cervix in pregnancy at term. Endocrinol Jpn 1975; 22:445–8.
15. Shimizu T, Endo M, Yosizawa Z. Glycoconjugates (glycosaminoglycans and glycoproteins) and glycogen in the human cervix uteri. Tohoku J Exp Med 1980; 131:289–99.
16. Theobald PW, Rath W, Kühnle H, Kuhn W. Histological and electron-microscopic examinations of collagenous connective tissue of the non-pregnant cervix, the pregnant cervix, and the pregnant prostaglandin-treated cervix. Arch Gynecol 1982; 231:241–5.
17. Minamoto T, Arai K, Hirakawa S, Nagai Y. Immunohistochemical studies on collagen types in the uterine cervix in pregnant and nonpregnant states. Am J Obstet Gynecol 1987; 156:138–44.
18. Rath W, Adelmann-Grill BC, Schauer A, Kuhn W. Morphologische und Biochemische Aspekte der Prostaglandininduzierten Zervixreifung. Z Geburtshilfe Perinatol 1987; 191:21–8.
19. Di Lieto A, Catalano D, Campanile M et al. The morphological characteristics and ultrastructural aspects of cervical ripening induced by sulprostone. Acta Eur Fertil 1988; 19:33–6.
20. Owman C, Rosengren E, Sjöberg N-O. Adrenergic innervation of the human female reproductive organs: a histochemical and chemical investigation. Obstet Gynecol 1967; 30:763–73.
21. Fried G, Meister B, Rådestad A. Peptide-containing nerves in the human pregnant uterine cervix: an immunohistochemical study exploring the effect of RU 486 (mifepristone). Hum Reprod 1990; 5:870–6.
22. Bryman I, Sahni S, Norström A, Lindblom B. Influence of prostaglandins on contractility of the isolated human cervical muscle. Obstet Gynecol 1984; 63:280–4.
23. Conrad JT, Ueland K. Reduction of the stretch modulus of human cervical tissue by prostaglandin E_2. Am J Obstet Gynecol 1976; 15:218–23.
24. Bakke T. Cervical consistency in women of fertile age measured with a new mechanical instrument. Acta Obstet Gynecol Scand 1974; 53:293–302.
25. Soden PD, Kershaw I. Tensile testing of connective tissues. Med Biol Eng 1974; 7:510–18.
26. Hulka JF, Lefler HT, Anglone A, Lachenbruch PA. A new electronic force monitor to measure factors influencing cervical dilatation for vacuum curettage. Am J Obstet Gynecol 1974; 120:166–73.
27. Liu DTY, Black MM, Melcher DH, Melville HAH, Cameron S, Morgon J. Dilatation of the parous non-pregnant cervix. Br J Obstet Gynaecol 1975; 82:246–51.
28. Fisher J, Anthony GS, McManus TJ, Coutts JRT, Calder A. Use of a force measuring instrument during cervical dilatation. J Med Eng Technol 1981; 5:194–5.
29. Rath W, Kühnle H, Theobald P, Kuhn W. Objective demonstration of cervical softening with a prostaglandin $F_{2\alpha}$ gel during first trimester abortion. Int J Gynaecol Obstet 1982; 20:195–9.
30. Richardson W, Smith DC, Evans AL, Anthony GS. A novel cervical dilator force measurement instrument. J Med Eng Techn 1989; 13:220–1.
31. Cabrol D, Jannet D, Le Houezec R, Dudzik W, Bonoris E, Cedard L. Mechanical properties of the pregnant human uterine cervix. Use of an instrument to measure the index of cervical distensibility. Gynecol Obstet Invest 1990; 29:32–6.
32. Hulka JF, Higgins G. Tears of the internal cervical os during dilation for routine curettage. Am J Obstet Gynecol 1961; 82:913–19.
33. Hulka JF. Pratt dilators: resistance at 9 mm is an instrumentation artifact. Am J Obstet Gynecol 1988; 159:871–3.
34. Kiwi R, Neuman MR, Merkatz IR, Selim MA, Lysikiewicz A. Determination of the elastic properties of the cervix. Obstet Gynecol 1988; 71:568–74.
35. Anthony GS, Fisher J, Coutts JRT, Calder AA. The effect of exogenous hormones on the resistance of the early pregnant human cervix. Br J Obstet Gynaecol 1984; 91:1249–53.
36. Ott ER. Pregnancy termination: cervical dilatation – a review. Popul Rep 1977; 6:85–103.
37. Johnson N. Intracervical tents: usage and mode of action. Obstet Gynecol Surv 1989; 44: 410–20.
38. Jonasson A, Larsson B. Biochemical changes in human cervical connective tissue during pretreatment with Laminaria tents in legal first trimester abortions. Int J Gynaecol Obstet 1989; 28:361–4.
39. Grimes DA, Ray IG, Middleton CJ. Lamicel versus laminaria for cervical dilatation before early second-trimester abortion: a randomized clinical trial. Obstet Gynecol 1987; 69:887–90.
40. Atienza MF, Burkman RT, King TM. Use of osmotic dilators to facilitate induced midtrimester abortion: clinical evaluations. Contraception 1984; 30:215–23.
41. Hillier K, Coad N. Synthesis of prostaglandins by the human uterine cervix in vitro during passive mechanical stretch. J Pharm Pharmacol 1982; 34:262–3.

42. Norström A, Bergman I, Hansson HA. Cervical dilatation by Lamicel before first trimester abortion: a clinical and experimental study. Br J Obstet Gynaecol 1988; 95:372–6.
43. Crankshaw DJ, Crankshaw J, Branda LA, Daniel EE. Receptors for E type prostaglandins in the plasma membrane of non-pregnant myometrium. Arch Biochem Biophys 1979; 198:70–7.
44. WHO Prostaglandin Task Force. Randomized comparison of different prostaglandin analogues and laminaria tent for preoperative cervical dilatation. Contraception 1986; 34:237–51.
45. Gréen K, Christensen NJ, Bygdeman M. The chemistry and pharmacology of prostaglandins, with reference to human reproduction. J Reprod Fertil 1981; 62:269–81.
46. Uldbjerg N, Ekman G, Malmström A, Sporrong B, Ulmsten U, Wingerup L. Biochemical and morphological changes of human cervix after local application of prostaglandin E_2 in pregnancy. Lancet 1981; ii:267–8.
47. Uldbjerg N, Ekman G, Herltoft P, Malmström A, Ulmsten U, Wingerup L. Human cervical connective tissue and its reaction to prostaglandin E_2. Acta Obstet Gynecol Scand [Suppl] 1983; 113:163–6.
48. Philibert D, Moguilewsky M, Mary I, Lecaque D, Tournemine C, Secchi J, Deraedt R. Pharmacological profile of RU 486 in animals. In: Segal SJ, Baulien EE, eds., The antiprogestin steroid RU 486 and human fertility control. New York: Plenum Press, 1985; 49–68.
49. Moguilewsky M, Philibert D. RU 38486: potent antiglucocorticoid activity correlated with strong binding to the cytosolic glucocorticoid receptor followed by an impaired activation. J Steroid Biochem 1984; 20:271–6.
50. Heikinheimo O. Summary of a doctoral thesis: Antiprogesterone steroid RU 486. Pharmacokinetics and receptor binding in humans. Acta Obstet Gynecol Scand 1990; 69:357–8.
51. Philibert D, Hardy M, Gaillard-Moguilewsky M, Nique F, Tournemine C, Nédélec L. New analogues of mifepristone with more dissociated antiprogesterone activities. J Steroid Biochem 1989; 34:413–17.
52. Bygdeman M, Swahn ML. Progesterone receptor blockage. Effect on uterine contractility and early pregnancy. Contraception 1985; 32:45–51.
53. Couzinet B, Le Strat N, Ulmann A, Baulieu EE, Schaison G. Termination of early pregnancy by the progesterone antagonist RU 486 (mifepristone). N Engl J Med 1986; 315:1565–70.
54. Mishell DRJ, Shoupe D, Brenner PF et al. Termination of early gestation with the anti-protestin steroid RU 486: medium versus low dose. Contraception 1987; 35:307–21.
55. Birgerson L, Odlind V. The antiprogestational agent RU 486 as an abortifacient in early human pregnancy: a comparison of three dose regimens. Contraception 1988; 38:391–400.
56. Swahn ML, Bygdeman M. The effect of antiprogestin RU 586 on uterine contractility and sensitivity to prostaglandin and oxytocin. Br J Obstet Gynaecol 1988; 95:126–34.
57. Silvestre L, Dubois C, Renault M, Rezvani Y, Baulieu EE, Ulmann A. Voluntary interruption of pregnancy with mifepristone (RU 486) and a prostaglandin analogue. N Engl J Med 1990; 322:645–8.
58. UK Multicentre Trial. The efficacy and tolerance of mifepristone and prostaglandin in first trimester termination of pregnancy. Br J Obstet Gynaecol 1990; 97:480–6.
59. Rådestad A, Christensen NJ, Strömberg L. Induced cervical ripening with mifepristone in first trimester abortion. A double-blind randomized biomechanical study. Contraception 1988; 38:301–12.
60. Durlot F, Dubois C, Brunerie J, Frydman R. Efficacy of progesterone antagonist RU 486 (mifepristone) for pre-operative cervical dilatation during first trimester abortion. Hum Reprod 1988; 3:583–4.
61. De Grandi P, Giudici G. Administration orale d'un antiprogesterone (Mifepristone, RU 486) pour la préparation du col utérin à l'interruption de grossesse au cours du premier trimestre. J Gynecol Obstet Biol Reprod 1989;18:801–8.
62. Lefebvre Y, Proulx L, Elie R, Poulin O, Lanza E. The effects of RU-38486 on cervical ripening. Am J Obstet Gynecol 1990; 162:61–5.
63. Gupta JK, Johnson N. Effect of mifepristone on dilatation of the pregnant and non-pregnant cervix. Lancet 1990; 335:1238–40.
64. Johnson N, Bryce FC. Could antiprogesterones be used as alternative cervical ripening agents? Am J Obstet Gynecol 1990; 162:688–90.
65. WHO Task Force on Post-ovulatory Methods for Fertility Regulation. The use of mifepristone (RU 486) for cervical preparation in first trimester pregnancy termination by vacuum aspiration. Br J Obstet Gynaecol 1990; 97:260–6.
66. Rådestad A, Bygdeman M, Gréen K. Induced cervical ripening with mifepristone (RU 486) and bioconversion of arachidonic acid in human pregnant uterine cervix in the first trimester. A double-blind randomized biomechanical and biochemical study. Contraception 1990; 41:283–92.

67. Abel MH, Baird DT. The effect of beta-estradiol and progesterone on prostaglandin production by human endometrium maintained in organ culture. Endocrinology 1980; 106:1599–606.
68. Kelly RW, Healy DL, Cameron MJ, Cameron IT, Baird DT. The stimulation of prostaglandin production by two antiprogesterone steroids in human endometrial cells. J Clin Endocrinol Metab 1986; 62:1117–23.
69. Jeremy JY, Dandona P. RU 486 antagonises the inhibitory action of progesterone on prostacyclin and thromboxane A$_2$ synthesis in cultured rat myometrial explants. J Endocrinol 1986; 19:655–60.
70. Norman JE, Wu WX, Kelly RW, Glasier AF, McNeilly AS, Baird DT. Effects of mifepristone in vivo on decidual prostaglandin synthesis and metabolism. Contraception 1991; 44:89–98.
71. Cabrol D, Carbonne B, Bienkiewicz A, Dallot E, Alj AE, Cedard L. Induction of labor and cervical maturation using mifepristone (RU 486) in the late pregnant rat. Influence of a cyclooxygenase inhibitor (Diclofenac). Prostaglandins 1991; 42:71–9.
72. Stiemer B, Elger W. Cervical ripening of the rat in dependence on endocrine milieu; effects of antigestagens. J Perinatol Med 1990; 18:419–29.
73. Hegele-Hartung C, Chwalisz K, Beier HM, Elger W. Ripening of the uterine cervix of the guinea-pig after treatment with the progesterone antagonist onapristone (ZK 98,299): an electron microscopic study. Hum Reprod 1989; 4:369–77.
74. Uldbjerg N, Ulmsten U. The physiology of cervical ripening and cervical dilatation and the effect of abortifacient drugs. Baillère Tindall, Clin Obstet Gynaecol, 1990; 4:263–82.

Discussion

Calder: A point about laminaria. Dr Rådestad was suggesting that the effect of laminaria may be a mechanical one. But Stubbelfield in Boston, who has very large experience of laminaria, says that it is never his experience to find that a laminaria is difficult to remove from the cervix, it always just slides out, which suggests that the cervix dilates in advance of the swelling Laminaria. But I could not agree more that that kind of approach using swelling devices which at the same time release active agents has got to be the way forward in terms of the cervix.

Amy: One word of caution on the use of a combination of prostaglandin and hypotonic solution. There have been malpractice cases in the United States where practitioners have been prosecuted after saline abortions, very late abortions, where the fetus was born alive and survived. It is not an absolute guarantee that the fetus will be born dead.

MacKenzie: That is obviously right. My major concern is to suggest that there is a place for it, but given the problems associated with hypotonic solutions it is really only for that reason.

Husslein: What is the reason for the high rate of late second trimester abortions? Are these all medically indicated? Can something not be done to cut this unnecessarily high figure down?

MacKenzie: The proportion of second trimester abortions?

Husslein: The proportion of second trimester in comparison to first trimester and the proportion of late second in comparison to early second. We are talking about specific problems of late second trimester abortion and one way to solve those problems would be to reduce the number of necessary second trimester late abortions. That would be much more efficient than saline or whatever.

MacKenzie: An attempt was made through Parliament to stop abortions being done beyond 18 weeks and that did not come to pass, and most people believe that it was good that it did not.

I did not show the breakdown of abortions by gestation beyond 12 or 13 weeks, but the number of abortions performed at 20 weeks and over is about 1.5% of the total. The proportion of second trimester abortions in England and Wales has halved and has gradually been coming down, albeit very slowly, and as Dr Husslein is implying perhaps not fast enough. It is certainly not that most of the abortions that are done in the second trimester are for medical reasons. Most are still what we would all agree are social.

Can someone suggest how we might reduce the numbers?

Keirse: Probably by getting the referral system moving more quickly. Would that be part of the problem?

MacKenzie: That might reduce the number that are done at 14 or 15 weeks, but there is still a fairly large proportion in the second trimester that are done at 16, 17 and 18 weeks, and I do not think the referral delay is a significant factor.

Drife: Late social abortions are more a matter of ambivalence on the part of women going to their doctors rather than a delay in referral by the doctors. They may be under-age girls who have been afraid to admit that they are pregnant, or people whose circumstances have changed. The social problems that the patients have tend to be fairly marked.

MacKenzie: There has been a tendency to suggest that if a woman is to have a prostaglandin abortion when she is 13 or 14 weeks, it should be delayed to 16 weeks. The evidence, from the literature and from our own data, is that there is no advantage in delaying it by a week. The results are no better.

Cameron: To go back to the intra-amniotic story. Clearly one can understand the wish to use intra-amniotic techniques to avoid delivering a live fetus, but is the mobidity much greater with intra-amniotic than vaginal routes so that perhaps we should be favouring vaginal in any case?

MacKenzie: Having dealt with numbers of late abortions, including intra-amniotic, I have found that there is nothing more frightening than with the needle into the amniotic sac injecting the prostaglandins, the woman suddenly collapses. It is almost certainly because the needle is not quite where one thought it was, despite every attempt to ensure it, and one has injected 1, 2 or 3 mg of PGE_2 into the systemic circulation. That is what I think is the greatest worry and if one can avoid it by using vaginal PGs, then although it is more costly, for me that must be the biggest reason for doing so.

Cameron: I think I would agree.

Amy: I have a second objection to the use of intra-amniotic prostaglandins. There may be an increased incidence of isthmic rupture with the use of PGs intra-amniotically compared with the other routes.

MacKenzie: Isthmic rupture being rupture of the cervix. I am not sure that that is supported by fact. It is an impression that one gets and there have been a number reported in the literature. But the problem with trying to work out the true incidence is that there is no denominator. Certainly the national statistics do not break down how prostaglandins appear.

Calder: But there was a strong impression that it was much more common with $PGF_{2\alpha}$ than with PGE_2 intra-amniotically.

MacKenzie: That was something we noted. But a number of those cases were from the USA where there was a tendency to use $PGF_{2\alpha}$ and the intra-amniotic route. I am not sure that one could really blame $PGF_{2\alpha}$ rather than PGE_2. My inclination is to agree with Professor Amy that it is another risk, and an even greater risk if one combines a hypertonic solution where very powerful contractions can be generated and it is as though the cervix does not have the time to open up before the contractions get under way.

Greer: When he did the study in which the cervix was biopsied before and after RU486 and a comparison showed no change, what histological parameters was Dr Rådestad looking at and how did he assess it?

Rådestad: We looked at the numbers of monocytes and leukocytes, the vascularity, the number of capillaries ingrown through the tissue.

Greer: Did someone look at collagen or proteoglycan composition? and was there no difference in collagen or proteoglycans?

Rådestad: Yes but not with this method. It was not a morphometric method.

Greer: Dr Rådestad also alluded to the fact that he thought that RU486-induced ripening was a non-prostaglandin-mediated event. Last year he published a report of work in which he looked at radiolabelled arachidonic acid incorporated into biopsies and looked at PG production. Did he see anything else, a non-prostaglandin product? Did he look for it? Did he see an increase in leukotrienes, for example, which would go along with it being an inflammatory type reaction?

Rådestad: In that study we did not look for lipoxylase products, but we have looked at it in another study where we showed that the early pregnant cervix is capable of producing both leukotrienes and hydroxy acids. But it is not related to mifepristone administration.

Parturition

Chapter 10

A Pathway for the Regulation of Prostaglandins and Parturition

D. M. Olson, T. Zakar, Z. Smieja, E. A. MacLeod and
S. L. Brown

Introduction

Parturition is the culmination of dual physiological processes, both of which develop in parallel at the end of gestation (Fig. 10.1). They are the change in sensitivity or responsiveness that occurs with the target organs such as the myometrium, enabling it to respond to activators of contraction with coordinated, synchronous activity; and the generation of effector molecules which elicit the alterations of physiological state of the target organs. This chapter will deal with the second part of this process and will focus on the generation of prostaglandins, compounds which have been assigned a central role in eliciting the final events of parturition.

Defining the Problem

Prostaglandins have been characterised as the trigger for parturition. Although there is strong evidence to support this concept in certain species [1], it remains controversial, especially in relation to human parturition [2]. This is largely due to the fact that there is still much which is not known about the tissue source(s) of prostaglandins, the mechanisms regulating prostaglandin synthesis, and whether prostaglandins are synthesised before or as a consequence of labour. Adding to the complexity of these questions are the difficulties in performing controlled experiments in human subjects. It is not the intention of this chapter to address

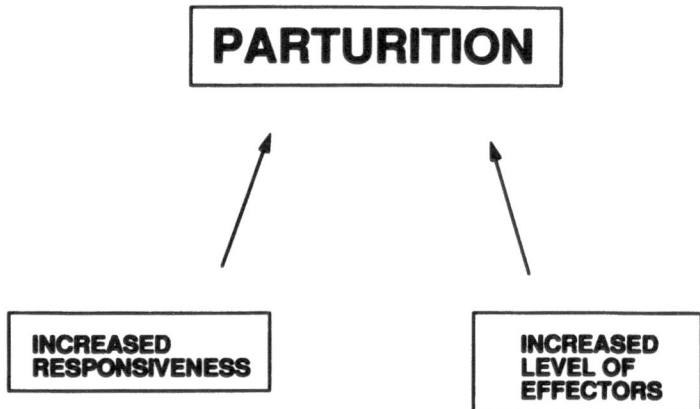

Fig. 10.1. Dual physiological processes for parturition.

these issues directly, but rather to suggest an approach which can be useful and to demonstrate its application.

In their study of animal models of parturition, investigators have enjoyed significant success in determining the sequence of events that give rise to the changes in prostaglandin concentrations and increased myometrial activity at the end of gestation [3,4]. However, there are a number of discrepancies in the events leading to labour between humans and most commonly studied experimental animal models, especially the sheep [1]. These include the tissue sources of prostaglandins [1,3,5–7] and the role of steroid hormones [1,8] in eliciting changes in prostaglandin concentrations. In spite of this, there are commonalities in the nature of the events leading to enhanced prostaglandin levels. Fig. 10.2

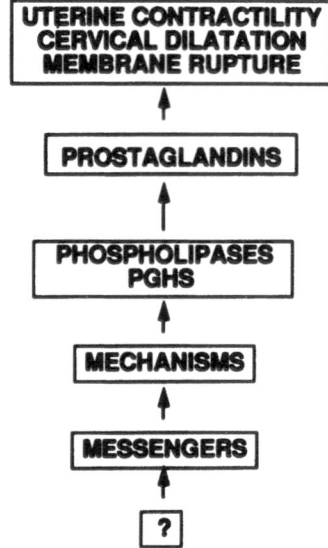

Fig. 10.2. Proposed pathway leading to parturition.

illustrates a suggested pathway leading to enhanced prostaglandin synthesis and parturition which contains features common to all species. This pathway is described in reverse order, that is from the known final events of parturition to those which precede it. We suggest that it is possible to answer certain critical questions, including whether prostaglandins are a cause or a consequence of labour, by identifying changes which occur in the sequence of events leading to labour.

The first step is to define the pathway. It begins with enhanced myometrial contractility, cervical dilatation and membrane rupture, three physiological endpoints for which data exist that suggest a role for prostaglandins (for reviews see [1,9,10]). Next the pathway describes increases in the circulating and tissue levels of prostaglandins as the cause leading to these three physiological events. There are ample examples from animal studies which describe increases in prostaglandin levels in amniotic fluid, fetal or maternal plasma, or intrauterine tissue prior to the initiation of the final events of parturition [1,3,5,11]. In sheep the apparent source of these prostaglandins is vascularized tissue close to the myometrium, e.g. fetal cotyledon and chorioallantois [3,5,6].

The increased prostaglandin levels are due to increased activity of the two enzymes responsible for prostaglandin synthesis, phospholipases (A_2 and C) and prostaglandin endoperoxide H synthase (PGHS, frequently called cyclo-oxygenase) [3,12–14]. The pathway in Fig. 10.2 now becomes less certain, as those mechanisms and messengers responsible for causing the changes in the activities of these enzymes are less well defined. Rice [14] has reported an increase in the mass of PGHS in ovine cotyledon with increasing gestation. Certainly, there is little argument that there is some role for changes in the steroids of pregnancy, progesterone and oestradiol, as factors responsible for altering prostaglandin synthetic enzyme activity [1,4]. However, their precise role is not defined. Those events which lead to alteration in the relative levels of the pregnancy steroids and other messengers would include activation of the hypothalamic–pituitary–adrenal axis and increased fetal circulating cortisol levels [3,15]. Although our knowledge of all steps to ovine parturition is incomplete, enough information is available to define the major points of the pathway. We are now able to apply this scheme to other species, including human, to identify the events associated with each major point of the pathway.

Using the Pathway

Model

Our laboratory has chosen to address the problem of understanding the sequential events of prostaglandin synthesis in relation to parturition using the human amnion as a model. There are a number of good reasons why the amnion serves this purpose well. It synthesizes PGE_2 nearly exclusively [1,5,16,17] and the content or output of PGE_2 increases with the onset of labour [7,18–21]. The amnion is responsive, both as fresh tissue and in culture, to a large number of effectors which modify PGE_2 output (summarised in [22]). Also, it is composed of a single layer of epithelial cells, plus associated fibroblasts in the connective tissue layer under the epithelial layer, which are relatively easy to disperse and study directly or to grow in culture. These factors, together with its relative ease of procurement, have made it the most studied human intrauterine tissue for prostaglandin synthesis regulation. This is not to say, however, that other intrauterine tissues need not be studied for their term prostaglandin synthetic capacities. Indeed, decidua vera has frequently demonstrated an increase in PGE_2 or $PGF_{2\alpha}$ content or output with the onset of labour [18,23]. Sullivan et al. [24] have indicated that this increase is due to stromal cells, which, when isolated from other decidual cells by percoll gradients, produce approximately 30 times more PGE_2 with the onset of labour. Additionally, more attention needs to be directed at the capacity and regulation of placental prostaglandin production. From a number of studies, it has become obvious that placental prostaglandin has an important role in fetal development, such as regulating fetal breathing movements [25] and possibly serving as a source of prostaglandins for the development and differentiation of the fetal lung [26,27]. It is our hope that the elucidation of the regulatory mechanisms responsible for controlling amnion prostaglandin synthesis will lead to the rapid understanding of the regulation of prostaglandin synthesis in the other intrauterine tissues.

Synthetic Enzymes

There are two points of control over the synthesis of prostaglandins for parturition, namely, the enzymes, phospholipases A_2 and C and prostaglandin H synthase (PGHS) [12–14]. Because we have directed our efforts mostly toward PGHS, this will be considered in the remainder of this chapter. In order to gain some insight into the role of PGHS, studies performed in animals are examined. In general, these studies demonstrate a significant increase in the activity of PGHS during the third trimester. Eliot et al. [28] described a linear, tenfold increase in prostaglandin synthesis by rabbit amnion from day 20 to day 30 gestation (term = 31 days). Nodem et al. [29], measuring O_2 consumption as an index of enzyme activity, obtained similar results in rabbit amnion, although the increase in activity was 38-fold and increased more sharply on days 29 and 30 of gestation. In sheep, cotyledonary enzyme activity is low up to day 100 of gestation, increasing somewhat to day 120 and then more rapidly to term (day 147) [3,30]. In parallel with this increase in enzyme activity, Rice et al. [14] demonstrated an increase in PGHS mass in cotyledons using western transfer and immunoblotting techniques. These data suggest that the increased mass is responsible for the increased activity. It remains to be shown that this reflects new enzyme synthesis.

Amnion PGHS

The presence of PGHS protein in human fetal membranes and decidua has been identified from early in gestation to term by immunocytochemistry [31,32]. It is localised in the amnion epithelium and the cytoplasm of fibroblast-like cells in the subepithelial connective tissue. It is also found in the villus and chorionic cytotrophoblast, villus syncytiotrophoblast, and decidualised stroma. The decidua has the most intense staining. However, the amnion epithelium has a hetero-geneous staining pattern; most epithelial cells are stained intensely with some adjacent areas with no staining. There does not appear to be any change in the percentage of cells with positive staining from the first trimester to term, and there is no difference in the staining pattern or intensity with onset of labour.

Prostaglandin synthase activity in fetal membranes and placenta was described in earlier reports. Kinoshita et al. [16] studied the activity in term amnion, chorion, decidua and placental villi following spontaneous delivery. They observed that radiolabelled arachidonic acid was converted into radiolabelled PGE_2, but only in the presence of the cofactors, reduced glutathione, haemoglobin and 1-adrenaline. There was no enzyme activity in the mitochondrial or cytosolic fractions, only in the microsomal fraction obtained by centrifugation (80 000 g) of tissue homogenate. Each tissue had enzyme activity, and eicosatrienoic acid and arachidonic acid were converted into PGE_1 and PGE_2, respectively. Microsomes from decidua had greater specific activity than those from amnion in 10 min incubations. The specific activity of the amnion microsomes was 2.2 pg PGE_2 μg protein^{-1} min^{-1}. Changes in enzyme activity with onset of labour were not described. Duchesne et al. [33] described the conversion of radiolabelled arachidonic acid into prostaglandins in placental and fetal membrane (amnion and chorion together) microsomes. In assays which were well characterised, they observed that fetal membranes produced PGE_2 nearly exclusively. The activity of prostaglandin synthase in fetal membranes was 2.6 pg PGE_2 μg protein^{-1} min^{-1} which was 4–5-fold greater than that of placenta. The K_m for fetal membranes was 7 μM.

A different approach for studying prostaglandin synthase in fetal membranes and placenta was used by Ohel et al. [34]. One product formed by the peroxidation of arachidonic acid is malondialdehyde, which can be quantitated spectrophotometrically. A concentration-dependent increase in malondialde-hyde formation was evident with increasing arachidonic acid and was highest in amnion and chorion microsomes. This was inhibited with indomethacin treat-ment in amnion and chorion, but not in placenta, possibly indicating the presence of other arachidonate metabolising enzymes in the placental preparation.

Prostaglandin synthase activity was studied at term with the onset of labour in amnion, chorion, and decidua tissue by Okazaki et al. [17]. Using whole tissue homogenates and radiolabelled arachidonic acid, they determined that prosta-glandin synthase activity was highest in amnion and that only amnion demon-strated a 2.4 fold increase in enzyme activity with labour. While this approach provided important information regarding prostaglandin synthase activity, it was not possible to determine whether changes in enzyme activity were due to substrate affinity or enzyme velocity.

We therefore developed a specific enzyme assay for amnion PGHS to test for differences in PGHS K_d and V_{max} with labour (Smieja et al., unpublished observation). A significant increase in the V_{max} of the enzyme occurs with the onset of labour ($P=0.012$) from 11±8 (caesarean section (CS)) to 19±4 (spontaneous labour (SL)) pg PGE_2 μg protein^{-1} min^{-1} (mean±SD). There was no change in the K_m of the enzyme, 1.4±1.2 μM (CS) vs. 2.4±1.3 μM (SL). On the surface it appears that even though the catalytic velocity of PGHS increases with the onset of labour in human amnion, we are no closer to understanding the sequential changes which precede labour, if indeed there are any. Further, it is difficult to test whether there are longitudinal changes in tissue enzyme activity with gestation in humans.

Although we cannot sample human amnion sequentially before labour onset, the data presented above do suggest, indirectly, that PGHS activity is increasing before the onset of labour. It is usually assumed that the variance of a population increases with increasing mean values. However, a close examination of the data shows that the variance is smaller in the SL group, which has a higher mean V_{max} than the CS group. By comparing the F ratio of the variances (4.0), it is observed that there is a significant difference ($P<0.05$) in the variances of the two patient populations ($F_{\alpha\ 0.05[9,8]}=3.39$). This suggests that the enzyme activity is more variable in the CS group of the patients. One plausible explanation for this is that PGHS activity is changing in this population. Because the mean values are increasing from CS to SL patient groups, the data would suggest that PGHS activity is increasing before the onset of labour.

Mechanisms

Further understanding of the sequential events leading to enhanced prostaglandin synthesis at term by the amnion requires the examination of the cause of the increased PGHS activity observed at term. This has been addressed by Gaffney et al. [35] who irreversibly inactivated formed PGHS with aspirin in tissue explants obtained from chorioamnions and placentas of women at term before the onset of labour (CS) and following spontaneous onset of labour at term (SL). The experiment was designed to determine the time required for the aspirin-treated tissues to regain their full prostaglandin synthetic capacity. It was observed that the half-time of recovery was substantially less (about one-fifth) in SL tissues than it was in CS tissues, suggesting a faster rate of PGHS synthesis following labour onset.

How can this observation be explained? Clearly, there are several possibilities: decreased turnover of the enzyme (PGHS has a short half-life, less than 1 h [36]); increased transcription and/or translation; or increased stability of the mRNA species. At this time answers to these questions in the fetal membranes do not exist. However, we have begun to address some of these issues in minced amnion tissue obtained from SL patients immediately after delivery.

RNA Synthesis Independence

Examination of the PGE_2 output from fresh, minced SL amnion showed that it was 3.97 ± 1.13 ng $PGE_2\ \mu g\ DNA^{-1}\ 14\ h^{-1}$ (mean $\pm$ SEM, $n = 19$ patients). This corresponds to 2.62 ± 0.75 ng $PGE_2/10^5$ cells/14 h, based on 6.6 pg DNA per human diploid cell. This level of output is 10–100 times greater than that observed with cultured amnion cells under serum-depleted conditions [37]. The RNA synthesis inhibitor, actinomycin D ($0–4\ \mu g\ ml^{-1}$), was added to the tissue incubations to test the possibility that this prostaglandin output was dependent on constant RNA synthesis. The conditions of this and subsequent experiments consisted of pretreating the tissue with agonists or inhibitors, washing the tissue, and adding 10 μM arachidonic acid for 2 h. The media from this 2 h incubation were collected and assayed for PGE_2. Although not a direct assay for PGHS, this approach is an effective means of assessing its activity. Actinomycin D did not inhibit PGE_2 output, but instead increased the output of prostaglandin approximately twofold, suggesting that perhaps a transcription-dependent inhibitor of PGHS was present (Zakar et al., unpublished observation). Regardless of the presence of any such inhibitor, the basal output of PGE_2 is not dependent on the synthesis of new RNA.

Protein Synthesis Dependence

To test whether PGHS activity in fresh amnion tissue depends on protein synthesis, tissue pieces were incubated with cycloheximide ($0-40\,\mu\,ml^{-1}$), washed and then incubated with fresh medium containing arachidonic acid ($10\,\mu M$) for 2 h (Zakar et al., unpublished observation). The results indicated a significant and complete dose-dependent inhibition of arachidonate-dependent basal amnion PGE_2 output. These data indicate that constant protein synthesis is required to sustain PGHS activity in fresh amnion tissue, and imply the presence of a stable mRNA species coding for PGHS.

To summarise the observations so far, PGHS activity increases with the onset of, and quite possibly before, labour. This is due to an increase in the rate of PGHS synthesis. In postlabour fresh amnion tissue, PGHS activity is dependent on constant protein synthesis from preformed RNA. An RNA synthesis-dependent inhibitor of PGHS activity (or synthesis) may also exist, although this inhibitor is not absolute. There are no data which preclude the possibility that the expression of a mRNA for PGHS is an early event in the sequence of events leading to enhanced PGHS activity, occuring before the tissue was obtained after SL delivery at term.

Messengers

We examined the next step shown in Fig. 10.2 which leads to enhanced prostaglandin synthesis for labour, the messengers (extracellular and intracellular) which activate amnion to produce prostaglandins. Although many factors have been identified with the ability to alter prostaglandin synthesis in amnion [22], much of this work has been performed on cultured cells and needs confirmation in fresh tissue. One intracellular mediator which may be a common pathway for several extracellular initiators in terms of amnion PGE_2 synthesis is protein kinase C [37]. Recently, $10^{-7}M$ 12-O-tetradecanoylphorbol 13-acetate (TPA), a phorbol ester activator of protein kinase C, has been shown to stimulate the conversion of arachidonic acid into PGE_2 3–4-fold in fresh, minced SL amnion tissue. The inhibitor of protein kinase C, staurosporine ($0-1\,\mu M$), blocked arachidonate-enhanced PGE_2 output induced by TPA in a dose-dependent fashion (Zakar et al., unpublished observations). Staurosporine alone had no effect on the basal or unstimulated prostaglandin output, suggesting that the sustained basal output of PGE_2 was not dependent on constant protein kinase C activity.

The initiators which may activate protein kinase C have not been identified. Two possible factors include vasopressin and oxytocin, which increase PGE_2 output in fresh amnion tissue, early or confluent cell cultures [38–40]. Although there is no definitive evidence showing a direct activation of protein kinase C in mediating the action of an effector on amnion prostaglandin synthesis, there is a high probability that protein kinase C is involved. In addition to the evidence provided above that activators and inhibitors of protein kinase C modulate PGE_2 output, we have evidence which illustrates the translocation of protein kinase C from cytosol to membranes which occurs in confluent cultured amnion epithelial cells upon activation with TPA (Zakar et al., unpublished observation). Further, Dr Kathleen Eyster of the University of South Dakota, who recently discovered an endogenous stimulator of protein kinase C activity in rat ovarian cytosol (unpublished observation) has found, in collaboration with our laboratory, a stimulator of protein kinase C activity in the cytosol of both human term amnion and placenta (unpublished observation). This factor, which stimulates partially purified rat brain protein kinase C about twofold, is unmasked with prior heat treatment in placenta (80–90°C, 2 min) but is evident without prior heating in the amnion. There is no significant difference in the activity of the factor between CS and SL amnions or placentas. The ovarian activator is approximately 100 kDa and is not soluble in petroleum ether, chloroform:methanol or acidified chloroform:methanol. Further characterisation of this factor is being carried out. More will be described regarding the action of protein kinase C in fresh, minced SL amnion later in this chapter.

Another group of messengers which have been regarded as having an important role in regulating prostaglandin synthesis for labour are the steroid hormones of pregnancy [1,3,4]. A number of steroid hormones have been tested on fresh, minced SL amnion for their ability to influence arachidonate-enhanced PGE_2 output (unpublished observation). All pretreatments were for 14 h in the absence or presence of test compounds before washing and subsequent 2 h treatment in the presence of 10 μM-arachidonic acid. Cycloheximide nearly completely blocked PGE_2 output, as described earlier. There was no effect from several of the steroids tested: oestradiol-17β, progesterone, dehydroepiandrosterone sulphate, testosterone and 17-hydroxy progesterone (all at 10^{-7}M). Each of the glucocorticoids tested, cortisol (10^{-7}M) and dexamethasone (10^{-7}M), inhibited the output of PGE_2 up to about 55%.

The inhibition of arachidonic acid conversion into PGE_2 is an unusual effect for glucocorticoids, having been described only once before in amnion [41] and infrequently in other cells and tissues [42]. We therefore tested it further, alone and in the presence of the protein kinase C stimulator, TPA, to ascertain the apparent level of synthesis regulation that it affects. In this experiment, minced SL amnion was first treated with acetylsalicylic acid to irreversibly inactivate preformed PGHS. The tissue was washed and incubated in the absence or presence of test compounds for 14 h. Again, the tissue was washed and incubated for a further 2 h in the presence of 10 μM-arachidonic acid to test for recovery of PGHS activity. It was observed that cortisol (10^{-7}M) inhibited the recovery of PGHS activity by approximately 80%. However, when cortisol was coincubated with actinomycin D (1 μM), the inhibitory activity of cortisol was completely lost, suggesting that the cortisol effect is to stimulate transcription of an inhibitory factor for PGHS activity or synthesis. Actinomycin D alone had no effect on the recovery of PGHS activity, confirming our earlier experiment and further supporting the concept that new PGHS synthesis is dependent upon a preformed mRNA. Activation of protein kinase C with TPA (10^{-7}M) enhanced the conversion of arachidonic acid into PGE_2 as described earlier, and coincubation of TPA with actinomycin D returned the PGE_2 output to control levels. These data suggest that protein kinase C promotes transcription of PGHS mRNA.

When cortisol and TPA were coincubated, a partial, but significant, inhibition of PGE_2 output was observed so that values were intermediate between control and TPA alone. This is consistent with the inhibitory action of cortisol seen earlier. However, it is important to note that the inhibitory effect of cortisol was only partial, even at maximally effective concentrations, and that the conversion of arachidonate to PGE_2 was still increased by TPA activation of protein kinase C. When actinomycin D was coincubated with cortisol and TPA, neither the inhibitory effect of cortisol nor the stimulatory effect of TPA/protein kinase C could be expressed, and the result was no different from controls (Zakar et al., unpublished observations).

Implications for Human Parturition

The results reported here and our interpretation of their implications for the control of amnion prostaglandin synthesis are based mainly on tissue obtained after the spontaneous onset of labour at term. We can only suggest possible steps within pathway events from the approaches employed in these studies. More definitive proof of the steps proposed must come from direct studies.

Nevertheless, a scenario can be proposed which is testable and ties together many of the observations we and others have made (Fig. 10.3). This scenario is only partial, as it does not include the role of phospholipases or intracellular messengers, other than protein kinase C. Maturition of a paracrine communication system within the uterus generates local factors (cytokines, peptide hormones) which have the potential to bind receptors on amnion and other cells,

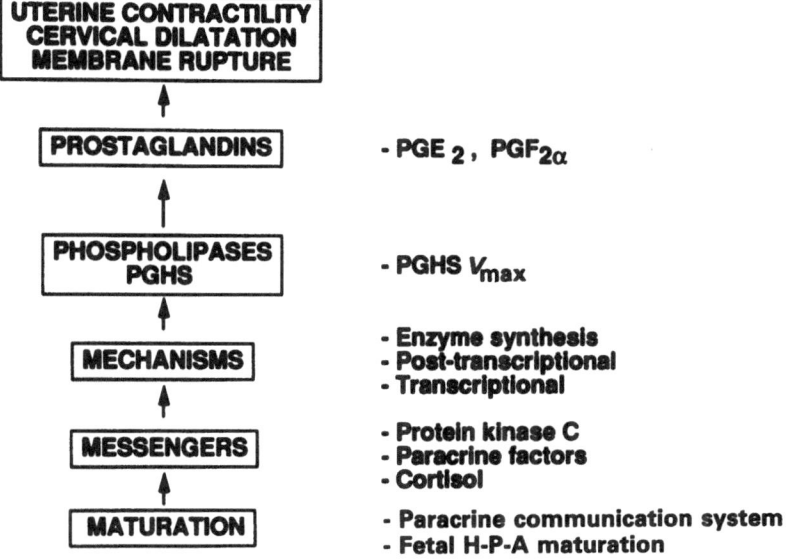

Fig. 10.3. Suggested events in human amnion associated with pathway leading to parturition.

including decidual stromal cells, activate phospholipase C, generate diacylglycerol and stimulate the activity of protein kinase C. Protein kinase C, in turn, stimulates gene expression and the transcription of a stable messenger RNA coding for PGHS. This accelerates the rate of PGHS synthesis, leading to an increase in activity and increased prostaglandin synthesis. Meanwhile, maturation of the fetal hypothalamic–pituitary–adrenal axis results in the generation of fetal cortisol. This contributes to an increase in amniotic fluid cortisol levels [43,44] where the free, unbound levels [45] can reach 40 nM or more. These are concentrations which are effective in modulating amnion PGE_2 output. This cortisol may have a partial inhibitory effect on PGHS synthesis or action, preventing errant or preterm increases in intrauterine paracrine factors from stimulating PGHS synthesis. But it does not have the ability completely to prevent protein kinase C mediated increases in PGHS synthesis. A second role for fetal cortisol may be to promote maturation of the intrauterine paracrine communication system [46]. Additionally, cortisol contributes to the maturation of the fetal lung [47], promoting the synthesis of surfactant and its associated apoproteins, which are discharged into the amniotic fluid, where they can bind to and stimulate amnion cell PGE_2 output [48]. In these ways, fetal cortisol may contribute to the fine tuning of the timing of parturition [49].

Identification of the steps in the pathway which occur before the onset of labour would confirm an important role for prostaglandins in the initiation of labour.

References

1. Challis JRG, Olson DM. Parturition. In: Knobil E, Neill JD, eds. The physiology of reproduction, vol. 2. New York: Raven Press, 1988; 2177–216.
2. Casey ML, Cox SM, Word RA, MacDonald PC. Cytokines and infection-induced preterm labour. In: Salamonsen LA, Healy DL, Brennecke SP, eds. Prostaglandins and pregnancy. Australia: CSIRO, 1990; 83–93.
3. Rice GE, Thorburn GD. The gestational development of ovine placental prostaglandin-synthesizing capacity. In: Gluckman PD, Johnston BM, Nathanielsz PW, eds. Advances in fetal physiology: reviews in honor of G.C. Liggins. Ithaca, NY: Perinatology Press, 1989; 387–407.
4. Nathanielsz PW. The regulation of the switch from myometrial contractures to contractions in late pregnancy: studies in the pregnant sheep and monkey. In: Gluckman PD, Johnston BM, Nathanielsz PW, eds. Advances in fetal physiology: reviews in honor of G.C. Liggins. Ithaca, NY: Perinatology Press, 1989; 409–20.
5. Olson DM, Lye SJ, Skinner K, Challis JRG. Prostanoid concentrations in maternal/fetal plasma and amniotic fluid and intrauterine tissue prostanoid output in relation to myometrial contractility during the onset of ACTH-induced preterm labor in sheep. Endocrinology 1985; 116:389–97.
6. Olson DM, Lye SJ, Challis JRG. Prostaglandin concentrations in ovine maternal and fetal tissues at late gestation. Pediatr Res 1986; 20:83–6.
7. Mitchell MD. Sources of eicosanoids within the uterus during pregnancy. In: McNellis D, Challis J, MacDonald P, Nathanielsz P, Roberts J, eds. The onset of labor: cellular and integrative mechanisms. Ithaca, NY: Perinatology Press, 1988; 165–81.
8. Mitchell BF, Challis JRG. Estrogen and progesterone metabolism in human fetal membranes. In: Mitchell BF, ed. The physiology and biochemistry of the human fetal membranes. Ithaca, NY: Perinatology Press, 1988; 5–28.
9. Calder AA, Greer IA. Prostaglandins and the biological control of cervical function. In: Salamonsen LA, Healy DL, Brennecke SP, eds. Prostaglandins and pregnancy. Australia: CSIRO, 1990; 43–9.
10. Bryant-Greenwood GD, Greenwood FC. The human membranes and decidua as a model for

paracrine interactions. In: McNellis D, Challis J, MacDonald P, Nathanielsz P, Roberts J, eds. The onset of labor: cellular and integrative mechanisms. Ithaca, NY: Perinatology Press 1988; 253–73.

11. Ducsay CA, McNutt CM. Circadian uterine activity in the pregnant rhesus macaque; do prostaglandins play a role? Biol Reprod 1989; 40:988–93.

12. Bleasdale JE, DiRenzo GC. Fetal influence on parturition. In: Rodeck C, ed. Fetal medicine, Vol. 1. London: Blackwell, 1989; 242–88.

13. Wilson T. Phospholipase in human parturition. In: Salamonsen LA, Healy DL, Brennecke SP, eds. Prostaglandins and pregnancy. Australia: CSIRO, 1990; 95–105.

14. Rice GE. Labour: a process dependent upon prostaglandin G/H synthase. In: Salamonsen LA, Healy DL, Brennecke SP, eds. Prostaglandins and pregnancy. Australia: CSIRO, 1990; 107–17.

15. Challis JRG, Hooper S. Birth: outcome of a positive cascade. Bailliere's Clin Endocrinol Metab 1989; 3:781–93.

16. Kinoshita K, Satho K, Sakamoto S. Biosynthesis of prostaglandin in human decidua, amnion, chorion and villi. Endocrinol Jpn 1977; 24:343–50.

17. Okazaki T, Casey ML, Okita JR, MacDonald PC, Johnston JM. Initiation of human parturition. XII. Biosynthesis and metabolism of prostaglandins in human fetal membranes and uterine decidua. Am J Obstet Gynecol 1981; 139:373–81.

18. Willman EA, Collins WP. Distribution of prostaglandins E_2 and $F_{2\alpha}$ within the fetoplacental unit throughout human pregnancy. J Endocrinol 1976; 68:413–19.

19. Olson DM, Skinner K, Challis JRG. Prostaglandin output in relation to parturition by cells dispersed from human intrauterine tissues. J Clin Endocrinol Metab 1983; 57:694–9.

20. Kinoshita K, Satoh K, Sakamoto S. Human amnion membrane and prostaglandin biosynthesis. Biol Res Pregnancy Perinatol 1984; 5:61–7.

21. Lopez Bernal A, Hansell DJ, Alexander S, Turnbull AC. Prostaglandin E production by amniotic cells in relation to term and preterm labour. Br J Obstet Gynaecol 1987; 94:864–9.

22. Olson DM, Zakar T, Potestio FA, Smieja Z. Control of prostaglandin production in human amnion. News Physiol Sci 1990; 5:259–63.

23. Skinner KA, Challis JRG. Changes in the synthesis and metabolism of prostaglandins by human fetal membranes and decidua at labor. Am J Obstet Gynecol 1985; 151:519–23.

24. Sullivan MHF, Khan H, Ishihara O, Elder MG. Changes in decidual stromal cell prostaglandin E_2 production and cyclooxygenase enzyme in labour. 2nd European Congress on Prostaglandins in Reproduction 1991; 102 (Abstract).

25. Adamson SL, Kuipers IM, Olson DM. Umbilical cord occlusion stimulates breathing independent of blood gases and pH. J Appl Physiol 1991; 70:1796–809.

26. Acarregui MJ, Snyder JM, Mitchell MD, Mendelson CR. Prostaglandins regulate surfactant protein A (SP-A) gene expression in human fetal lung in vitro. Endocrinology 1990; 127:1105–113.

27. Ballard PL, Gonzales LW, Williams MC, Roberts JM, Jacobs MM. Differentiation of type II cells during explant culture of human fetal lung is accelerated by endogenous prostanoids and adenosine 3', 5'-monophosphate. Endocrinology 1991; 128:2916–24.

28. Eliot WJ, McLaughlin LL, Block MH, Needleman P. Arachidonic acid metabolism by rabbit fetal membranes of various gestational ages. Prostaglandins 1984; 27:27–36.

29. Nodem PA, Smith WL, DeWitt DL, Roux JF. Prostaglandin forming cyclooxygenase activity in rabbit amnion, yolk sac splanchnopleure, decidua and uterus at 20 to 30 days' gestation. Biol Reprod 1981; 24:1042–7.

30. Rice GE, Wong MH, Hollingsworth S, Thorburn GD. Prostaglandin G/H synthase in ovine cotyledons: a gestational profile. Eicosanoids 1991; 3:231–6.

31. Bryant-Greenwood GD, Rees MCP, Turnbull AC. Immunohistochemical localization of relaxin, prolactin and prostaglandin synthase in human amnion, chorion and decidua. J Endocrinol 1987; 114:491–6.

32. Price TM, Kaumma SW, Curry TE, Jr, Clark MR. Immunohistochemical localization of prostaglandin endoperoxide synthase in human fetal membrane and decidua. Biol Reprod 1989; 41:701–5.

33. Duchesne MJ, Thaler-Dao H, Crastes de Paulet A. Prostaglandin synthesis in human placenta and fetal membranes. Prostaglandins 1978; 15:19–41.

34. Ohel G, Kisselevitz R, Margalioth EJ, Schenker JG. Ascorbate-dependent lipid peroxidation in the human placenta and fetal membranes. Gynecol Obstet Invest 1985; 19:73–5.

35. Gaffney RC, Rice GE, Brennecke SP. Is human labor triggered by an increase in the rate of synthesis of prostaglandin G/H synthase? Reprod Fertil Dev 1991; 3: 483–88.

36. Raz A, Wyche A, Siegel N, Needleman P. Regulation of fibroblast cyclooxygenase synthesis by interleukin-1. J Biol Chem 1988; 263:3022–8.
37. Zakar T, Olson DM. Stimulation of human amnion prostaglandins E_2 production by activators of protein kinase C. J Clin Endocrinol Metab 1988; 67:915–23.
38. Fuchs A-R, Husslein P, Fuchs F. Oxytocin and the initiation of human parturition II. Stimulation of prostaglandin production in human decidua by oxytocin. Am J Obstet Gynecol 1981; 141:694–7.
39. Bala GA, Thakur NR, Bleasdale JE. Characterization of the major phosphoinositide-specific phospholipase C of human amnion. Biol Reprod 1990; 43:704–11.
40. Moore JJ, Dubyak GR, Moore RM, VanderKooy D. Oxytocin activates the inositol-phospholipid-protein kinase-C system and stimulated prostaglandin production in human amnion cells. Endocrinology 1988; 123:1771–7.
41. Gibb W, Lavoie J-C. Effects of glucocorticoids on prostaglandin formation by human amnion. Can J Physiol Pharmacol 1990; 68:671–6.
42. Bailey JM, Makheja AN, Pash J, Verma M. Corticosteroids suppress cyclooxygenase messenger RNA levels and prostanoid synthesis in cultured vascular cells. Biochem Biophys Res Commun 1988; 157:1159–63.
43. Murphy BEP, Patrick J, Denton RL. Cortisol in amniotic fluid during human gestation. 1975; 40:164–7.
44. Fencl MD, Tulchinsky D. Total cortisol in amniotic fluid and fetal lung maturation. N Engl J Med 1975; 292:133–7.
45. Challis JRG, Bennett MJ. Cortisol binding in human amniotic fluid. Am J Obstet Gynecol 1977; 129:655–61.
46. Jones SA, Brooks AN, Challis JRG. Steroids modulate corticotrophin-releasing hormone in human fetal membranes and placenta. J Clin Endocrinol Metab 1989; 68:825–30.
47. Ballard PL, Gonzales LW. Hormonal factors in lung maturation. In: Gluckman PD, Johnston BM, Nathanielsz PW, eds. Advances in fetal physiology: reviews in honor of G. C. Liggins. Ithaca, NY: Perinatology Press, 1989; 103–21.
48. Lopez Bernal A, Newman GE, Phizackerly PJR, Turnbull AC. Surfactant stimulates prostaglandin E production in human amnion. Br J Obstet Gynaecol 1988; 95:1013–17.
49. Nory MJ, Walsh SW. Dexamethasone and estradiol treatment in pregnant rhesus macaques: effects on gestational length, maternal plasma hormones, and fetal growth. Am J Obstet Gynecol 1983; 145:920–30.

Chapter 11

Myometrial Function

P. W. N. Nathanielsz and M. B. O. M. Honnebier

Methods of Recording Myometrial Activity In Vivo

Myometrial function can be recorded experimentally using invasive techniques in pregnant animal models by the placement of sensors within the uterine cavity to record intra-amniotic pressure (IAP), strain gauges on the uterine wall to measure alterations in length and tension of the myometrium during periods of activity, and electrodes sewn into the uterine muscle to record extracellular potential changes as the myometrial electromyogram (EMG). Each of these methods provides data that reflect slightly different features of myometrial function. In addition they are each subject to different types of recording artifact. When reviewing the available data on myometrial function it is necessary to use methods that can quantify different types of myometrial activity in a way that reflects physiological and pathophysiological features of mechanistic importance.

The animal species in which myometrial activity throughout pregnancy has been most often studied in vivo for long periods are the pregnant sheep and pregnant non-human primates, such as the rhesus monkey and baboon. The majority of work reported in this chapter is taken from studies undertaken by our colleagues and myself on pregnant non-human primates.

Different Types of Myometrial Activity: Contractures and Contractions

In the last few years there has been considerable interest in the study of myometrial activity that occurs throughout pregnancy. In 1872 Braxton Hicks [1] described low-grade epochs of myometrial activity that he observed from midgestation onwards in women. We and several other groups of investigators have used invasive techniques to demonstrate that myometrial contractility occurs throughout pregnancy in a wide range of species. In all species studied to date, periodic epochs of contractility lasting several minutes occur through the majority of pregnancy. These epochs of activity have been demonstrated in sheep [2], pigs [3], dogs [4], horses [5], cows [6], goats [7], cynomolgus monkeys [8], rhesus monkeys [9] and baboons [10].

Myometrial activity throughout pregnancy has been most extensively studied in sheep and non-human primates. In pregnant sheep from 60 days of pregnancy (term 150 days) to a few hours before they deliver, these epochs of myometrial contractility occur at relatively regular intervals of about one every 40–90 min [11,12]. We have called these epochs contractures. Contractures are clearly distinguished from labour and delivery contractions by two major characteristics. First, contractures are of much longer duration (up to 15 min) than contractions, which last less than 1 min. Second, contractures generate much smaller increments in IAP than contractions. Typically a contracture only raises IAP by 5–10 mmHg whereas at labour a contraction raises IAP by 20–40 mmHg. As mentioned above, contractures have been shown to be present for a major portion of pregnancy in at least nine mammalian species. We have recently used power spectral analysis to provide a very rapid assessment of whether the myometrium is in the contractures or contractions mode (Figs. 11.1–11.3) [13].

It is clearly impossible to record invasively from pregnant women over a prolonged period of time. However, epochs of myometrial activity that are clearly more similar to contractures than contractions as recorded in experimental animals can be seen on pressure recordings obtained invasively in pregnant women following placement of intra-amniotic pressure catheters. Similar epochs may occasionally be registered non-invasively using the guard ring tocodynamometer. In addition, ultrasonographers have reported that they regularly see long-lasting thickenings of the uterine wall prior to amniocentesis before any needle has been introduced through the pregnant woman's skin.

This chapter will focus on the factors that regulate contractures and that are responsible for the switch from contractures to contractions that must occur for labour and delivery to take place. A firm understanding of the regulation of the switch from contractures to contractions is important before we are able to predict, diagnose and treat the problems of term, preterm and post-term delivery.

Factors that Regulate Contractures

Prostaglandins

Very few studies have directly addressed the role of prostaglandins in the regulation of the frequency and intensity of contractures in any species. When indomethacin was used to inhibit labour contractions in a pregnant rhesus monkey, contractures were also completely abolished [13]. In pregnant sheep we have demonstrated that prostaglandin synthetase inhibitors will greatly decrease, and in some cases completely abolish, contractures [14]. Thus the frequency with which contractures occur may be influenced by the endogenous level of prostaglandin production.

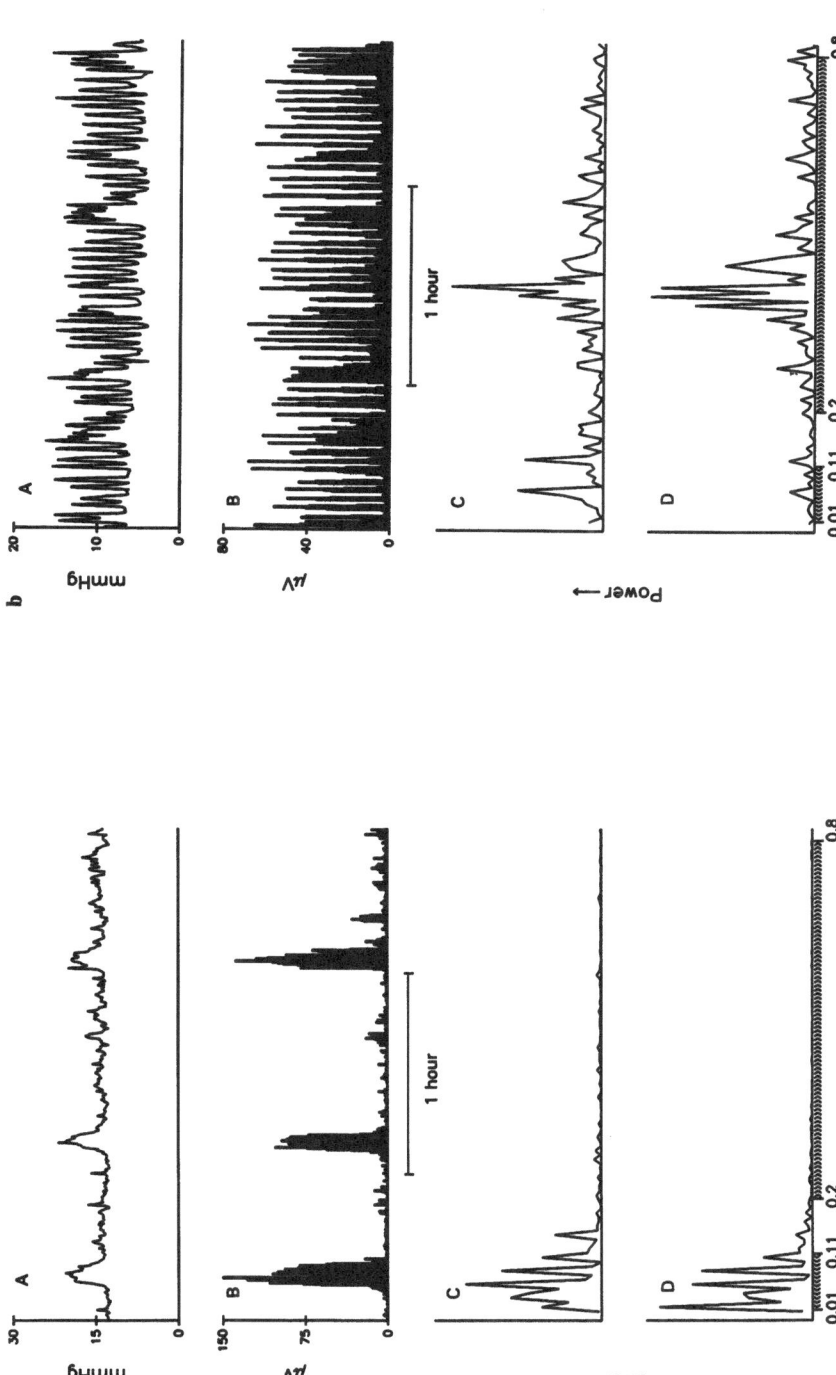

Fig. 11.1. a Contracture-type and **b** contraction-type of myometrial activity pattern in a pregnant sheep. A, Intrauterine pressure recording; calibration bar 10 mmHg. B, Myometrial electromyogram at the same time as A; calibration bar 50 μV. C, Power spectral analysis of intrauterine pressure recording in A. D, Power spectral analysis of electromyogram recording in B.

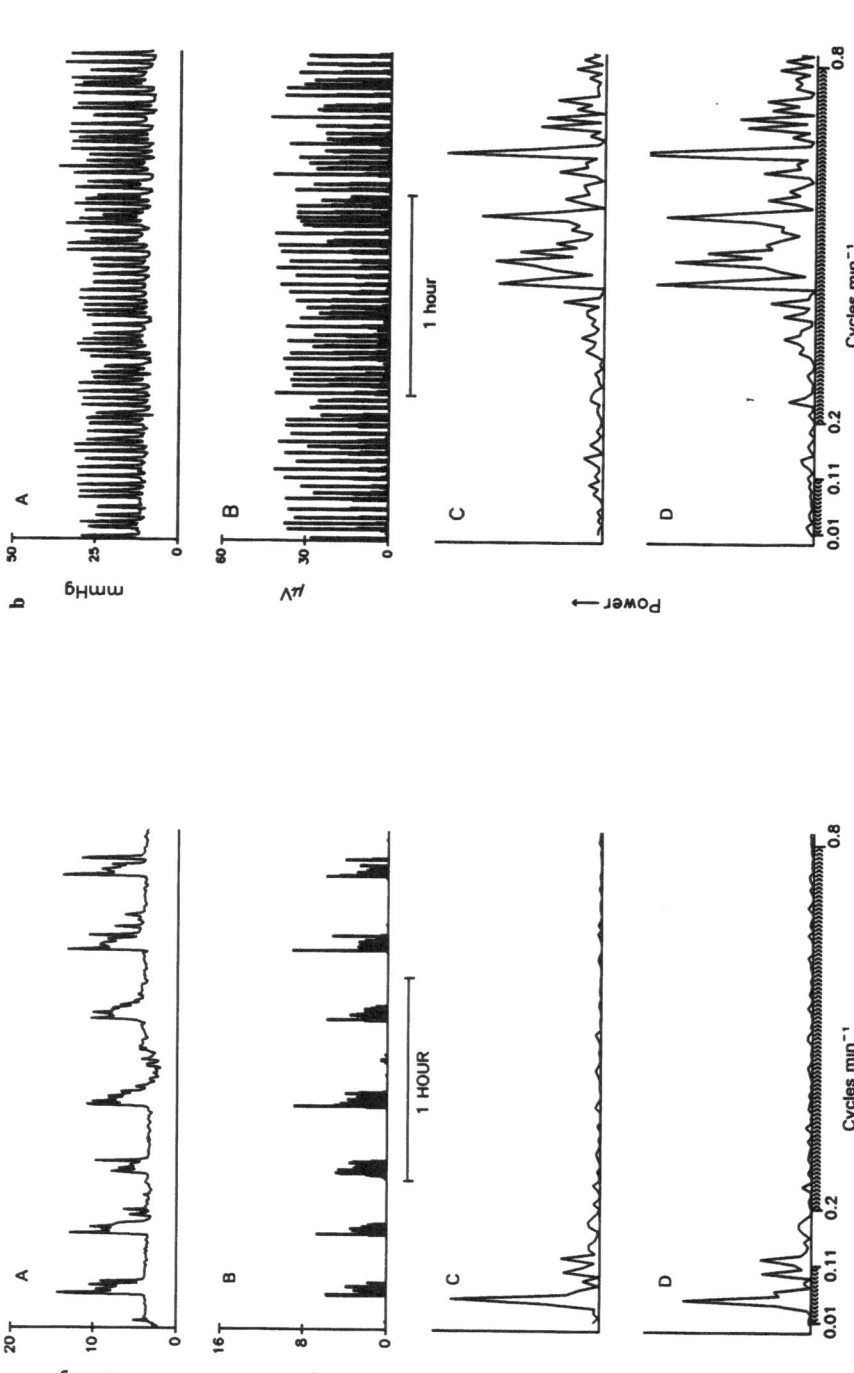

Fig. 11.2. a Contracture-type and **b** contraction-type of myometrial activity pattern in a pregnant monkey. A, Intrauterine pressure recording; calibration bar 10 mmHg. B, Myometrial electromyogram at the same time as A; calibration bar 50 μV. C, Power spectral analysis of intrauterine pressure recording in A. D, Power spectral analysis of electromyogram recording in B.

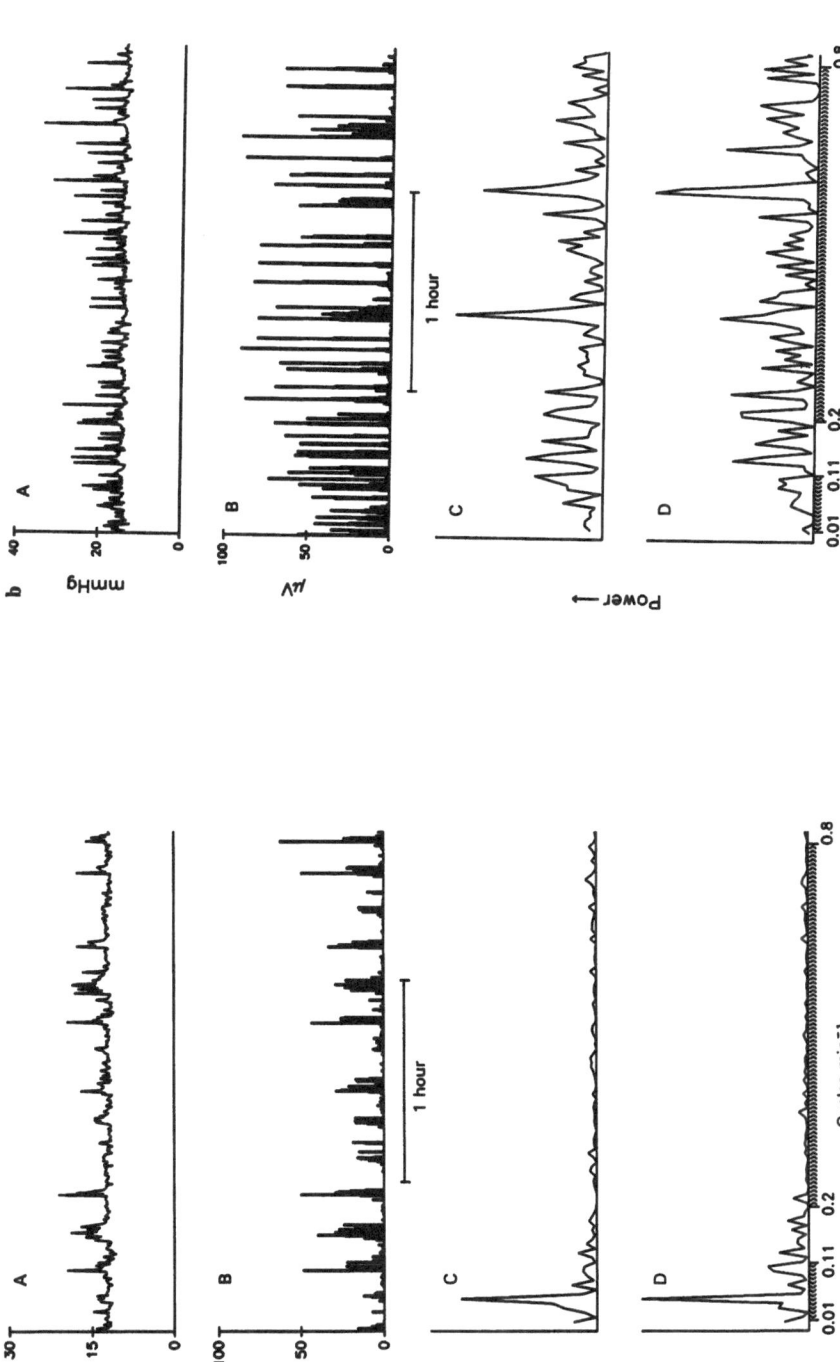

Fig. 11.3. a Contracture-type and **b** contraction-type of myometrial activity pattern in a pregnant baboon. A, Intrauterine pressure recording; calibration bar 10 mmHg. B, Myometrial electromyogram at the same time as A; calibration bar 50 µV. C, Power spectral analysis of intrauterine pressure recording in A. D, Power spectral analysis of electromyogram recording in B.

Removal of food from pregnant sheep late in gestation increases myometrial activity [15]. If pregnant sheep are deprived of food in the last week or so of pregnancy, the increased myometrial activity that occurs may lead to premature delivery. However, if the food withdrawal challenge occurs at 125–135 days of pregnancy (term 150 days), the increased contractility is solely in the form of contractures [16]. This increase in myometrial activity is accompanied by an increased production of prostaglandins by the tissues supplied by the utero-placental vascular bed [15,17]. The increased prostaglandin production can be reversed by maintaining fetal normoglycaemia in the presence of maternal hypoglycaemia indicating that the signal to increase prostaglandin production in response to food withdrawal may be of fetal origin [16,18].

Oxytocin

In pregnant sheep, contracture frequency is diminished 15%–20% by administration of oxytocin antagonists [19]. Contractures are the expression of the spontaneous contractility exhibited by all smooth muscle. The frequency and strength of this spontaneous contractility of the myometrium is probably determined by the circulating milieu of many factors including oxytocin. The extent of contracture activity will thus be influenced by circulating as well as paracrine influences. Recently, Chibbar et al. have made the interesting observation that the oxytocin gene is expressed in the decidua and fetal membranes in pregnant women [20].

Uterine Stretch

To date no systematic studies have been conducted to determine the factors that regulate contractures in pregnant non-human primates. However, it has been demonstrated that stretching the uterine cavity by the infusion of saline increases contracture frequency. If the stretch is increased contractures switch to contractions.

The Switch from Contractures to Contractions

As mentioned above, contractures are the predominant form of activity throughout the whole of pregnancy in all species studied to date. In the pregnant sheep and cow contractures normally switch to contractions only once, about six hours before delivery.

The pattern of contractures and contractions which we have observed around the time of delivery is very different in pregnant non-human primates [9]. In pregnant rhesus monkeys and baboons in which the uterine cavity is not incised at the time of instrumentation, contractures are usually the only form of myometrial activity observed throughout pregnancy right up to the time at which contractures switch to contractions a few days before delivery occurs. The first switch from

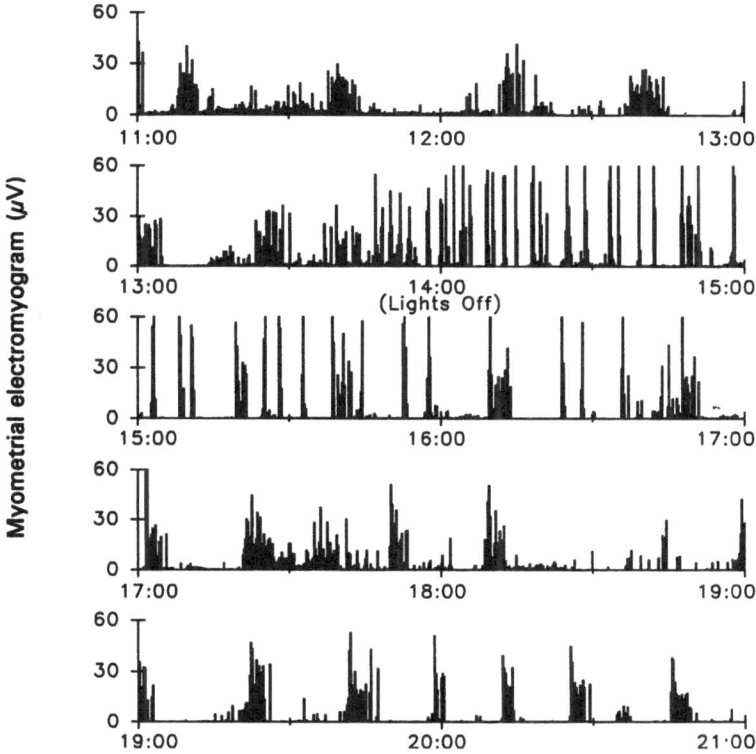

Fig. 11.4. The switch from contractures to contractions in a pregnant baboon recorded as myometrial electromyogram. Lights went off in the room at 1400 h.

contractures to contractions that precedes term labour is observed around the time the lights go off in the animal's environment and usually lasts only an hour or so before contractions switch back to contractures [9]. The switch from contractures to contractions recurs on the following and subsequent nights, each time at around the time the lights went off. On each occasion the contractions occur with greater intensity and last for a longer period of time until delivery occurs. Fig. 11.4 shows that the switch from contractures to contractions is a very dramatic event.

Is The Switch from Contractures to Contractions a True Circadian Rhythm?

Several investigators have demonstrated that there are 24 h patterns in various features of pregnancy in non-human primates. These include blood flow rhythms [21], plasma hormone concentrations [22] and myometrial contractility [9,23].

We have recently shown that this 24 h periodicity in the switch from contractures to contractions is a true circadian rhythm. In this study pregnant

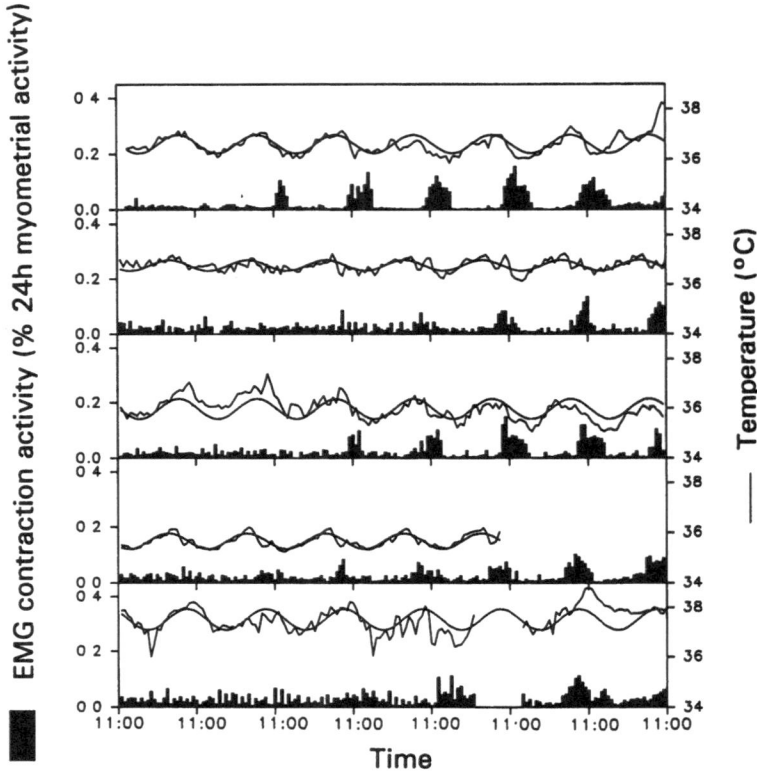

Fig. 11.5. Intra-abdominal temperature (−) and myometrial EMG activity (■) expressed as contraction activity in the power spectrum for each hour expressed as a percentage of the full 24 h day over the last 7 days before delivery in five pregnant rhesus monkeys kept at 5 lux from 61–77 days' gestation until delivery.

rhesus monkeys were maintained in a constant low-level light environment from 60 days of pregnancy until they delivered spontaneously at around 160 days [24]. These animals showed that when contractures switched to contractions they did so on a cycle that was approximately 24 h and bore a fixed phase relationship to well-known circadian rhythms such as maternal body temperature [24]. The cycle was idiosyncratic for each monkey. This was true even when pregnant monkeys were maintained in the same room in full view of each other, suggesting that the frequency was driven by an endogenous oscillator in each animal (Fig. 11.5).

Factors that Regulate the Switch from Contractures to Contractions

In studies in instrumented pregnant rhesus monkeys we have demonstrated that contractures switch to contractions in several situations.

1. Major surgery involving uterine incision and manipulations
2. Administration of pulses of oxytocin to the mother at any time during pregnancy
3. Infusions of androgens into the maternal circulation to produce an increase in plasma oestrogen concentrations in the mother
4. The stress of food withdrawal from the pregnant monkey which is also accompanied by an increase in maternal oestrogen
5. The stress of maternal haemorrhage
6. Normal term labour and delivery
7. Following the administration of endotoxin to monkeys in which the fetus had been removed but the placenta left in situ for other experiments

What Factors are Responsible for the Periodicity of the Switch?

Rhythms in Maternal and Fetal Steroid Hormones

Marked 24 h rhythms have been demonstrated in circulating concentrations of cortisol, androgens, oestrogens and progesterone in both the pregnant rhesus monkey and baboon [22,25]. It is likely that the changes in these hormones play an important role in regulating the recurring switch from contractures to contractions. It is not possible to deduce a causal relationship from temporal relationships. However, the production of oestrogens probably plays an important role in the periodicity of this myometrial switch. The evidence for this conclusion comes from studies in which it has been possible to inhibit the postsurgical myometrial contractions by administration of the aromatase inhibitor 4-hydroxyandrostenedione [26] or conversely to precipitate the switch by intravenous administration of androstenedione to pregnant rhesus monkeys to stimulate oestrogen production [27].

Oestrogens are powerful stimulants of contraction activity in the myometrium of non-pregnant ewes [28]. The timing of the tides of oestrogen in the peripheral blood to changes in myometrial contractility must be approached with caution. If the actions of oestrogens are systemic, e.g. alterations of oxytocin secretion, then consideration of the peripheral blood changes will be of importance. If the significant changes are due to altered production of oestrogens within the placenta and fetal membranes then the time relationships may well be obscured. It should be noted that oestrogens can produce genomic changes within a matter of minutes [29].

Progesterone may also play a role in the changing patterns of myometrial activity. Recent studies using the progesterone receptor blocker RU 486 in the pregnant rhesus monkey suggest that whereas myometrial activity increases following RU 486 administration, the predominant form of activity is of the contractures type [30].

Glucocorticoids have been implicated as regulators of prostaglandin synthesis.

Some studies have shown that glucocorticoids will stimulate and others that they will inhibit prostaglandin production [31,32].

Changes in Sensitivity of the Myometrium

We have demonstrated a change in sensitivity of the pregnant rhesus monkey myometrium to oxytocin pulses administered at different times of the day [33] (Fig. 11.6). Myometrial sensitivity is greatest in the early hours of darkness. We have also shown that a similar 24 h variability occurs in sensitivity of the pregnant human myometrium to oxytocin in the last few weeks of pregnancy [34]. These observations suggest that one of the critical factors in the 24 h rhythmicity of the switch from contractures to contractions is the change in myometrial sensitivity to oxytocin or some other uterotonin. This change in sensitivity may be related to the tides in plasma concentrations of maternal hormones, particularly oestrogens.

Oxytocin is the most potent uterotonic agent currently available. Receptors for oxytocin exist both on the endometrium and the myometrium [35]. At the cellular level, oxytocin acts by increasing intracellular inositol phosphates [36] and increasing the intracellular free calcium [37]. In pregnant non-human primates pulses of oxytocin switch contractures to contractions when administered during the second half of pregnancy [33]. It is interesting to note that large doses of oxytocin administered to pregnant sheep at the same stage of gestation only give rise to contractures. This response pattern is consistently maintained until a few hours before delivery, when the sensitivity of the myometrium is increased and a contraction response is obtained.

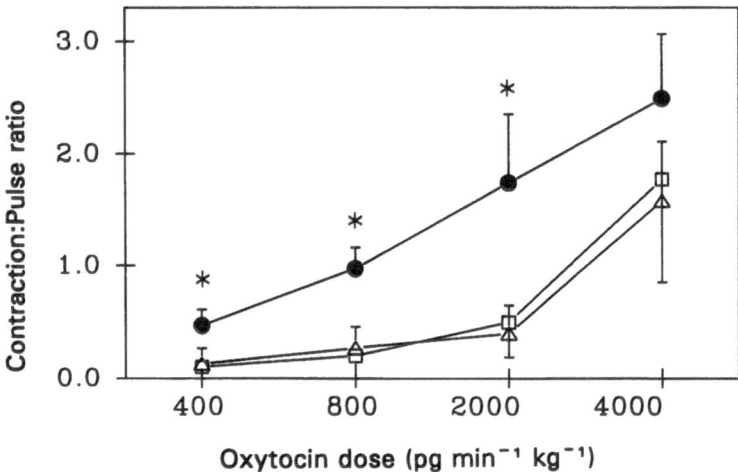

Fig. 11.6. Contraction to pulse ratio for oxytocin challenge in which one pulse of oxytocin at the dose given (abscissa) was administered to the pregnant monkey over one minute every five minutes. After six pulses, the dose was increased. The oxytocin challenge was conducted at night-time (●), in the afternoon (△) and the morning (□); mean ± SD for five animals. *$P<0.05$ compared with the other two times of the day.

Rhythms in Maternal Oxytocin Physiology

A well-defined 24 h pattern has been shown in circulating plasma concentrations of oxytocin in the later stages of pregnancy in the monkey. The peaks of plasma oxytocin concentration correspond well to the time of the switch from contractures to contractions. The possibility that these changes in maternal plasma oxytocin play a role in the periodicity of the switch from contractures to contractions is supported by studies in which oxytocin antagonists have successfully inhibited the switch [38,39]. The rhythm in influence of oxytocin on the pregnant myometrium may be regulated at two levels. First, by maternal oestrogens acting at the hypothalamic level to regulate oxytocin secretion, and second at the level of the myometrium by increasing the level of oxytocin receptors.

Use of Oxytocin Antagonists to Inhibit the Switch from Contractures to Contractions

Recently there has been much interest in the potential of various oxytocin antagonists to reduce myometrial contractility with a view to their use in the treatment of premature labour [40]. We have been particularly interested in the ability of oxytocin antagonists to reverse the switch from contractures to contractions. The first antagonist used was a vasotocin analogue kindly synthesised by Dr Jean Rivier [39]. Two other oxytocin antagonists, a compound ZK 139 (Schering) and Atosiban (Ortho), will inhibit the switch from contractures to contractions in various situations in which the switch has occurred. These agents have great potential in returning the myometrial contractile pattern from a contraction type pattern to contractures (Fig. 11.7).

The efficacy of oxytocin antagonists in regulating myometrial contractility in any particular physiological or pathological situation presumably depends on the extent of the role of oxytocin receptors in the stimulation of the increased contractility at that specific time. One initial and somewhat restricted experience is that oxytocin antagonists have limited effectiveness in controlling the contractions that occur following intrauterine surgery (unpublished observation). Atosiban was, however, very effective in controlling the contractions that occurred apparently randomly and infrequently in the early hours of darkness in pregnant baboons (Fig. 11.7). Surprisingly, Atosiban also had an inhibitory effect in one fetectomized rhesus monkey in which myometrial activity was increased by the administration of endotoxin though it did not have any effect in another fetectomized monkey similarly treated with endotoxin. Clearly if oxytocin antagonists are to be used effectively in the treatment of premature labour, then we must know more about the factors that have caused the switch from contractures to contractions in each of the several different situations that may precipitate premature labour. Oxytocin antagonists may have an important role to play in the regulation of the switch from contractures to contractions [38,39]. Although studies in the human clinical situation are promising, control patients must be included for full evaluation. In addition, more knowledge is required of the interactions of oxytocin with other uterotonins such as prostaglandins.

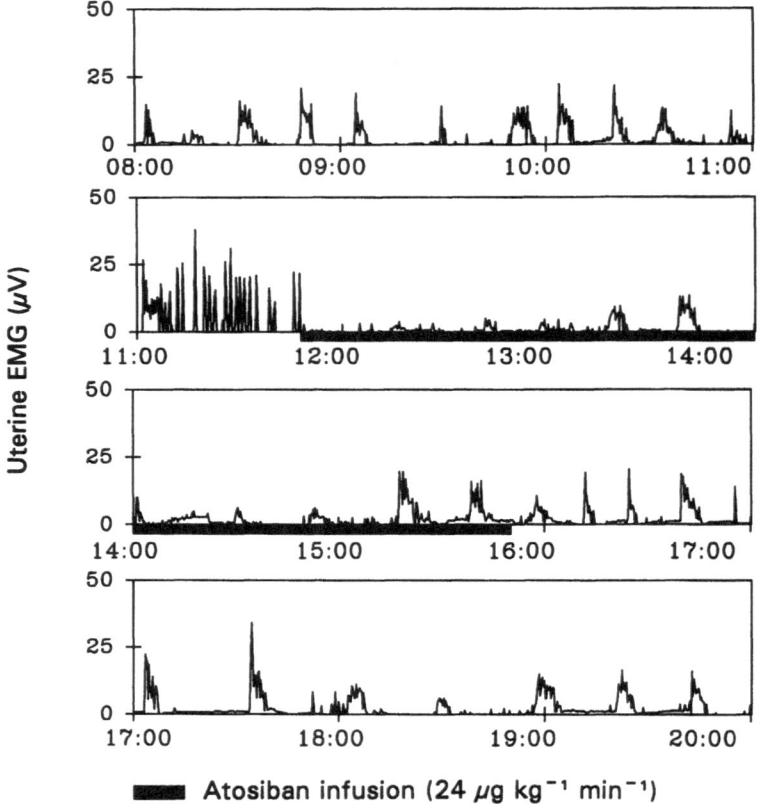

Fig. 11.7. The effect of Atosiban (24 μg kg^{-1} min^{-1}) administered i.v. to a pregnant baboon, 1 h after uterine activity had switched from contractures to contractions.

Oestrogens

We have demonstrated that contractures switch to contractions in several different physiological situations in which oestrogens are elevated: postsurgery [9]; following administration of androgens to increase endogenous oestrogen production [27]; during food withdrawal [16]; and prior to delivery [9].

Prostaglandins

One of the central issues regarding the mechanism of action of any uterotonic agent is whether the uterotonin in question plays a role in initiating the switch from contractures to contractions in any physiological or pathological condition. It is important to distinguish actions that initiate this switch from those that support the process of labour once it has begun. To date all the data available support a role for prostaglandins in normal term labour that is purely supportive. In situations such as infection, however, cytokine stimulation of prostaglandin production may be central to the switch from contractures to contractions that occurs under these conditions [41,42].

Progesterone

Progesterone is classically considered to be a restraining influence on myometrial contractility. In certain species progesterone block is considered to be one of the major factors in maintaining pregnancy. In these species, such as sheep, there is a clear and pronounced progesterone withdrawal at the time of labour and delivery. In pregnant women there is no equivalent withdrawal of progesterone from the peripheral plasma. It is uncertain whether local changes in progesterone within uterine tissues may play a role. Administration of the progesterone receptor blocker RU486 induces myometrial activity in pregnant rhesus monkeys but the pattern of activity differs from term labour and the cervix fails to dilate [30]. Thus delivery in human pregnancy may not require withdrawal of progesterone and parturition may consist simply of an increase in activity of factors which stimulate the myometrium without the necessity for a decrease in factors that inhibit myometrial activity. Clearly the overall activity of the myometrium will depend on the balance of stimulatory and inhibitory factors. One issue that comparative studies in different animals clearly demonstrate is that the myometrium of primates is very much more sensitive to changes in the environment than the myometrium of sheep and other ruminant species. Thus, in pregnant primates, the elements of progesterone block can apparently be easily overcome.

How Can an Understanding of Patterns of Myometrial Activity Assist in the Management of the Problems of Labour?

Several groups of researchers have demonstrated 24 h rhythms in myometrial activity during pregnancy in non-human primates. The study of these rhythms benefits from careful attention to the type of myometrial activity, contractures or contractions, rather than a restricted analysis of the quantity of activity regardless of its quality. Contractures are innocuous in relation to the possibility of impending labour whereas the presence of contractions must always raise suspicions that delivery may be imminent. A further consideration that needs to be faced is the interpretation of data from tissues obtained from patients or experimental animals in which the exact state of activity of the myometrium is not known. Clearly changes are occurring over several days before delivery in monkeys and baboons both at term and preterm. It is important to understand the functional significance of these prodromal changes.

Summary

Parturition is a multifactorial system of interconnected positive feed-forward and negative feedback loops which occur normally according to a precise temporal sequence. It is, thus, imperative in the management of premature labour that the vicious cycle of abnormal activity be broken early. To be most effective, oxytocin antagonists should probably be administered prophylactically in women at risk if they are to be successful in inhibiting uterine contractility.

Obstetricians are familiar with patients' histories of repeated bouts of nocturnal abdominal cramps for several nights before delivery. In addition, there is a large body of data to show that the onset of the final stages of labour occurs at night [43]. It must be remembered that low level myometrial activity may not reach the level of perception. Until we have recordings of myometrial activity in pregnant women that are as precise as the EMG and IAP data obtained from monkeys and baboons the similarity between these experimental models and pregnant women will remain uncertain. However, there are many marked similarities in both the hormonal changes and chronobiology of uterine contractility of pregnant women and pregnant non-human primates. If we can understand the mechanisms that regulate the switch from contractures to contractions, we will be more able to manage many of the problems of labour, including prematurity and postmaturity.

Acknowledgements. This work was supported by a grant from the National Institute of Child Health and Human Development HD 21350. We are grateful to our many colleagues who have worked with us on the studies reported here. We would like particularly to acknowledge the design of our data acquisition systems by Dr Robin Poore, the current management of the data by Dr Richard Wentworth and help with the data analysis from Susan Jenkins. Dr Xiu-Ying Ding helped with the surgery on the monkeys and baboons that often had to take place at antisocial hours. Finally we would like to thank Drs Jorge Figueroa, Barbera Honnebier, Zbigniew Binienda and Mark Morgan for various collaborations mentioned within this chapter and Karen Moore who helped with the preparation of the manuscript.

References

1. Hicks JB, Lond MD. On the contractions of the uterus throughout pregnancy: their physiological effects and their value in the diagnosis of pregnancy. Trans Obstet Soc Lond 1872; 13:216–31.
2. Nathanielsz PW, Ratter S, Thomas AL, Rees L, Jack PMB. The role and regulation of corticotropin in the fetal sheep. In: Knight J, ed. The fetus and birth. Amsterdam: Elsevier, 1976: 73–91.
3. Taverne MAM. Myometrial activity during pregnancy and parturition in the pig. In: Cole DJA, Foxcroft GR, eds. Control of pig reproduction. London: Butterworths, 1982:419–36.
4. van der Weyden GC, Taverne MAM, Dieleman SJ, Wurth Y, Bevers MM, van Oord HA. Physiological aspects of pregnancy and parturition in dogs. J Reprod Fertil Suppl 1989; 39:211–24.
5. Dudan FE, Figueroa JP, Frank DA, Elias B, Poore ER, Lowe JE, Nathanielsz PW. Frequency distribution and daily rhythm of uterine electromyographic epochs of different duration in pony mares in late gestation. J Reprod Fertil Suppl 1987; 35:725–7.
6. Janszen BPM, Knijn H, van der Weyden GC, Bevers MM, Dieleman SJ, Taverne MAM. Flumethason-induced calving is preceded by a period of myometrial inhibition during luteolysis. Biol Reprod 1990; 43:466–71.
7. Taverne MAM, Scheerboom JEM. Myometrial electrical activity during pregnancy and parturition in the pygmy goat. Res Vet Sci 1985; 38:120–3.

8. Germain G, Cabrol D, Visser A, Sureau C. Electrical activity of the pregnant uterus in the cynomolgus monkey. Am J Obstet Gynecol 1982; 142:513–19.

9. Taylor NF, Martin MC, Nathanielsz PW, Seron-Ferre M. The fetus determines circadian oscillation of myometrial electromyographic activity in the pregnant rhesus monkey. Am J Obstet Gynecol 1983; 146:557–67.

10. Morgan MA, Silavin SL, Wentworth RA, Figueroa JP, Honnebier MBOM, Fishburne JI, Jr, Nathanielsz PW. Different patterns of myometrial activity and 24 h rhythms in myometrial contractility in the gravid baboon during the last third of pregnancy. Biol Reprod 1991.

11. Jansen CAM, Krane EJ, Thomas AL et al. Continuous variability of fetal PO_2 in the chronically catheterized fetal sheep. Am J Obstet Gynecol 1979; 134:776–83.

12. Harding R, Poore ER, Bailey A, Thorburn GD, Jansen CAM, Nathanielsz PW. Electromyographic activity of the nonpregnant sheep uterus. Am J Obstet 1982; 142:448–57.

13. Hsu HW, Figueroa JP, Honnebier MBOM, Wentworth R, Nathanielsz PW. Power spectrum analysis of myometrial electromyogram and intrauterine pressure changes in the pregnant rhesus monkey in late gestation. Am J Obstet Gynecol 1989; 161:467–73.

14. El Badry A, Figueroa JP, Poore ER, Sunderji S, Levine S, Mitchell MD, Nathanielsz PW. Effect of fetal intravascular 4-aminoantipyrine infusions on myometrial activity (contractures) at 125–143 days gestation in the pregnant sheep. Am J Obstet Gynecol 1984; 150:474–81.

15. Fowden AL, Harding R, Ralph MM, Thorburn GD. The nutritional regulation of plasma prostaglandin E concentrations in the fetus and pregnant ewe during late gestation. J Physiol 1987; 394:1–12.

16. Binienda Z, Massmann A, Mitchell MD, Gleed RD, Figueroa JP, Nathanielsz PW. The effect of food withdrawal on arterial blood glucose and plasma 13,14-dihydro-15-keto-prostaglandin $F_{2\alpha}$ (PGFM) concentrations and nocturnal myometrial electromyograph activity in the pregnant rhesus monkey in the last third of gestation: a model for preterm labor? Am J Obstet Gynecol 1988; 160:746–50.

17. Fowden AL, Silver M. The effect of the nutritional state on uterine prostaglandin F metabolite concentrations in the pregnant ewe during late gestation. Q J Exp Physiol 1983; 68:337–49.

18. Binienda Z, Rosen ED, Kelleman A, Sadowsky DW, Mitchell MD, Nathanielsz PW. Maintaining fetal normoglycemia prevents the increase in myometrial activity and uterine 13,14-dihydro-15-keto- prostaglandin $F_{2\alpha}$ production during food withdrawal in late pregnancy in the ewe. Endocrinology 1990; 127(6):307–351.

19. Owiny JR, Chavin LC, Mitchell MD, Nathanielsz PW. Effect of 48 hour infusion of oxytocin antagonist (OTA) on myometrial activity of pregnant sheep at 139 days gestation age (dGA). 38th Annual Meeting of the Society for Gynecologic Investigation. Abstract 101. 1991.

20. Chibbar R, Miller FD, Mitchell BF. Oxytocin is synthesized in human fetal membranes. 38th Annual Meeting of the Society for Gynecologic Investigation. Abstract 7. 1991.

21. Harbert GM, Croft BY, Spisso KR. Effects of biorhythms on blood flow distribution in the pregnant uterus (Macaca mulatta). Am J Obstet Gynecol 1979; 135:828–42.

22. Walsh SW, Ducsay CA, Novy MJ. Circadian hormonal interactions among the mother, fetus and amniotic fluid. Am J Obstet Gynecol 1984; 150:745–53.

23. Harbert GM, Jr, Spisso KR. Biorhythms of the primate uterus (Macaca mulatta) during labor and delivery. Am J Obstet Gynecol 1980; 138:686–96.

24. Honnebier MBOM, Jenkins SL, Wentworth RA, Figueroa JP, Nathanielsz PW. Temporal structuring of delivery in the absence of a photoperiod: preparturient myometrial activity of the rhesus monkey is related to maternal body temperature and depends on the maternal circadian system. Biol Reprod 1991; 45:617–25.

25. Wilson L, Parsons MT, Flouret G. Forward shift in the initiation of the nocturnal estradiol surge in the pregnant baboon: Is this the genesis of labor? Am J Obstet Gynecol 1991; 165:1487–98.

26. Nathanielsz PW, Poore ER, Brodie A, Taylor NF, Pimentel G, Figueroa JP, Frank D. Update on molecular events of myometrial activity during pregnancy. In: Nathanielsz PW, Parer JT, eds., Research in perinatal medicine. Ithaca NY: Perinatology Press, 19:87–111.

27. Figueroa JP, Honnebier MBOM, Binienda Z, Wimsatt J, Nathanielsz PW. Effect of 48 hour intravenous 4A androstendione infusion on the pregnant rhesus monkey in the last third of gestation: changes in maternal plasma estradiol concentrations and myometrial contractility. Am J Obstet Gynecol 1989; 161:481–6.

28. Lye SJ, Wathes DC, Porter DG. Oestradiol-17β both inhibits and stimulates myometrial activity in ewes in vivo. J Reprod Fertil 1983; 67:335–41.

29. Loose-Mitchell DS, Chiappetta C, Stancel GM. Estrogen regulation of c-fos messenger ribonucleic acid. Mol Endocrinol 1988; 2:946–51.

30. Haluska GJ, West NB, Novy MJ, Brenner RM. Uterine estrogen receptors are increased by

RU486 in late pregnant rhesus macaques but not after spontaneous labor. J Clin Endocrinol Metab 1990; 70:181–6.

31. Potestio FA, Zakar T, Olson DM. Glucocorticoids stimulate prostaglandin synthesis in human anmion cells by a receptor-mediated mechanism. J Clin Endocrinol Metab 1988; 67:1205–10.

32. Casey ML, MacDonald PC, Mitchell MD. Despite a massive increase in cortisol secretion in women during parturition, there is an equally massive increase in prostaglandin synthesis. A paradox? J Clin Invest 1985; 75:1852–7.

33. Honnebier MBOM, Figueroa JP, Nathanielsz PW. Variation in myometrial response to pulsatile intravenous oxytocin administration – a pulsatile oxytocin challenge test at different times of the day in the pregnant monkey at 121 to 138 days gestational age. Endocrinology 1989; 125:1498–503.

34. Main DM, Honnebier MBOM, Grandberry P, Reganstein A, Nathanielsz PW. The use of a pulsatile oxytocin (OT) challenge test to determine variation in myometrial response to OT at different times of day in the human at 30–40 weeks gestation. 37th Annual meeting of the Society for Gynecologic Investigation. Abstract no. 395, 1990.

35. Soloff MS. The role of oxytocin in the initiation of labor, and oxytocin–prostaglandin interactions. In: McNellis D, Challis JRG, MacDonald PC, Nathanielsz PW, Roberts JM, eds. The onset of labor: cellular and integrative mechanisms. Ithaca, NY: Perinatology Press, 1988; 87–124.

36. Marc S, Leiber D, Harbon S. Carbachol and oxytocin stimulate the generation of inositol phosphates in guinea pig myometrium. FEBS Lett 1986; 201:9–14.

37. Anwer K, Hovington JA, Sanborn BM. Antagonism of contractants and relaxants at the level of intracellular calcium and phosphoinositide turnover in the rat uterus. Endocrinology 1989; 124:2995–3002.

38. Wilson L, Jr, Parsons MT, Flouret G. Inhibition of spontaneous uterine contractions during the last trimester in pregnant baboons by an oxytocin antagonist. Am J Obstet Gynecol 1990; 163:1875–82.

39. Honnebier MBOM, Figueroa JP, Rivier J, Vale W, Nathanielsz PW. Studies on the role of oxytocin in late pregnancy in the pregnant rhesus monkey (I): plasma concentrations of oxytocin in the maternal circulation throughout the 24 h day and the effect of the synthetic oxytocin antagonist [1-β- Mpa (β-(CH2)5)1,) Me)Tyr2,Orn8] OT on spontaneous nocturnal myometrial contractions. J Dev Physiol 1989; 12:225–33.

40. Akerlund M, Stromberg P, Hauksson A, Anderson LF, Lyndrup J, Trojnar J, Melin P. Inhibition of uterine contractions of premature labour with an oxytocin analogue. Results from a pilot study. Br J Obstet Gynaecol 1987; 94:1040–4.

41. Romero R, Avila C, Brekus CA, Mazor M. The role of systemic and intrauterine infection in preterm parturition. In: Garfield RE, ed. Uterine contractility. Norwell, MA: Serono Symposia, USA, 1990; 319–53.

42. Romero R, Emamian M, Wan M, Grzyboski C, Hobbins JC, Mitchell MD. Increased concentrations of arachidonic acid lipoxygenase metabolites in amniotic fluid during parturition. Obstet Gynecol 1987; 70:849–51.

43. Malek J. The manifestation of biological rhythms in delivery. Gynaecologia 1952; 133:365–72.

Discussion

Elder: We have had two interesting and contrasting chapters which illustrate the point that biochemistry and physiology need to be considered in parallel and not separately.

Lumsden: What happens to these monkeys' sleep patterns when they are kept on constant light?

Nathanielsz: I could not answer that but it is an extraordinarily good question. We have no method of monitoring those sleep patterns. My colleague says that she does go in there and finds them asleep, but we have not monitored them in any great detail. My gut reaction is that they would retain some sort of rhythm in their sleep patterns.

Lumsden: That might possibly be related to some change in the activity.

Nathanielsz: The current thinking about circadian rhythms is that they are driven by the endogenous oscillator in the suprachiasmatic nucleus, which presumably drives the temperature, the blood pressure and the sleep/wakefulness patterns. I would imagine that they would still have the same rhythms.

Greer: Anecdotally, obstetric residents will report that at two o'clock in the morning three or four women will come into the labour ward in labour; some of them settle and some do not. Is there any objective evidence in the human as to timing of parturition or pseudo-parturition? The impression of those who are still on the "shop floor" in obstetrics is that they occur after the hours of darkness.

Nathanielsz: I know of no objective evidence. I would love to have some monitor. One of my goals is to try and find some monitor of myometrial activity in pregnancy which is slightly better than the tocodynamometer. I realise that I cannot leave in intra-amniotic pressure catheters from 30 weeks: that would be a nice way of doing it but there is a slight risk of infection. I do not think anybody has objective data.

Husslein: The switch from contracture to contraction was well described. I believe there is another switch that is very relevant in clinics: the switch from those contractions a couple of days before delivery to much the same type of contractions that suddenly lead to delivery. We see it in the clinics. In premature labour the labour patterns are similar, with contractions that do not lead to premature delivery and then much the same pattern that suddenly leads to premature delivery.

What governs the switch from contractions that do not lead to cervical dilatation to the same contractions that lead to cervical dilatation?

Nathanielsz: I do not know. I always think of Leger's experiments with the sheep in Oxford and Michael Hollingsworth's with the rat, where if the cervix is isolated from the uterus, the cervix still softens and dilates. To some extent they are almost two separate issues. There can be good uterine contractions for several days but it is only after five or six days that the cervix begins to dilate.

Rådestad: Was there any change in the behaviour of these monkeys when they changed from contracture to contraction? And what about their awareness of pain?

Nathanielsz: That is related to the last question. My colleague observes them very much more closely than I do and may be able to give a better answer. When I have watched them on those four or five nights – the prodromal nights – they do not seem to have any behavioural changes or give any outward expression of pain. But on the last night they do. There is something different on that night when they eventually go into labour and when the cervix dilates.

Lopez-Bernal: From a therapeutic point of view, the difficulty of treating preterm labour is that it is difficult to predict. There are systems, quite popular in America, that measure contractility: one can ring in and find out what is happening. If we had a way of measuring contractility accurately, would that be the best predictor for preterm labour?

Nathanielsz: It would not be the best predictor. Our monkeys are a very heterogeneous group and the more we look at them the more we find. We have one now that, probably like some patients, is throwing bouts of contractions. She is about 30 days away from delivery, and one night she will have some contractions and the next night she will not. She has been doing this for two or three weeks. She is like some of the preterm labour patients who go on to deliver at term, which is fully what I expect her to do. Having a hard copy readout of what the equivalent patient could be doing could hardly be anything but useful.

What treatments might one use? This is the opportunity for me to say that I really do believe that oxytocin antagonists have a real role to play. Even though this is a Study Group on prostaglandins, one is entitled to talk about oxytocin because, as we have seen, oxytocin works and one of its mechanisms is probably working through PGs. We have had a lot of success stopping these early prodromal contractions with oxytocin antagonists and there is a trial currently ongoing in the United States. But if they are used in clinical practice, in my view they have to be used prophylactically. We get a lot of this activity postsurgery and oxytocin antagonists will not touch it. When the monkey is on the fourth or the fifth day of the switch, the oxytocin antagonists will not touch it. I presume that is because now she is generating a lot of endogenous prostaglandins. If oxytocin antagonists are ever to have any use – and I was asked what I would recommend as a way of stopping the switch – then that form of therapy should be used prophylactically and might be very efficacious.

Greer: Could the oxytocin concept be an epi-phenomenon and not at all related to labour? I accept that oxytocin induces uterine contractility and we use it effectively, but is that really why oxytocin is there physiologically? Surely it is there for purposes of lactation and we are utilising a side effect of its lactational effects on the uterus.

It could be that the data we saw with the pulses relate to an endogenous central force of oxytocin which is designed for postpartum use, for uterine retraction and for breastfeeding, and that what we are seeing is an epi-phenomenon in the uterus. The switch then comes about, and the uterus switches on its own contraction system, stimulating labour. We could equally well measure the intramammary pressure and probably get the same pulses.

Nathanielsz: Which is what Dr Olson's first slide showed. We have got to consider the factors that prepare the uterus and have it in a responsive mode.

I do not totally understand what an epi-phenomenon is. It is a marvellous word. Professor Greer might be suggesting, as many others have done, that oxytocin is a supportive feature once things start. Oxytocin physiology is a graveyard of scientific reputations. Oestrogens stimulate oxytocin release. Oestrogens stimulate oxytocin receptors. Uterine contractility stimulates oxytocin release by the Ferguson reflex. Oxytocin stimulates prostaglandin production. It is very difficult to take the whole thing apart and find out where it starts.

My view is that if we look in the monkey and the baboon, we get this nice gentle rise in oestrogens over the last 10 or 15 days and I think that is preparing the whole system. That indeed may be why stimulating an increase in oxytocin receptors starts off a response to oxytocin, even if the concentration does not rise, by stimulating prostaglandin synthesis. But then what is the evidence that oestrogens stimulate PG synthesis? It may be tissue specific. Are we looking in the right tissues?

I certainly cannot discount oxytocin as playing a role, so I would not consider it an epi-phenomenon in the sense that I understand the word. Whether it is the signal to labour and to switch from contractures to contractions, I do not know at this stage.

Smith: Is it not true that another group of workers are also using the oxytocin antagonist and getting a reduction in uterine contractions? The responses in the human are similar.

The second point about oxytocin is that data from Canada presented this year suggest that it is synthesised and released locally within the decidua.

Third, oxytocin in vasopressin is linked to a phospholipase C so to dissociate that out of the mechanism of PGs seems to be extremely complicated and extremely difficult.

Does anyone know what promotor sequences are present in the upstream 5' end of the cyclo-oxygenase? If I am right, that would explain many of the phenomena that were described.

Olson: If those data are known they are very new and I am not aware of them.

Nathanielsz: As somebody who works with the sheep and the non-human primate and does so intentionally, I am often forced to focus my attention on the differences between these two species. When we look at the results we are finding with cortisol inhibiting amniotic PG synthesis, then that is human amnion not sheep.

One of the interesting things here is the difference between the way the fetus initiates these systems. I am a firm believer that the work in the sheep will translate to the human. I know that some obstetricians feel that the human fetus does not have the same regulation over initiation of term labour as the sheep does; I feel very strongly that it does, but in a different way. Whereas the fetal sheep secretes a lot of cortisol which goes to the placenta and stimulates the cascade of enzyme productions, in the human and in the non-human primate it is androgen. Those changes in the placental tissue are not cortisol-driven in the human.

Olson: Dehydroepiandrosterone had no effect on the amnion production of prostaglandin in the way that we did it.

This whole oestrogen issue is one that needs more examination. No one has described the mechanism of oestrogen action in increasing prostaglandin synthesis. There have been examples in the literature of oestrogens driving prostaglandin synthesis but the mechanism is still undefined.

The possibility of looking at other tissues was mentioned. The decidua might be another target tissue that needs to be more closely examined. I published a paper a few years ago saying that oestradiol 17β and catechol oestrogen did increase prostaglandin coming from the decidua and inhibit prostacyclin production from that tissue as well. We need to look at mechanisms, but we did not try to define the mechanism in that paper.

As to the cortisol action, we find it to be a dichotomy. On the one hand we have always thought that increasing cortisol from the fetus might lead to prostaglandin synthesis ultimately, and yet our data suggest that perhaps it inhibits, and that the block is not a complete block. And there are other things that fetal cortisol might be doing which we may have to look at. For instance, cortisol could be maturing – as we all know, it matures fetal lungs. Dr Lopez-Bernal has indicated that surfactant coming from the fetal lungs through the amniotic fluid stimulates amnion prostaglandin synthesis, so this might be an indirect way in which cortisol has an effect. Also, there is evidence from more than one laboratory suggesting that cortisol might be able to mature the paracrine communication system within the fetal membranes and the decidua. In particular, it increases the levels of corticotropin releasing factor (CRF) that are found in the chorion and the CRF from these tissues can stimulate prostaglandin synthesis from amnion.

The third thing that cortisol might be doing is acting as a brake. It is not a complete inhibitor of PG synthesis but it might be a brake which prevents lesser stimuli from eliciting preterm birth when some other agonist effector comes along.

Kelly: Some studies have shown that if epostane is added to a preparation of antiprogestin in the guinea pig, then instead of working together, the inability of the antiprogestin is lost. The antiprogestin in question, OK98735, does not have very good anticorticoid activities and induces labour quite well on its own. Adding that with epostane reduces the activity to a baseline of almost zero. The author's interpretation of this is that it is an inhibition of oestrogen synthesis, so removing the ability to produce oestrogen removes the trigger mechanism. It does not affect the ripening, the increase in sensitivity, but it does remove the trigger mechanism.

Can I ask about cortisol? Is there any evidence whether cortisol, or even progesterone for that matter, changes the stability of the message of cyclo-oxygenase?

Olson: We have not done those experiments.

Kelly: Is it possible that cortisol could be acting as an antiprogestin in some circumstances? In the sheep, for instance?

Olson: That possibility exists. We have used RU486 in various circumstances and in one instance it seems to act as a blocker of glucocorticoid receptors and in another it seems to act as a corticoid agonist. So that possibility is certainly within the realm of reality.

Nathanielsz: In the whole organism there is a very interesting relationship of cortisol and progesterone insofar as they displace from the binding protein. But that is at a different level.

Chapter 12

Prostaglandins for Induction of Labour

P. Husslein

Improved diagnosis of possible intrauterine fetal risks and also the development of more effective and less hazardous methods of induction of labour have considerably enlarged the range of indications for premature termination of pregnancy in recent years. Table 12.1 gives a summary of the causes for premature termination of pregnancy accepted today, divided into maternal and fetal causes. Since induction of labour represents an interference in a natural process, such an indication is mandatory.

Table 12.1. Indications for induction of labour [12]

Maternal indications
Preeclampsia
Diabetes mellitus
Pyelonephritis
Premature rupture of the membranes
Other diseases of the mother

Fetal indications
Chronic placental insufficiency
Fetal growth retardation
Rh-incompatibility
Prolonged gestation
Diabetes-related fetopathy
Chorioamnionitis

The effectiveness of induction of labour depends predominantly on the duration of pregnancy and the cervical state [1–3], both of which correlate with the sensitivity of the myometrium towards labour-inducing agents [4,5]. When labour is induced prematurely or at a time when the cervix is not ripe, the rate of failure or surgical delivery is high and, moreover, labour is frequently protracted. Therefore, the criteria for patient selection in such cases must be very strict. On the other hand, a high success rate may be expected when the condition for induction is favourable, occasionally duration of labour may even be reduced and there will hardly be any inconvenience for the pregnant woman. In such cases the wishes expressed by the pregnant woman and her husband should be taken into consideration, even when there are no clear-cut medical indications.

In all cases, induction of labour requires information about the family concerned as well as careful evaluation of the basic obstetric situation (external clinical examination, cardiotocography, assessment of the cervical score). When the duration of pregnancy is not clear, labour should be initiated only in cases of maternal or fetal emergency in order to avoid problems with fetal maturity, in particular pulmonary maturity.

In principle there are no specific contraindications to induction of labour apart from an existing contraindication to vaginal delivery. However, if the fetal risk is very high and the conditions are very unfavourable for induction, primary surgical delivery should be preferred.

Every induction of labour leads to an at-risk labour, which requires intensive obstetric monitoring. The extent of monitoring will depend on the individual clinical case, but in all cases labour may only be induced under clinical observation in a hospital.

Methods of Induction of Labour

Apart from mechanical manoeuvres such as detaching the inferior pole of the fetal membranes during vaginal examination and artificial rupture of the membranes, the most widespread methods are the use of the labour-inducing hormones oxytocin and prostaglandins (PG). Since it has been shown that all manipulations of the cervix including artificial rupture of the membranes act only via endogenous prostaglandin synthesis [6] and that direct administration of PGE is possible, mechanical measures should play only a subordinate role; in particular because early rupture of the membranes may lead to an adverse pressure of time during the further course of labour [7].

Appreciation of the complex mechanism of childbirth makes it obvious that induction of labour shortly before the onset of spontaneous labour, i.e. at term or near term, when the cervix is ready for delivery, is more promising and associated with fewer complications than early induction long before term, when the cervix is not yet ripe. Therefore, these two clinical situations must be strictly differentiated.

Induction of Labour in Women with a Favourable Cervical Score

In such a clinical situation we may assume that the natural ripening processes are about to be completed so that there is a high susceptibility to labour-inducing agents. Until recently, oxytocin was the classical labour-inducing agent.

An intravenous infusion of a solution of 5 IU oxytocin in 500 ml 5%–10% glucose solution is recommended. When the cervix is favourable (and susceptibility to oxytocin is high), doses between 2 and 10 mIU/min will be sufficient to induce and maintain labour.

Understanding the mechanism of labour leads to the conclusion that oxytocin should be administered only for induction of labour at full term when the cervix is favourable – at a time when a sufficient number of oxytocin receptors is assumed to be available in the myometrium [8].

In view of the circumstances (e.g. infusion, confinement to bed) which frequently conflict with the wish of the mother for childbirth to be as natural as possible, induction with oxytocin should only be carried out when there is a definite medical indication. In such cases the pregnant woman will usually understand the technical facilities necessary in view of a special medical risk.

In the 1970s the era of prostaglandins in obstetrics began. Prostaglandins are hormones central to the human mechanism of labour [9]. They lead to myometrial contractions and to a series of biochemical effects on the uterine cervix leading to an increase in cervical compliance and they induce "gap junctions" (intermyometrial cell connections apparently necessary for the propagation of coordinated myometrial contractions [10]), effects that go together ideally to expel the fetus [5,11] (Fig. 12.1)

Twenty years of use have allowed basic rules for the use of prostaglandins for induction of labour to be developed [12].

1. As synthetic prostaglandin derivatives with a longer half-life would be expected to reduce the controllability of induction of labour and since

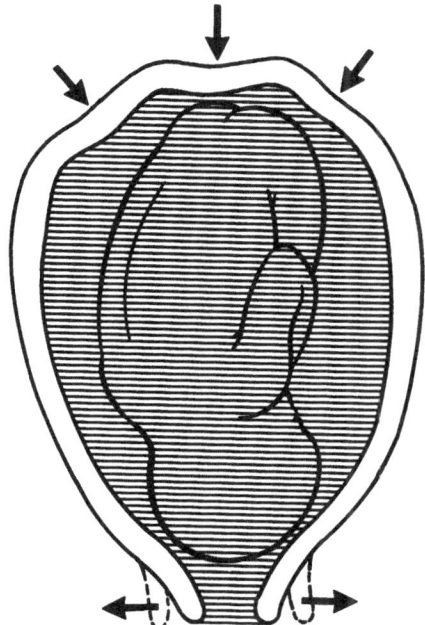

Fig. 12.1. Effects of prostaglandins on the pregnant uterus.

prostaglandins passing into the fetus could cause side effects in the fetus, only natural prostaglandins should be used for induction of labour with a living fetus.

2. Prostaglandins should be applied locally in order to exert maximal local and reduced systemic effects [13,14].

3. Since PGE_2 exerts a stronger effect on the cervical region and its superiority is supported by clinical evidence [15], it should be preferred to $PGF_{2\alpha}$ for cervical ripening or induction of labour.

4. Account must be taken of the marked increase of prostaglandin sensitivity during the course of pregnancy. Consequently, induction regimens for the third trimester and for delivery at or after term are not transferable to earlier periods of pregnancy.

5. Regimens for induction of labour must consider the pharmaceutical characteristics of prostaglandin preparations. Absorption from PGE_2-containing gel, for example, is much faster than absorption from ovules or tablets.

Intravaginal application of a tablet containing 3 mg PGE_2 or a gel with 2 mg PGE_2 has become generally accepted for induction of labour when the cervix is favourable [16–18].

If labour is induced by intravaginal application of a tablet containing 3 mg PGE_2, the tablet is placed into the posterior vaginal fornix during a vaginal examination (Fig. 12.2). The patient may get up immediately afterwards. Because of the delayed absorption labour occurs 2–3 h later, and it is recommended that a first routine cardiotocograph is performed after about 2 h or when the patient experiences back pain or labour pains. Application of another tablet after an interval of 6–12 h depending on the clinical situation may be appropriate.

Comparative studies of induction of labour with PGE_2 and oxytocin in favourable cervical states have shown that although the interval between induction and delivery is shorter when oxytocin is used, overall the two

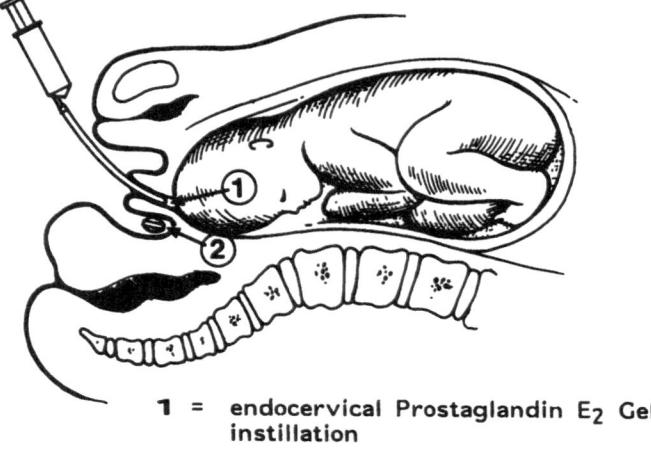

1 = endocervical Prostaglandin E_2 Gel instillation

2 = intravaginal Prostaglandin E_2 tablet insertion

Fig. 12.2. Schematic representation of anatomically correct instillation of the PGE_2-containing gel (1) and application of the PGE_2 vaginal tablet (2)

Table 12.2. Induction of labour at term: Possibilities in patients with favourable cervical states [12]

	Effectiveness	Fine control	Acceptance
Oxytocin IV	++	+	–
Prostaglandin E_2 vaginal tablet	++	–	+

procedures are medically equivalent. However, the acceptance of the prostaglandin tablet is considerably higher, because the pregnant woman remains mobile [12,16,18] (Table 12.2).

A special advantage of induction of labour by means of vaginal application of a tablet is the short interval between rupture of the membranes and delivery. This may be expected to reduce the rate of infection. Moreover several studies have also indicated (though without any control group) that the rate of surgical intervention in delivery has been reduced since the introduction of vaginal application of prostaglandin [16,18]. Since application of prostaglandin tablets in patients with favourable cervical states is a safe and effective procedure (hyperstimulations were reported, but are extremely rare [19]) patient selection in such cases can be more liberal after appropriate information has been given to the pregnant women. In this connection it was demonstrated that induction of labour with a vaginal PGE_2 tablet at full term, when there are no risks and the cervical score is favourable, is at least equivalent to supervised waiting for spontaneous onset of labour, so that the situation offers the opportunity of complying with the wishes of the patient and involving her in the decision-making process [20].

Induction of Labour in Women with an Unfavourable Cervical Score

Induction of labour in patients with unfavourable cervical states is associated with a higher failure rate, more complications and a higher incidence of protracted labour and thus is a far more crucial interference with the natural course of childbirth (Table 12.3). For these reasons and since labour is initiated before full term in most of these cases, the procedure requires a much stricter patient selection.

If parturition were initiated in patients with unfavourable cervical states by induction of labour alone, there would be an associated high rate of cervical dystocia, long duration of labour, maternal exhaustion and quite often fetal

Table 12.3. Induction of labour at term: Possibilities in patients with unfavourable cervical states [12]

	Effectiveness	Controllability	Risk potential	General side effects	Acceptance
Prostaglandin (gel intracervical)	+++	–	++	–	+
Prostaglandin (vaginal tablet)	++	–	+++	–	++
Prostaglandin (i.v.)	+	++	+	+++	–
Oxytocin (i.v.)	(+)	+++	+	–	–

distress. Therefore, cervical priming is – at least theoretically – appropriate in order to reduce cervical resistance and to mimic the course of events programmed by nature before the onset of spontaneous labour.

After initial studies with the extra-amniotic approach [2] endocervical instillation of 0.5 mg PGE_2-containing gel has been found to be the method of choice because the risk of infection is lower than with extra-amniotic application and the cervical changes can be induced – at least theoretically – without myometrial stimulation [21–24] (Fig. 12.2). At 12–24 h after prostaglandin application, an intravenous infusion of oxytocin may follow in order to induce labour when the cervix has reached a favourable state. However, depending on the duration of pregnancy and the cervical score, a single PGE_2 instillation is followed by regular contractions and progressive dilatation of the cervix either subsequent to or simultaneously with cervical ripening in 30%–60% of cases [2,25–27].

Special Features and Complications of Induction of Labour with Prostaglandins

Spontaneous rupture of the membranes is in principle not a contraindication to local application of PGE_2 [28]. Especially in unfavourable cervical states the success rate of induction of labour may be considerably increased by endocervical instillation of a PGE_2 gel [29]. The theoretically increased risk of infection does not appear to play a role here. When vaginal preparations are used, however, account must be taken of the fact that a change in the local physiological condition of the vagina by the leaking of amniotic fluid may lead to increased absorption of PGE_2.

A previous delivery by caesarean section is not a contraindication to induction of labour with prostaglandins, but such an induction should be performed only when there is a definite indication for it and strict monitoring is guaranteed. It was demonstrated that local application of PGE_2 gel markedly reduced the rate of new caesarean sections [30]. Simultaneous administration of oxytocin and prostaglandins frequently leads to hyperstimulation due to an increase of oxytocin sensitivity caused by prostaglandin and should be strictly avoided. Therefore, no oxytocin should be given, until at least 6 h after the last prostaglandin application. Despite this precaution, hyperstimulation may occur when one of the labour-inducing agents is used alone [19]. At least intermittent cardiotocographic monitoring is therefore imperative in any induction of labour. In particular, local application of PGE_2 in unfavourable cervical states may lead in up to 10% of cases to uterine contractions of high frequency and usually low amplitude, which mostly do not contribute to the progress of birth. Such hyperstimulation seems to occur more frequently if prostaglandins are applied into the extra-amniotic space. Therefore strict endocervical administration is recommended. Treatment of such hyperstimulation episodes is determined mainly by the fetal cardiogram. If there are no signs of hypoxia, a wait-and-see policy should be adopted; in most cases contractions will soon change to a pattern characterised by normal frequency, high amplitude and low basal tone. If fetal decelerations occur however, action must be taken depending on the clinical situation. Amniotomy may lead to normalisation of the pathological cardiotoco-gram, but if amniotomy is undesirable from a clinical point of view, intravenous administration of a betamimetic drug (e.g. slow intravenous infusion of 10 mg hexoprenaline or 20 mg fenoterol) will always interrupt the hyperkinetic labour pattern at least for a short period of time (Fig. 12.3). A single intravenous dose is frequently sufficient; only rarely will a continuous intravenous infusion be necessary. Only in very rare cases is such hyperstimulation the only indication for surgical delivery.

The rate of uterine hyperstimulation after endocervical PGE_2 administration is very low – as indicated earlier – provided application of the gel was strictly endocervical [27]. A study of 400 cases reported only two cases of hyperstimu-lation, in one of which a double dose was applied, i.e. 1.0 mg PGE_2 [11].

There has been much discussion in the literature over whether oxytocin or prostaglandin-induced uterine contractions are similar to or different from those after spontaneous onset. Such comparative studies are handicapped by the fact that the physiological conditions, e.g. concerning maturity of the mechanism of

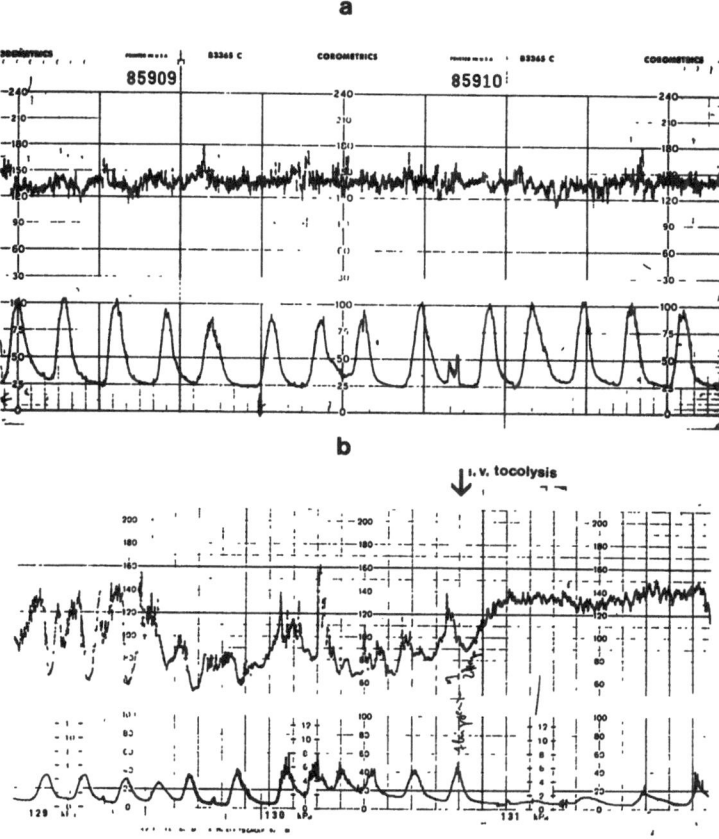

Fig. 12.3. Hyperstimulation after local application of PGE_2. **a** Frequent contractions without fetal distress; **b** Frequent contractions with acute fetal distress; decrease of labour activity and immediate improvement of the cardiogram after intravenous administration of a betamimetic agent.

labour, are by definition not the same at induction of labour, otherwise spontaneous labour would have started already. Most studies have shown that uterine contractions induced during the active stage of labour cannot be differentiated from spontaneous labour. Intrauterine pressure measurement has demonstrated that there was no difference between $PGF_{2\alpha}$-induced labour and spontaneous labour, but that uterine contractions induced by oxytocin were of somewhat shorter duration [31]. Intrauterine pressure measurements were also used to study the question of why average delivery time is shorter after induction of labour with a 3 mg PGE_2 vaginal tablet than after spontaneous onset of labour, in particular when the cervix is not ripe. The waveform of prostaglandin-induced contractions was similar to that of contractions after spontaneous onset or oxytocin induction, but in total, higher Montevideo units were achieved after PGE_2 induction [32]. A final assessment of the problem appears to be difficult since too many factors may influence the study results (time of induction of labour, type of medication, dose, form of applications, cervical state, parity).

Rupture of the uterus is extremely rare after prostaglandin administration. No case of a ruptured uterus after endocervical instillation of PGE_2 gel has been reported so far. A few reports of such accidents after vaginal application of prostaglandins have been published [33]. Upon detailed examination, however, it becomes apparent that excessively high doses were given in most of these cases (e.g. 20 mg PGE_2 in the form of suppositories); frequently these patients were women who already had a history of caesarean section.

It has been claimed that the incidence of postpartum haemorrhage is higher after induction of labour, but this is not yet clear [34].

Although it is known that PGE_2 may cause an increase in body temperature [35], the doses used for induction of labour, in particular for local application, are not large enough to produce such an effect. Therefore if a rise in body temperature is observed after local application of PGE_2, this must not be attributed to the medication, but the possibility of an infection should be considered. In view of the small amount of prostaglandins absorbed after local application for induction of labour, the general contraindications to prostaglandin application (e.g. bronchial asthma) are not relevant in this situation.

Follow-up of Children after Induction of labour

It has been postulated that induction of labour with prostaglandin is associated with a lower rate of neonatal hyperbilirubinaemia than induction of labour with oxytocin [36]. However, the incidence may well depend more on fetal maturity than on the labour-inducing agent [37].

The influence of induction of labour and in particular of prostaglandins on the vital functions of the newborn has been studied [38]. Psychomotor follow-up has been done up to 30 months after birth, but no pathological findings have been obtained [39].

In summary, the introduction of prostaglandins for cervical ripening and/or induction of labour can be considered an improvement of the therapeutic possibilities of modern obstetrics. Since prostaglandins are potent drugs their use should be limited to specialists with knowledge of their advantages and potential risks.

References

1. Bishop EH. Pelvic scoring for elective induction. Obstet Gynecol 1964; 24:266–8.
2. Calder AA. Cervical ripening. In: Bydgeman M, Berger G, Keith L, eds. Prostaglandin and its inhibitors in clinical obstetrics and gynecology. Lancaster: MTB Press, 1986.
3. Lange AP, Secher NJ, Westergaard JC, Skovgard, I. Prelabor evaluation of inducibility. Obstet Gynecol 1982; 60:137–47.
4. Kofler E, Husslein P, Langer M, Fuchs AR, Fuchs F. Die Bedeutung der Oxytocinempfindlichkeit für den spontanen Wehenbeginn beim Menschen. Geburtshilfe Frauenheilk 1983; 43:533–7.
5. Huszar G, Cabrol D, Naftolin E. The relationship between myometrial contractility and cervical maturation in pregnancy and labor. In: Huszar G, ed. The physiology and biochemistry of the uterus in pregnancy and labor. Boca Raton: CRC Press, 1986.
6. Husslein P. Die Bedeutung von Oxytocin und Prostaglandinen für den Geburtsmechanismus beim Menschen. Wien Klin Wochenschr suppl 1984; 155:1–32.
7. Turnbull AC, Anderson ABM. Induction of labour. J Obstet Gynecol Br Cwlth 1967; 74:8–19.
8. Fuchs AR, Fuchs F, Husslein P, Soloff MS. Oxytocin receptors in the human uterus during pregnancy and parturition. Am J Obstet Gynecol 1984; 150:734–41.
9. Lundin-Schiller S, Mitchell MD. The role of prostaglandins in human parturition. Prostaglandins Leukotrienes Essential Fatty Acids 1990; 39:1–10.
10. Garfield RE, Hayashi RH. Appearance of gap junctions in the myometrium of women during labor. Am J Obstet Gynecol 1981; 140:254–60.
11. Ulmsten U. The cervix. In: Bydgeman M, Berger G, Keith L, eds. Prostaglandins and their inhibitors in clinical obstetrics and gynecology. Lancaster: MTP Press, 1986.
12. Husslein P. Use of prostaglandins for induction of labor. Semin Perinatol 1991; 15:173–81.
13. Husslein P, Reichel R, Goeschen K, Rasche M, Sinzinger H. Plasma concentration of 13,14-dihydro-15-keto-PGE$_2$ (PGEM) after various ways of cervix ripening with PGE$_2$. Prostaglandins 1984; 28:209–15.
14. O'Brien WF, Knuppel RA, Cohen GR. Plasma prostaglandin metabolite levels after use of prostaglandin E$_2$ gel for cervical ripening. Am J Obstet Gynecol 1986; 155:1037–40.
15. MacKenzie IZ. A comparison of PGE$_2$ and PGE$_{2alpha}$ vaginal gel for ripening the cervix before induction of labor. Br J Obstet Gynaecol 1979; 86:167–70.
16. Kofler E, Egarter CH, Husslein P. Erfahrungen bei 2149 Geburtseinleitungen mit 3 mg PGE$_2$-Vaginaltabletten. Geburtshilfe Frauenheilkd 1986; 46:863–8.
17. Macer J, Buchanan M, Yonekura L. Induction of labor with prostaglandin E$_2$ vaginal suppositories. Obstet Gynecol 1984; 63:664–8.
18. Gordon-Wright AP Elder, M. Prostaglandin E$_2$ tablets used intravaginally for induction of labor. Br J Obstet Gynaecol 1979; 86:32–6.
19. Egarter CH, Husslein P, Rayburn WF. Uterine hyperstimulation after low-dose prostaglandin E$_2$ therapy: tocolytic treatment in 181 cases. Am J Obstet Gynecol 1990; 163:794–6.
20. Husslein P, Egarter Ch, Sevelda P, Genger H, Salzer H, Kofler E. Geburtseinleitung mit 3 mg Prostaglandin-E$_2$-Vaginaltabletten. Eine Renaissance der programmierten Geburt. Geburtshille Frauenheilkd 1986; 46:83–7.
21. Thiery M, Decoster JM, Parewijck W et al. Endocervical prostaglandin E$_2$-gel for preinduction cervical softening. Prostaglandins 1984; 27:429–39.
22. Ulmsten U, Kirstein-Pedersen A, Stenberg P et al. A new gel for intracervical application of prostaglandin E$_2$. Acta Obstet Gynaecol Scand 1979; 84:19–21.
23. Forman A, Ulmsten U, Baynat J et al. Evidence for a local effect of intracervical prostaglandin E$_2$ gel. Am J Obstet Gynecol 1982; 143:756–9.
24. Granström L, Ekman G, Ulmsten U. Myometrial activity after local application of prostaglandin E$_2$ for cervical ripening and term labor induction. Am J Obstet Gynecol 1990; 162:691–4.
25. Ekman GA, Forman K, Marsal U et al. Intravaginal versus intracervical applications of

prostaglandin E_2 in viscous gel of cervical priming and induction of labor at term in patients with an unfavourable cervical state. Am J Obstet Gynecol 1983; 147:657–61.

26. Rayburn WF. Prostaglandin E_2 gel for cervical ripening and induction of labor: a critical analysis. Am J Obstet Gynecol 1989; 160:529–34.

27. Husslein P. et al. Pre-induction intracervical application of a highly viscous prostaglandin E_2-gel in pregnant women with an unripe uterine cervix: a double-blind placebo-controlled trial. Eur J Obstet Gynecol 1991.

28. Ekman-Ordeberg G, Uldbjerg N, Ulmsten U. Comparison of intravenous oxytocin and vaginal prostaglandins E_2 gel in women with unripe cervices and premature rupture of the membranes. Obstet Gynecol 1985; 66:307–10.

29. Goeschen K, Fuchs AR, Fuchs F et al. Vorzeitiger Blasensprung: Einfluß von intrazervikaler PGE_2-Gabe auf Oxytocin-PGFM- und PGEM-Plasmakonzentrationen bei Mutter und Kind. Geburtshilfe Frauenheilkd 1984; 42:772–6.

30. MacKenzie IZ, Bradley S, Embrey MR. Vaginal PG and labour induction for patients previously delivered by caesarean section. Br J Obstet Gynaecol 1984; 91:7–10.

31. Seitschik J, Chatkoff ML, Hayashi H. Intrauterine pressure waveform characteristics of spontaneous and oxytocin-or prostaglandin F_{2alpha}-induced labor. Am J Obstet Gynecol 1977; 127:223–7.

32. Egarter Ch, Philipp K, Skodler D, Kofler E. Uterusaktivität bei Geburtseinleitung durch vaginale Applikation von PGE2-Tabletten. Z Geburtshilfe Perinatol 1986; 190:129–32.

33. Claman P, Carpenter RJ, Theobald C, Reiter A. Uterine rupture with the use of vaginal PGE_2 for induction of labor. Am J Obstet Gynecol 1984; 150:889–90.

34. MacKenzie IZ. Induction of labour and postpartum haemorrhage. Br Med J 1979; 1:750.

35. Nelson GH, Bryans CI. Body temperature recordings during oral prostaglandin E_2 induction of labor. Obstet Gynecol 1979; 54:585–7.

36. Grünberger W, Coadello H, Huber J, Husslein P. Postpartale kindliche Serum-Bilirubinspiegel nach Geburtseinleitung mit Prostaglandinkappe oder Oxytocin. Z Geburtshilfe Perinatol 1981; 185:116–20.

37. Beazeley JM, Aldermann B. Neonatal hyperbilirubinaemia following the use of oxytocin in labour. Br J Obstet Gynaecol 1975; 82:265–71.

38. Lange AP. Induction of labor. In: Bydgeman M, Berger G, Keith L, eds. Prostaglandins and their inhibitors in clinical obstetrics and gynecology. Lancaster: MTP Press, 1986.

39. deCoster W, Goethals A, Vandierendonck A et al. Labor induction with prostaglandin F_{2alpha}: influence on psychomotor evaluation of the child in the first 40 months. Prostaglandins 1976; 12:559–64.

Chapter 13

Cervical Ripening

I. A. Greer

Cervical ripening, whether physiological or pharmacological, is the conversion of the rigid "sphincter" associated with maintenance of pregnancy into a compliant and easily dilating structure which allows uterine contractility easily to effect the transport of the fetus through the birth canal. Since the ripeness of the cervix governs the ease and success of induction of labour [1], making it a prerequisite to induction *per se*, we should consider the physiological mechanism of cervical ripening and study pharmacologically those agents which control or effect this process, as the aim of pharmacological ripening is to mimic the physiological process as closely as possible.

The Physiology of Ripening

Connective Tissue Remodelling

Collagen fibrils bound together into dense bundles confer on the cervix the rigidity which is characteristic of its non-pregnant and early pregnant state. The ground substance consists of large molecular weight proteoglycan complexes containing a variety of glycosaminoglycans (GAGs). Glycosaminoglycans are long chains of highly negatively charged repeating disaccharides containing one hexosamine (glucosamine or galactosamine) and one uronic acid (glucuronic or iduronic). There are a variety of GAGs, such as heparin and heparan sulphate and dermatan and chondroitin sulphate. These vary in their composition with regard to the exact combination of hexosamine and uronic acid residues and each varies intrinsically with regard to chain length. The predominant GAGs found in the cervix are chondroitin and dermatan sulphate [2,3]. As well as forming the ground substance of the tissue, proteoglycans invest collagen fibrils [4] with their protein cores attaching to the collagen. The GAG side chains of the proteoglycan can then interact with further collagen molecules and with each other. This relationship is important in orientating the collagen fibrils and thus providing mechanical strength [4–6]. The binding affinity of GAGs to collagen increases with increasing chain length and charge density. Hyaluronic acid, which is not found in proteoglycans but exists as a free GAG or linked to proteoglycans forming proteoglycan complexes typical of cartilage, therefore binds least strongly of the GAG molecules and will act to destabilise the collagen fibrils. GAGs containing iduronic as opposed to glucuronic acid such as dermatan sulphate bind strongly and promote tissue stability [7]. Changes in the proteoglycans/GAG composition can therefore alter the collagen binding and facilitate collagen breakdown. In the non-pregnant state, the cervix consists of around 80% water [8]. This increases to around 86% in late pregnancy [2]. As GAGs are hydrophilic, these molecules may be important in controlling tissue hydration, with increased hydration destabilising the collagen fibrils and promoting ripening. The collagen fibrils and GAGs are produced by fibroblasts which constitute the major cellular component of the cervical connective tissue. A small amount of elastin is also present within the cervix and there is a reduction in cervical elastin during pregnancy [9]. However, the changes in elastin fibre concentration and distribution in physiological and pharmacological cervical ripening have yet to be established. Elastin may also be important in returning the cervix to a non-pregnant shape following delivery.

The changes associated with cervical ripening include a reduced collagen concentration within the tissue, an increase in water content, and a change in the proteoglycan/GAG content. Fibroblast activation occurs and local prostaglandin production increases. An inflammatory infiltrate also occurs at term in parallel with this ripening process and the stroma becomes oedematous and highly vascularised. However, the mechanism whereby these changes occur is unclear.

Although there is an increase in the total collagen content of the cervix at term, the collagen concentration is reduced [10–12] and the cervical connective tissue at term shows widely scattered and dissociated collagen fibrils with an increase in the ground substance when compared to the early pregnant or non-pregnant cervix [13]. In addition, the collagen fibrils are reduced in size [13]. The cervical collagen concentration measured biochemically also decreases [14–16], but this change in collagen concentration appears to be more marked when studied histologically using stains specific for polymerised collagen, as it seems that a much lower proportion of the collagen exists as intact fibres in the dilated cervix at term [7]. Several mechanisms have been postulated to explain these changes in collagen composition; essentially, these are increased enzymatic collagen degradation and/or alteration in the proteoglycan/GAG composition of the ground substance.

Collagen is amenable to breakdown by collagenase produced by fibroblasts and leukocytes and leukocyte elastase produced by macrophages, polymorphs and eosinophils. Collagenase is secreted in a latent form, procollagenase, which is activated by cleavage of the proenzyme by plasmin or stromelysin to the active form which specifically breaks down the triple helix of the collagen fibril by hydrolysing peptide bonds while elastase acts on the telpeptide non-helical domains [18,19]. Collagenase will degrade collagen types I, II and III. The predominant types of collagen found in the human cervix are type I (66%) and type III (33%) [20]. Elastase can break down not only elastin and collagen, but also proteoglycans. It may act synergistically with collagenase on collagen. The collagen fragments produced by these enzymes can be further broken down by non-specific proteases. As the cervical collagen content decreases through pregnancy the leukocyte elastase and collagenase activity increase [15]. In addition, the amount of soluble collagen, reflecting partly degraded collagen, in the tissue increases in parallel with the increased enzyme activities [15,21]. There is evidence from animal models that collagen degradation fragments are found in the cervix at parturition [22]. Thus there appears to be a remodelling of collagen during pregnancy and parturition. Mature collagen with many cross links may be broken down during pregnancy and replaced with new collagen which is more amenable to rapid breakdown at the time of parturition, having fewer cross links. The importance of collagen content to the progress of labour is illustrated by Ekman et al. [23] who showed that among women in spontaneous labour there were significantly higher cervical collagen concentrations in those with low cervical scores (i.e. less cervical ripeness) compared to those with high cervical scores. Once labour is established, there is a major increase in circulating collagenase [24] and collagenase activity in cervical tissue. Increased levels of collagenase activity have been reported in cervical biopsies obtained at 6–8 cm dilatation during labour compared to biopsies from non-pregnant and pregnant non-labouring subjects [25]. Rajabi et al. [26] have reported an increase in cervical collagenase activity of 13–14 times over that obtained in tissue from women at term not in labour.

Procollagenase production in the cervix, at least in animal models, appears to be under the control of steroid hormones and prostaglandins, with increased procollagenase production and gene expression being found in response to physiological (10^{-7}–10^{-9}M) concentrations of oestrogen and progesterone [27]. Furthermore, there is evidence that this oestrogen-stimulated increase in procollagenase is associated with an increase in collagen degradation reflecting active collagenase activity [22]. In addition to a direct effect on procollagenase production [28], prostaglandins may act as the intermediary in oestrogen-induced procollagenase production, as indomethacin (an inhibitor of prostaglandin production) inhibits the effect of oestrogen [27]. Paradoxically progesterone, which might have been expected to inhibit procollagenase production, increased the production of this protease at physiological concentrations. However, this may be important for tissue remodelling during pregnancy or to increase stores of this latent form of the protease in anticipation of activation at the time of parturition. Pharmacological concentrations of progesterone (10^{-4}M) inhibit procollagenase production and gene expression in response to oestrogen [27]. This change in collagenolytic activity may also be reflected in the further increase in soluble collagen seen at term and during labour [16,29]. However, Granstrom et al [16] have shown no difference in collagenolytic activity between women at term not in labour and women at term in labour, although both groups had significantly and substantially higher collagenolytic activities compared to the non-pregnant cervix. Although there are conflicting data on collagenase activity in the cervix in relation to parturition, it would appear that there is a remodelling of collagen in the cervical connective tissue which occurs as pregnancy advances.

The physiological basis of this would appear to be to facilitate ripening during the processes of parturition.

The changes of cervical ripening do not appear to be due simply to collagen breakdown as there are also changes in the proteoglycan, GAG and water content. The total GAG content of the cervix increases substantially by term, indicating active synthesis; however, the concentration of GAGs may remain relatively constant [6]. There may be a relative increase in hyaluronic acid and a relative decrease in chrondroitin and dermatan sulphate [3,6], compared to the non-pregnant cervix. However, other studies have not found any increase in hyaluronic acid concentration [2,10,30]. It has been suggested that tissues become more rigid with increasing chondroitin sulphate concentration. Thus, a reduction in the chondroitin sulphate concentration might result in increased compliance whereas increased hyaluronic acid (if this occurs), or an increase in the hyaluronic acid available to bind water may be associated with an increase in tissue hydration, and increased tissue deformability. Such a change in hyaluronic acid concentration/availability could at least partly explain the increased water content of the cervix which is seen during pregnancy [2,21] and more particularly the marked increase seen just prior to term [31]. The accumulation of hyaluronic acid and water between collagen fibrils will disperse them and increase distensibility. In addition, in view of the role of GAGs in orientating the collagen fibrils and protecting them from breakdown, a decrease in chondroitin sulphate concentration is likely to reduce the mechanical strength of collagen fibrils, and make them more amenable to breakdown by proteolytic enzymes. The increase in total GAGs is likely to reflect increased production by fibroblasts which become increasingly active as pregnancy advances [17,32]. Alternatively (or additionally), the increased hyaluronic acid content and associated increase in hydration could reflect breakdown of the proteoglycan complexes to provide free hyaluronic acid and proteoglycans. The proteases required for this could come from the activated fibroblasts, or the leukocytes which infiltrate the cervical connective tissue. In addition to providing these proteases, leukocytes could increase vascular dilatation and permeability and thereby enhance tissue hydration.

The lack of agreement as to whether GAG concentrations actually change during ripening, perhaps suggests that the alteration in the ground substance may be more subtle. It could reflect a change in the proteoglycan composition of the tissue which may not require a significant change in the concentration of GAGs, but rather in their organisation relative to proteoglycans. There are at least three proteoglycans relevant to cervical connective tissue: two small proteoglycans substituted with one (small proteoglycan 2 (PG-S2)) or two (PG-S1) dermatan sulphate chains and a large proteoglycan (PG-L) with chondroitin/dermatan sulphate side chains. PG-S2 is the predominant proteoglycan found in cervical tissue and avidly binds collagen [30,33]. PG-S1 appears not to bind collagen well due to its biglycan structure and could destabilise collagen fibrils. PG-L forms proteoglycan complexes linking to hyaluronic acid in a similar way to that in cartilage and could control tissue hydration. At term there is an increase in the ratio of PG-S2 to collagen and an increase in production of PG-S1 and PG-L [30,34]. Such an alteration in the proteoglycan composition of the ground substance could easily result in a major alteration of the biomechanical properties of the cervix. In the rat, a strong correlation exists between the cervical linear circumference and the small dermatan sulphate proteoglycan:collagen ratio [11] supporting this contention.

Physiological Control of Cervical Ripening

Cervical ripening appears to be an active process rather than a passive process consequent upon increased uterine activity. The latter possibility seems improbable in view of the changes which occur within the connective tissue and cellular components of the cervix during ripening, as these changes suggest significant activity within the tissue. Furthermore, in animal studies cervical ripening occurs even when the cervix is physically isolated from the uterus [35,36], and ripening can also occur in the absence of detectable uterine activity.

Prostaglandins undoubtedly play a role in the control of cervical ripening in the human. The main prostaglandins produced by the cervix are PGE_2, PGI_2, and to a lesser extent $PGF_{2\alpha}$ and their production increases at term [37]. In addition, amniotic fluid concentrations of PGE_2 and $PGF_{2\alpha}$ correlate directly with the cervical score in women at term who are not in labour [38]. Receptors for PGE_2 and $PGF_{2\alpha}$ can also be demonstrated in the cervix [39]. These data suggest that prostaglandins have a physiological role in ripening and a further increase accompanies parturition *per se*. There is no doubt that prostaglandins are effective pharmacological agents for ripening the cervix and natural and synthetic prostaglandins can ripen the cervix at any stage in pregnancy [38,40]. Much of our knowledge regarding the physiological properties of prostaglandins in cervical ripening has been inferred from pharmacological observations. There are essentially two possible ways in which prostaglandins might bring about ripening: first, they could induce collagen breakdown, and second, they could alter collagen binding and tissue hydration by altering the GAG/proteoglycan composition.

There is little doubt that PGE_2 treatment will reduce collagen concentration, promoting changes similar to those seen during physiological ripening [23,41], but there is disagreement as to whether PGE_2 will induce collagenolysis. Some studies have reported an increase in collagenase or collagenase-like hydrolytic activity following PGE_2 administration [42,43] and prostaglandins, as discussed above, appear to be involved in the control of procollagenase production in animal models [27,28]. Other studies have reported no change or a reduction in collagenase [44–46]. To some extent this may reflect methodological problems in assessing collagenase activity. However, Rath et al. [46] not only showed no change in collagenase activity, but also found an absence of collagen breakdown fragments on electrophoresis of tissue extracts taken from pregnant human cervices treated with the prostaglandin analogue sulprostone compared to placebo treated cervices. In this study significant cervical ripening occurred in the treated group. This evidence suggests that prostaglandin treatment may have no direct stimulatory effect on collagenase activity, at least in the human, in vivo. Furthermore, Hillier and Wallis [47] have shown that PGE_2 and $PGF_{2\alpha}$ have no effect on collagen breakdown in vitro.

In contrast, however, arachidonic acid, the substrate for prostaglandins and leukotrienes, increased collagen breakdown in similar experiments. Phospholipase inhibitors were found to block this response, whereas cyclo-oxygenase inhibitors were ineffective at concentrations which blocked prostaglandin production [47]. Despite this, cervical ripening in terms of tissue compliance occurs rapidly in vitro following treatment with PGE_2 [48]. This discrepancy may be explained by the findings that cervical tissues treated with PGE_2 and arachidonic acid produced an increase in unidentified arachidonic acid products which were not prostaglandins [49,50]. Thus, arachidonic acid-induced ripening may be a non-prostaglandin mediated effect perhaps due to leukotriene production which may also be stimulated by PGE_2. This possibility, however, remains speculative, but would be in keeping with the hypothesis [51] that cervical ripening is an inflammatory type process. Such an hypothesis is supported by the work of Ito et al. [52,53] who showed that cytokines markedly stimulate collagenase synthesis from macrophages and monocytes, that cervical explants from pregnant rats but not non-pregnant rats produce interleukin-1 like factors and that interleukin-1a can stimulate the production of elastase-like enzymes in human uterine cervical fibroblasts. Prostaglandins might also act in this manner to stimulate the production of chemotactic cytokines which would induce a neutrophil influx and possibly a release of leucocyte collagenase which is stored in granules within the neutrophil. As such a process is dependent on neutrophils being recruited to the tissue it would not be evident in vitro.

Prostaglandins may also act on the GAG composition and proteoglycan complexes in the cervical tissue [41,45]. In animal studies PGE_2 has been shown to induce an increase in hydration and hyaluronic acid concentration [54]. Paradoxically Cabrol et al. [55] found that in a rat model inhibition of prostaglandin production resulted in an increase in hyaluronic acid and suggested that this may be due to diversion of substrate towards the lipoxygenase pathway. PGE_2 can influence cervical fibroblast production of collagen and GAG. The production of these two substances is inversely related so that when collagen synthesis is reduced, an increase in GAG production occurs [56,57]. This increase in GAG production by prostaglandins may be due to induction of the enzyme hyaluronic acid synthetase within the fibroblasts resulting in a substantial increase in hyaluronic acid [58]. A further possible mechanism is that PGE_2 may induce proteolytic breakdown of proteoglycan complexes which could also cause the increase in free hyaluronic acid content. Some studies, however, do not support an increase in hyaluronic acid production in response to prostaglandins [45]. We have recently shown that in vivo PGE_2-induced cervical ripening at term will promote a substantial increase in circulating levels of chondroitin/dermatan sulphate and similar increases are seen in spontaneous labour (Greer, Johnston and Calder, unpublished observation). These increases in chondroitin/dermatan sulphate seen in labours induced with PGE_2 parallel PGE_2 absorption and increasing PGE metabolite levels. This suggests that PGE_2 induces proteoglycan breakdown and/or GAG production although the mechanism behind this is unclear. Thus, PGE_2 mediated cervical ripening might easily be explained by changes in GAG/proteoglycan content which will disperse and destabilise the collagen fibrils and increase tissue compliance as discussed above.

Other agents also act to control cervical structural changes. Oestradiol can stimulate prostaglandin production where there has been previous exposure to progesterone, and has been used to bring about cervical ripening in the clinical situation [59,60]. The mechanism underlying the effect of oestradiol may be due, at least in part, to induction of prostaglandin synthesis. These findings have also been reported in the sheep where oestradiol-induced ripening has been associated with increased cervical prostaglandin production along with an alteration in GAG synthesis [31]. In addition, oestradiol has been linked to an increase in collagenase activity [61] although this has not been confirmed by others [44,62]. Oestradiol might also be responsible for the influx of protease-producing leukocytes which could induce ripening and which would not be evident in vitro.

Progesterone appears to have an inhibitory effect on cervical ripening and parturition in animals where a decrease in progesterone at term results in ripening and labour. Such decrease does not occur in the human, but progesterone is a potent anti-inflammatory agent [63] and could still be an important physiological inhibitor of the ripening process in vivo by inhibiting neutrophil influx and activation [64]. This possibility is supported by the ripening effect of antiprogestins on the cervix prior to termination of pregnancy [65,66] and which is associated with a neutrophil influx in animal models [67]. However, antiprogestins might exert their effects through prostaglandins as they appear to stimulate prostaglandin synthesis and reduce catabolism in vitro [68,69]. This may also be the mechanism of uterine sensitisation to oxytocin seen with antiprogestin treatment. However, ex vivo studies of cervical biopsies treated with the antiprogestin RU 486 have shown no difference in prostaglandin production from radiolabelled arachidonic acid compared to placebo-treated cervices despite a significant objectively assessed ripening effect in the treated group [66]. Nonetheless, the marked success of antiprogestins in effecting cervical ripening and abortion suggest that they will provide a useful tool to help understand the physiological control of cervical ripening and perhaps also an effective agent for cervical ripening and induction of labour in clinical practice [70].

Relaxin has been shown to have some effect on cervical ripening in women [71] and it has been reported to increase collagenase activity [72]. Human fibroblasts exhibit relaxin receptors and relaxin has a mitogenic effect on fibroblasts [73]. Relaxin may therefore be involved in the ripening process but our understanding of this possible mechanism is far from clear. However, if relaxin were to prove an effective pharmacological agent for ripening in the clinical situation, it may, unlike the prostaglandins, be selective on the cervix and devoid of stimulatory effects on uterine contractility. Such a selective effect would be of value in induction, avoiding the stimulation of uterine activity prior to adequate cervical ripening.

Cervical Ripening in the Clinical Situation

The distinction between ripening and induction of labour is somewhat blurred, with ripening often merging into induction. However, it is an important distinction to make as embarking on induction when the cervix is not ripe is fraught with hazard especially in primigravidae. The increased risk of morbidity from the process of induction of labour is dependent not only on parity and the patient's past obstetric performance, but also on the degree of cervical ripeness which reflects how close the patient is to spontaneous labour [74]. The cervical ripeness can be quantified by cervical scoring systems [74,75] (Table 13.1). These are useful in providing an objective assessment of ripeness, which is essential for comparative studies on methods of cervical ripening and induction of labour. In addition they may to some extent predict the outcome of labour [76]; a ripe cervix is likely to be associated with a short and easy induction of labour with little additional stress to the fetus, whereas with a very unripe cervix the opposite will apply. Clearly, it is in the latter situation that pharmacological ripening has most to offer.

Table 13.1. Cervical score [75] modified from the pelvic score of Bishop [74]. The total score is derived from the summation of the scores for each parameter

Score	0	1	2	3
Dilatation (cm)	<1	1–2	2–4	>4
Length (cm)	>4	2–4	1–2	<1
Consistency	Firm	Average	Soft	–
Position	Posterior	Mid-anterior	–	–
Level	0–3	0–2	0–1; 0	–

There is no doubt that the pharmacological use of prostaglandins is the most effective means of effecting cervical ripening explored to date. Prior to the development of suitable prostaglandin preparations, a variety of methods, which were usually mechanical, were used. These have included bougies and laminaria, Foley catheter balloons and digital stretching of the cervix and stripping of the membranes from the lower segment of the uterus. However, the effectiveness of these physical methods is likely to depend, at least in part, on the local generation of prostaglandins from the traumatised tissues. In addition, a variety of other pharmacological techniques for cervical ripening have been explored. Prolonged intravenous infusions of oxytocin have been employed although the effectiveness of this practice is questionable [77]. Oestrogens [59] and relaxin [71] have been employed with some success, although their efficacy does not reach that of prostaglandins. In the future antiprogestagens may have an important role in this area as they have been used successfully in ripening prior to termination of pregnancy as discussed above and also for induction of labour with promising results [70]. Results of further clinical studies on these compounds are awaited with interest, but in the meantime the most effective and clinically proven agent for cervical ripening at term remains prostaglandin E_2.

Only prostaglandins E_2 and $F_{2\alpha}$ have been studied extensively for ripening at term. It is clear that both of these substances are involved in the process of parturition. Prostaglandins E_2 and $F_{2\alpha}$ and their metabolites increase during labour in both the amniotic fluid [78,79] and the peripheral circulation [80–82], although in the peripheral circulation PGF metabolites show the greatest change. Our own results have shown that in longitudinal studies throughout labour both PGE_2 and $PGF_{2\alpha}$ metabolites increase. However, the major increase in PGE_2 metabolites (PGEM) appears to occur prior to established labour whereas the major increase in $PGF_{2\alpha}$ metabolite occurs during labour and correlates directly with the duration of labour and inversely with the need for augmentation with oxytocin [83]. In cervical ripening and labour induced by prostaglandins, correlations between the increase in PGEM and the increase in cervical score have been noted [84,85]. These data suggest that the magnitude of increase in PGEM following cervical priming may be an important factor in the clinical response to PGE_2 administration. This effect may to some extent mimic spontaneous labour where PGE_2 is the important prostaglandin in early labour, possibly stimulating cervical ripening and sensitising the uterus by development of gap junctions, which transform the disparate myometrial cells into a functional syncytium, and oxytocin receptors. PGE_2 may also stimulate endogenous $PGF_{2\alpha}$ production from decidua by an as yet undefined mechanism, so switching on uterine activity. This would be in keeping with previous studies where PGE_2 has been suggested to be the dominant prostaglandin in early labour, with greater specificity for the cervix than $PGF_{2\alpha}$, whereas $PGF_{2\alpha}$ is the dominant prostaglandin in active labour [86,87]. Thus PGE_2 may be important for cervical ripening and perhaps uterine sensitisation whereas $PGF_{2\alpha}$ may be more important for generating and maintaining uterine contractility [88]. This hypothesis is supported by the work of Reddi et al. [89], who showed that amniotic fluid levels of $PGF_{2\alpha}$ were reduced in women with dysfunctional labour, and similar findings have been noted with regard to peripheral plasma metabolites of $PGF_{2\alpha}$ in our own studies (Johnston et al., unpublished data).

Although $PGF_{2\alpha}$ has been employed successfully for cervical ripening, PGE_2 is 5–10 times more potent and appears to be associated with fewer side effects than $PGF_{2\alpha}$. These features together with the ready availability of PGE_2 in pharmaceutical preparations have meant that PGE_2 is the major prostaglandin employed for cervical ripening. Its efficacy is borne out by a recent review of 27 prospective studies comparing PGE_2-induced ripening with placebo or no treatment prior to induction with oxytocin [90]. This review documented a reduced incidence of operative delivery and a shorter duration of labour in the treated groups, with minimal maternal side effects. Other extensive reviews have also documented the value and safety of PGE_2 for preinduction cervical ripening [91].

A variety of routes of administration have been used and local administration is favoured as it is associated with increased efficacy and fewer systemic side effects. Local administration can be achieved by extra-amniotic, endocervical or vaginal application using a variety of vehicles. The ideal preparation for cervical ripening would produce a satisfactory effect on the cervix while not stimulating myometrial activity. As the overall aim of such intervention is to induce labour, myometrial activity may not be a serious problem. However, myometrial activity in advance of a compliant cervix will result in increased stress for mother and fetus which may be particularly problematical in inductions where the fetus is compromised.

The extra-amniotic route was the first to be explored with regard to cervical ripening [92]. This involved the transcervical passage of a Foley catheter which was retained in the extra-amniotic space by the inflated catheter balloon. PGE_2 in a dose of 400–500 μg was then applied extra-amniotically, usually in a viscous gel such as Tylose. This technique is undoubtedly effective in significantly reducing the induction–delivery interval, caesarean section rate, maternal pyrexia rate and incidence of babies born with low Apgar scores in women subsequently induced with amniotomy and intravenous oxytocin, as shown in a number of controlled clinical studies [1]. The disadvantages of this technique are its invasiveness and perhaps a risk of infection and the possibility of bleeding into the choriodecidual space, which could lead to uterine hypertonus due to rapid uptake of the prostaglandin. Furthermore, patients may find the catheter placement an unpleasant procedure. Although this technique has been replaced almost entirely by vaginal and endocervical administration it may still be of value in the most unripe and difficult cases [93]. Although single applications of PGE_2 vaginally cannot achieve the same effects as extra-amniotic administration [93], repeated vaginal administration using two applications can produce similar ripening effects and clinical efficacy [94]. Repeated vaginal administration is also associated with less uterine activity and analgesic requirements than extra-amniotic administration, suggesting that it may provide a more selective action on the cervix [94]. The difference between extra-amniotic and vaginal PGE_2 is probably related to differences in absorption of the prostaglandin, with greater absorption being seen in the former where there is a rapid and substantial increase in PGE metabolites which correlates with the increase in cervical score [85]. Despite dramatic changes in prostaglandin metabolites there appears to be no significant effect on fetal wellbeing or umbilical artery blood flow following priming with PGE_2 [95].

Endocervical application of PGE_2 has also become increasingly popular following the studies by Ulmsten's group in Sweden [96–98]. A variety of vehicles has been employed but those most commonly used are the starch-based gel marketed in Europe as Cerviprost (Organon) and the triacetin-based gel marketed as Prepidil (Upjohn). The former is very viscous and sticky and so will tend to remain in the endocervical canal. The latter is more fluid and could potentially "run out" of the cervical canal if care is not taken in the application of the gel. The dose administered is 0.5 mg with each preparation. Although a degree of skill is required to effect the placement of the gel accurately in the canal, avoiding on the one hand placement into the extra-amniotic space and on the other leakage from the external os, the procedure is considered less invasive than the extra-amniotic route. Endocervical administration of PGE_2 for cervical ripening has been shown to have a more specific effect on the cervix compared to extra-amniotic or vaginal application; the latter two techniques result in significant uterine activity in the 90 min following PGE_2 administration compared to virtually absent uterine contractility with the endocervical gel as assessed by an extra-amniotic microtransducer pressure catheter [99]. Inadvertent extra-amniotic placement is likely to lead to increased myometrial activity thus losing the selective effect on the cervix which is the aim of such therapy. Double blind studies have confirmed that it is the PGE_2 which is effective rather than the physical effects of the gel in the canal. Ulmsten [100] has recently summarised his group's extensive experience with endocervical gel and reported that cervical ripening will occur in 40% of patients within 5–6 h and 65% will have a ripe cervix or be in labour or delivered within 24 h, 20% of patients will require a second application of gel and in about 15% no significant ripening effect will occur despite repeated applications of gel. As would be expected the outcome is dependent on the initial cervical score [101]. The triacetin gel preparation is also effective [102] and the response appears to correlate with the absorption of the PGE_2 [103]. There are also comparative data to suggest that endocervical administration is superior to vaginal administration [104,105].

Successful cervical ripening can be achieved in most patients with vaginal preparations in the form of tablets or gels. It would appear that gels provide greater efficacy and bioavailability than the tablets [84,106]. Furthermore, our own in vitro studies show that gel preparations have more rapid and reliable release of PGE_2 than the tablets and also that the release of PGE_2 can be influenced by pH and abolished if the preparation is coated with obstetric cream (unpublished data), factors which may be responsible for variable absorption and clinical responses in the clinical situation. A much larger dose of PGE_2 is required vaginally than that used extra-amniotically or endocervically and repeated applications may be required [93,94], although in the unfavourable cervix it appears that if ripening has not occurred after three applications of gel vaginally, then there is no benefit from further vaginal gel application (J Norman, personal communication). In this situation, sophisticated hydrogel polymers [107,108] which allow a slow sustained release of PGE_2 would appear to have a major role as they are easy to insert, and avoid the more invasive technique discussed above and possibily the need for repeated applications. A recently marketed commercially available hydrogel polymer providing sustained release of PGE_2 has been used successfully in primigravidae with unfavourable cervical scores for cervical ripening/induction of labour [83]. This device contained 10 mg of PGE_2 designed to be released at a constant rate over an 8 h period. Plasma PGEM levels obtained with this preparation reached a plateau at 2 h at concentrations compatible with, though slightly higher than, those seen in spontaneous labour. PGFM rose initially and again towards the end of the 8-h period. The peak change in PGEM correlated with the increase in cervical score whereas PGFM correlated inversely with the need for augmentation and the length of labour. These data again suggest that PGE_2 is important for cervical ripening whereas $PGF_{2\alpha}$ is important for uterine activity. However, this preparation has been the subject of apparent adverse events in the form of uterine hypertonus and difficulty in removing the pessary [109,110] although the former reports are anecdotal rather than from a controlled trial. The hypertonous effect may have reflected the different release characteristics obtained in vivo from the highly predictable release obtained in vitro [83] or may be due to poor patient selection as the dose may be too high for women with ripe cervices especially if they are parous. Nonetheless the clinical potential of such a preparation remains substantial in the situation of the unripe cervix providing that the potential for such adverse events can be avoided by modification to the product or dose of PGE_2 or improved patient selection such as restriction to those patients with unripe cervices.

References

1. Calder AA. Cervical ripening. In: Bygdeman M, Berger GS, Keith LG, eds. Prostaglandins and their inhibitors in obstetrics and gynaecology. Lancaster: MTP Press, 1986; 145–64.
2. Uldbjerg N, Ekman G, Malmstrom A. Ripening of the human uterine cervix related to changes in collagen, glycosaminoglycans and collagenolytic activity. Am J Obstet Gynecol 1983; 147:662–6.
3. von Maillot K, Stuhlsatz HW, Mohanaradhkrishan V et al. Changes in the glycosaminoglycan distribution pattern in the human uterine cervix during pregnancy and labour. Am J Obstet Gynecol 1979; 135:503–6.
4. Scott JE, Orford CR. Dermatan sulphate rich proteoglycan associates with rat tail tendon collagen at the d band in the gap region. Biochem J 1981; 197:213.
5. Lindahl U, Hook M. Glycosaminoglycans and their binding to biological macromolecules. Ann Rev Biochem 1978; 47:385.
6. Golichowski A. Cervical stromal interstitial polysaccharide metabolism in pregnancy. In: Naftolin F, Stubblefield PG, eds. Dilatation of the uterine cervix: connective tissue biology and clinical management. New York: Raven Press, 1980; 99–112.
7. Obrink B. A study of the interactions between monomeric tropocollagen and glycosaminoglycans. Eur J Biochem 1973; 33:387–400.
8. Liggins GC. Ripening of the cervix. Semin Perinatol 1978; 2:261.
9. Leppert PC, Yu SY, Keller S, Cerreta J, Mandl I. Decreased elastic fibres and desmosine content in incompetent cervix. Am J Obstet Gynecol 1987; 157:1134–9.
10. Fosang AJ, Handley CJ, Santer V, Lowther DA, Thorburn GD. Pregnancy-related changes in the connective tissue of the ovine cervix. Biol Reprod 1984; 30:1223–35.
11. Kokenyesi R, Woessner JR. Relationship between dilatation rate of the uterine cervix and a small dermatan sulfate proteoglycan. Biol Reprod 1990; 42:87–89.
12. Jeffrey JJ. Collagen and collagenase: pregnancy and parturition. Semin Perinatol 1991; 15:118–26.
13. Danforth DN, Buckingham JC, Roddick JW. Connective tissue changes incident to cervical effacement. Am J Obstet Gynecol 1960; 86:939–45.

14. Danforth DN, Veis A, Breen M et al. The effect of pregnancy and labor on the human cervix: changes in collagen, glycoproteins and glycosaminoglycans. Am J Obstet Gynecol 1974; 120:641–9.
15. Uldbjerg N, Ulmsten V, Ekman G. The ripening of the human uterine cervix in terms of connective tissue biochemistry. Clin Obstet Gynecol 1983; 26:14–26.
16. Granstrom L, Ekman G, Ulmsten U et al. Changes in the connective tissue of corpus and cervix uteri during ripening and labour in term pregnancy. Br J Obstet Gynaecol 1989; 96:1198–202.
17. Junqueira LCU, Zugaib M, Montes GS et al. Morphological and histochemical evidence for the occurrence of collagenolysis and for the role of neutrophilic polymorphnuclear leukocytes during cervical dilatation. Am J Obstet Gynecol 1980; 138:273–81.
18. Wooley DE. Mammalian collagenases. In: Piez KA, Reddi AH eds. Extracellular matrix biochemistry. New York: Elsevier, 1984; 119–57.
19. Stricklin GP, Hibbs MS. Biochemistry and physiology of mammalian collagenases. In: Nimni ME, ed. Collagen biochemistry, vol. 1. Boca Raton: CRC Press, 1988; 187–205.
20. Kleissl HP, van der Rest M, Naftolin F, Glorieux FH, De Leon A. Collagen changes in human cervix at parturition. Am J Obstet Gynecol 1978; 130:748–53.
21. Ito A, Kitamura K, Mori Y, Hirakawa S. The change in solubility of type 1 collagen in human cervix in pregnancy at term. Biochem Med 1979; 21:262–70.
22. Rajabi MR, Dodge GR, Solomon S, Poole AR. Immunochemical and immunohistochemical evidence of estrogen-mediated collagenolysis as a mechanism of cervical dilatation in the guinea pig at parturition. Endocrinology 1991; 128:371–8.
23. Ekman G, Malmstrom A, Uldbjerg N. Cervical collagen: an important regulator of cervical function in term labour. Obstet Gynecol 1986; 67:633–6.
24. Rajabi MR, Dean DD, Woessner Jr JF. Serum collagenase activity in pregnant parturient and postpartum women. Ann NY Acad Sci 1985; 460:492–3.
25. Osmers R, Rath W, Adelmann-Grill BC, Fittkow C, Severenyi M, Kuhn W. Collagenase activity in the cervix of non-pregnant and pregnant women. Arch Gynecol Obstet 1990; 248:75–80.
26. Rajabi MR, Dean DD, Beydoun SN et al. Elevated tissue levels of collagenase during dilatation of uterine cervix in human parturition. Am J Obstet Gynecol 1988; 159:971–6.
27. Rajabi MR, Solomon S, Poole AR. Hormonal regulation of interstitial collagenase in the uterine cervix of the guinea pig. Endocrinology 1991; 128:863–71.
28. Goshowaki H, Ito A, Mori Y. Effects of prostaglandins on the production of collagenase by rabbit uterine cervical fibroblasts. Prostaglandins 1988; 36:107–14.
29. von Maillot K, Zimmermann BK. The solubility of collagen of the uterine cervix during pregnancy and labour. Archiv Gynakol 1976; 220:275–80.
30. Uldbjerg N, Malmstrom A. The role of proteoglycans in cervical dilatation. Semin Perinatol 1991; 15:127–132.
31. Fitzpatrick RJ, Dobson H. Softening of the ovine cervix at parturition. In: Elwood DA, Anderson ABM, eds. The cervix in pregnancy and labour: clinical and biochemical investigations. Edinburgh: Churchill Livingstone, 1981; 40–56.
32. Parry DS, Ellwood DA. Ultrastructural aspects of cervical softening in sheep. In: Ellwood DA, Anderson ABM, eds. The cervix in pregnancy and labour: clinical and biochemical investigations. Edinburgh: Churchill Livingstone, 1981; 74–84.
33. Uldbjerg N, Danielsen CC. A study of the interaction between type I collagen and a small dermatan sulphate proteogylcan. Biochem J 1988; 251:643–8.
34. Uldbjerg N, Ulmsten U. The physiology of cervical ripening and cervical dilatation and the effect of abortificient drugs. Baillieres Clin Obstet Gynaecol 1990: 4:263–82.
35. Stys SJ, Clarke KE, Clewell WM, et al. Hormonal effects on cervical compliance in sheep. In: Naftolin F, Stubblefield PG, eds. Dilatation of the uterine cervix. New York: Raven Press, 1980; 147–56.
36. Ledger WL, Webster M, Harrison LP et al. Increase in cervical extensibility during labour induced after isolation of the cervix from the uterus in the pregnant sheep. Am J Obstet Gynecol 1985; 151:397–402.
37. Ellwood DA, Mitchell MD, Anderson ABM. The in vitro production of prostanoids by the human cervix during pregnancy: preliminary observations. Br J Obstet Gynaecol 1980; 87:210–14.
38. Calder AA. Pharmacological management of the unripe cervix in the human. In: Naftolin F, Stubblefield PG, eds. Dilatation of the uterine cervix. New York: Raven Press, 317–333. 1980.
39. Crankshaw DJ, Crankshaw J, Branda LA, Daniel EE. Receptors for E type prostaglandins in the plasma membrane of non-pregnant myometrium. Arch Biochem Biophys 1979; 198:459–65.

40. Calder AA, Greer IA. Pharmacological modulation of cervical compliance in the first and second trimesters of pregnancy. Semin Perinatol 1991; 15:162–72.
41. Uldbjerg N, Ekman G, Malmstrom A et al. Biochemical and morphological changes of human cervix after local application of prostaglandin E_2 in pregnancy. Lancet 1981; i:267–8.
42. Szalay S, Husslein P, Grunberger W. Local application of prostaglandin E_2 and its influence on collagenolytic activity of cervical tissue. Sing J Obstet Gynecol 1989; 12:15.
43. Ding JQ, Granberg S, Norstrom A. Clinical effects and cervical tissue changes after treatment with 16, 16 dimethyl-trans delta 2 PGE_1 methylester. Prostaglandins 1990; 39:281–5.
44. Ellwood DA, Anderson ABM, Mitchell MD et al. Prostanoids, collagenase and cervical softening in sheep. In: Ellwood DA, Anderson ABM, eds. The cervix in pregnancy and labour. Clinical and biochemical investigations. Edinburgh: Churchill Livingstone, 1981; 57–73.
45. Uldbjerg N, Ekman G, Malmstrom A, Ulmsten U, Wingerup L. Biochemical changes in human cervical connective tissue after local application of prostaglandin E_2. Gynecol Obstet Invest 1983; 15:291–9.
46. Rath W, Adelmann-Girill BC, Pieper U et al. The role of collagenases and proteases in prostaglandin induced cervical ripening. Prostaglandins 1987; 34:119–27.
47. Hillier K, Wallis RM. Prostaglandins, steroids and the human cervix. In: Ellwood DA, Anderson ABM, eds. The cervix in pregnancy and labour. Edinburgh: Churchill Livingstone, 1981; 144–62.
48. Conrad JT, Ueland K. Mediation of the stretch modulus of human cervical tissue by prostaglandin E_2. Am J Obstet Gynecol 1976; 126:218.
49. Christensen NJ, Bygdeman M. The effect of prostaglandins on the bioconversion of arachidonic acid in cervical tissue in early pregnancy. Prostaglandins 1985; 29:291–302.
50. Christensen NJ, Belfrage P, Bygdeman M, Floberg J, Miszuhashi N, Green K. Bioconversion of arachidonic acid in human pregnant uterine cervix. Acta Obstet Gynecol Scand 1985; 64:259–65.
51. Liggins GC. Adrenocortical-related maturational events in the fetus. Am J Obstet Gynecol 1976; 126:931.
52. Ito A, Hiro D, Sakyo K, Mori Y. The role of leukocyte factors on uterine cervical ripening and dilatation. Biol Reprod 1987; 37:511–17.
53. Ito A, Lippert P, Mori Y. Human recombinant interleukin-1a increases elastase-like enzyme in human uterine cervical fibroblasts. Gynecol Obstet Invest 1990; 30:239–41.
54. Cabrol D, Dubois P, Sedbon E et al. Prostaglandin E_2-induced changes in the distribution of glycosaminoglycans in the isolated rat uterine cervix. Eur J Obstet Gynecol 1987; 26:359–65.
55. Cabrol D, Dallot E, Bienkiewicz A, El Alj A, Sedbon E, Cedard L. Cyclooxygenase and lipoxygenase inhibitors induce changes in the distribution of glycosaminoglycans in the pregnant rat uterine cervix. Prostaglandins 1990; 39:515–23.
56. Norstrom A. The effects of prostaglandins on the biosynthesis of connective tissue constituents in the non-pregnant human cervix uteri. Acta Obstet Gynecol Scand 1984; 63:169–73.
57. Norstrom A, Bergman I, Lindblom B et al. Effects of 9 deoxo- 16,16 dimethyl-9-methylene PGE_2 on muscle contractile activity and collagen synthesis in the human cervix. Prostaglandins 1985; 29:337–46.
58. Murota S, Abe M, Otsuka K. Stimulatory effect of prostaglandins on the production of hexosamine-containing substances by cultured fibroblasts. (3) Induction of hyaluronise acid synthetase by prostaglandin $F_{2\alpha}$. Prostaglandins 1977; 14:983–91.
59. Gordon AJ, Calder AA. Oestradiol applied locally to ripen the unfavourable cervix. Lancet 1977; ii:1319–21.
60. Allen J, Uldbjerg N, Petersen LK et al. Intracervical 17-β-oestradiol before induction of second trimester abortion with a prostaglandin E_1 analogue. Eur J Obstet Gynecol Reprod Biol 1989; 32:123–7.
61. Mochizuki M, Tojo S. Effect of DHA sulphate on softening and dilatation of the uterine cervix in pregnant women. In: Naftolin F, Stubblefield PG, eds. Dilatation of the uterine cervix. New York: Raven Press, 1980; 267–86.
62. Wallis RM, Hillier K. Regulation of collagen dissolution in the human uterine cervix by oestradiol-17β and progesterone. J Reprod Fertil 1981; 62:55–61.
63. Sitteri PK, Febres F, Clemens LE et al. Progesterone and maintenance of pregnancy: is progesterone nature's immunosuppressant? Ann NY Acad Sci 1977; 286:384–97.
64. Jeffrey JJ, Koob TJ. Endocrine control of collagen degradation in the uterus. In: Naftolin F, Stubblefield PG, eds. Dilatation of the uterine cervix. New York: Raven Press, 1980; 135–45.
65. Gupta JK, Johnson N. Effect of mifepristone on dilatation of the pregnant and non-pregnant cervix. Lancet 1990; i:1238–40.
66. Rådestad A, Bygdeman M, Green K. Induced cervical ripening with mifepristone (RU 486) and

bioconversion of arachidonic acid in human pregnant uterine cervix in the first trimester. Contraception 1990; 41:283–92.

67. Chwalisz R. Cervical ripening and induction of labour with progesterone antagonists. XIth European Congress of Perinatal Medicine, Rome: CIG, 1988; 60.

68. Kelly RW, Healy DL, Cameron IT et al. The stimulation of prostaglandin production by two antiprogesterone steroids in human endometrial cells. J Clin Endocrinol Metab 1986; 62:1116–23.

69. Kelly RW, Bukman A. Antiprogestagenic inhibition of uterine prostaglandin inactivation: a permissive mechanism for uterine stimulation. J Steroid Biochem Mol Biol 1990; 37:97–101.

70. Frydman R. Baton C, Lelaidier C, Vial M, Bourget Ph, Fernandez H. Mefipristone for induction of labour. Lancet 1991; 337:488–9.

71. MacLennan AH. Cervical ripening and the induction of labour by vaginal prostaglandin $F_{2\alpha}$ and relaxin. In: Ellwood DA, Anderson ABM, eds. The cervix in pregnancy and labour: clinical and biochemical investigations. Edinburgh: Churchill Livingstone, 1981; 187–96.

72. von Maillot K, Weiss M, Nagelschmidt M et al. Relaxin and cervical dilatation during parturition. Archiv Gynakol 1977; 223:323–31.

73. McMurty JP, Floerscheim GL, Bryant-Greenwood GD. Characterization of the binding of ^{125}I-labelled succinylated porcine relaxin in human and mouse fibroblasts. J Reprod Fertil 1980; 58:43–9.

74. Bishop EH. Pelvic scoring for elective induction. Obstet Gynecol 1964; 24:266–8.

75. Calder AA, Embrey MP, Tait T. Ripening of the cervix with extraamniotic prostaglandin E_2 in viscous gel before induction of labour. Br J Obstet Gynaecol 1977; 84:264–8.

76. Calder AA. The human cervix in pregnancy: a clinical perspective. In: Ellwood DA, Anderson ABM, eds. The cervix in pregnancy and labour: clinical and biochemical investigations. Edinburgh: Churchill Livingstone, 1981; 103–22.

77. Lilienthal C, Ward J. Medical induction of labour. J Obstet Gynaecol Br Cwlth 1971; 78:317–22.

78. Hillier K, Calder AA, Embrey MP. Concentrations of prostaglandin $F_{2\alpha}$ in amniotic fluid and plasma in spontaneous and induced labours. J Obstet Gyaecol Br Cwlth 1974; 81:257–63.

79. Keirse MJNC. Endogenous prostaglandins in human parturition. In: Keirse MJNC, Anderson ABM, Bennebroek Gravenhorst J, eds. Human parturition. Leiden University Press: The Hague, 1979; 101–41.

80. Mitchell MD, Flint ADF, Bibby J, Brunt J, Arnold JM, Anderson ABM, Turbull AC. Plasma concentrations of prostaglandin during late human pregnancy: influence of normal and preterm labour. J Clin Endocrinol Metab 1978; 46:947–51.

81. Mitchell MD. The mechanism(s) of human parturition. J Dev Physiol 1984; 6:107–18.

82. Brennecke S, Castle BM, Demers LM, Turnbull AC. Maternal plasma prostaglandin E_2 metabolite levels during human pregnancy and parturition. B J Obstet Gynaecol 1985; 92:345–9.

83. Johnston TA, Greer IA, Kelly RW, Gallacher A, Calder AA. Plasma prostaglandin metabolites in human labour. 7th International conference on prostaglandins and related molecules, Florence, 1990; 165.

84. Greer IA, McLaren M, Calder AA. Plasma prostaglandin E_2 and prostaglandin $F_{2\alpha}$ metabolite levels following vaginal administration of prostaglandin E_2 for induction of labor. Acta Obstet Gynecol Scand 1990; 69:621–5.

85. Calder AA, Greer IA. Cervical physiology and induction of labour. In: Bonnar J, ed. Recent advances in obstetrics and gynaecology, vol. 17. London: Churchill Livingstone, 1991.

86. Keirse MJNC, Turnbull AC. E prostaglandins in amniotic fluid during pregnancy and labour. J Obstet Gynaecol Br Cwlth 1973; 80:970–3.

87. Keirse MJNC, Flint APF, Turnbull AC. F prostaglandins in amniotic fluid during pregnancy and labour. Obstet Gynaecol Br Cwlth 1974; 81:131–5.

88. Geirsson RT, Greer IA. Prostaglandins: a key factor in human labour. Acta Obstet Gynecol Scand 1990; 69:371–3.

89. Reddi K, Kambaran SR, Norman RJ, Joubert SM, Philphott RH. Abnormal concentrations of prostaglandins in amniotic fluid during labour in multigravid patients. Br Obstet Gynaecol 1984; 91:781–7.

90. Keirse MJ, van Oppen ACC. Preparing the cervix for induction of labour. In: Chalmers I, Enkins M, Keirse MJ, eds. Effective care in pregnancy and childbirth. Oxford: Oxford University Press, 1989; 988–1056.

91. Rayburn WF. Prostaglandin E_2 gel for cervical ripening and induction of labor: a critical analysis. Am J Obstet Gynecol 1989; 160:529–34.

92. Calder AA, Embrey MP. Prostaglandins and the unfavourable cervix. Lancet 1973; ii:1322.

93. Stewart P, Kennedy JH, Hillan E, Calder AA. The unripe cervix: management with vaginal or extraamniotic prostaglandin E_2. J Obstet Gynaecol 1983; 4:90–4.
94. Greer IA, Calder AA. Preinduction cervical ripening with extra-amniotic and vaginal prostaglandin E_2. J Obstet Gynecol 1989; 10:18–22.
95. Fairlie FM, Lang GD, Greer IA, McLaren M. Umbilical artery Doppler flow velocity waveforms and maternal prostaglandin E_2 and $F_{2\alpha}$ metabolite concentrations during cervical ripening with prostaglandin E_2. Eur J Obstet Gynecol Reprod Biol 1990; 37:7–13.
96. Ulmsten U. A new gel for intracervical application of PGE_2. Lancet 1979; i:377.
97. Ulmsten U, Wingerup L. Clinical experience with a new gel before therapeutic abortion or induction of term labor. Prostaglandins 1980; 20:533.
98. Ulmsten U, Kirstein-Pedersen A, Stenberg P, Wingerup L. A new gel for intracervical application of PGE_2. Acta Obstet Gynecol Scand [Suppl] 1979; 84:19–21.
99. Granstrom L, Ekman G, Ulmsten U. Myometrial activity after local application prostaglandin E_2 for cervical ripening and term induction of labour. Am J Obstet Gynecol 1990; 162:691–4.
100. Ulmsten U. Intracervical application of prostaglandin E_2. In: Egarter C, Husslein P, eds. Prostaglandins for cervical ripening and/or induction of labour. Vienna: Facultas, 1988; 42–5.
101. Ekman GA, Persson PH, Ulmsten N, Wingerup L. The impact on labor induction of intracervically applied PGE_2-gel related to gestational age in patients with an unripe cervix. Acta Obstet Gynecol Scand 1983; 113:173–5.
102. Wiqvist I, Norstrom A, Wiqvist N. Induction of labor by intracervical PGE_2 in viscous gel. Acta Obstet Gynecol Scand 1986; 65:485–92.
103. Kimball FA, Ruppel PL, Noah ML, Decoster JM, de la Fruente P, Castillo JM, Hernandez JM. The effect of endocervical PGE_2-gel (Prepidil) on plasma levels of 13,14-dihydro-15-keto-PGE_2 in women at term. Prostaglandins 1986; 32:527–36.
104. Ekman GA, Forman A, Marshal K, Ulmsten U. Intravaginal versus intracervical application of prostaglandin E_2 in viscous gel for cervical priming and induction of labour at term in patients with an unfavourable cervical state. Am J Obstet Gynecol 1983; 147:657–61.
105. Husslein P. Use of prostaglandins for induction of labour. Semin Perinatol 1991; 15:173–81.
106. Mahmood TA. A prospective comparative study on the use of prostaglandin E_2 gel and prostaglandin E_2 tablet for the induction of labour. Eur J Obstet Gynecol Reprod Biol 1989;33:169–75.
107. Embrey MP, Graham NB, McNeill ME. Induction of labour with a sustained release prostaglandin E_2 vaginal pessary. Br Med J 1980; 281:901–2.
108. Embrey MP, MacKenzie IZ. Labour induction with a sustained release prostaglandin E_2 polymer vaginal pessary. J Obstet Gynecol 1985; 6:38–41.
109. Khouzam MN, Ledward RS. Difficulties with controlled release prostaglandin E_2 pessaries. Lancet 1990; ii:119.
110. Bex P, Gunasekera PC, Phipps JH. Difficulties with controlled release prostaglandin E_2 pessaries. Lancet 1990; ii:119.

Discussion

Nathanielsz: Dr Husslein said something with which, from our experimental animal point of view, I would not agree: that if one tries to induce labour, there is a group that responds and a group that does not and this is related to the state of the cervix. He then went on to say that the situation in the cervix was a direct reflection of the oxytocin receptors. Is that correct?

Husslein: Since we do not do animal experiments, we can only make indirect correlations. There is a clearcut correlation between the cervical state and the sensitivity to oxytocin which is easy to measure by applying a very low dose of oxytocin and seeing whether or not the woman then has a contraction. We did this correlation. We measured the ripeness of the cervix by vaginal examination and did an oxytocin sensitivity test and we were able to show that there is almost a direct correlation. An unripe cervix has no oxytocin responsiveness of the uterus and a ripe cervix has a very nice sensitivity. Then in a single set of correlations we measured oxytocin receptor concentrations in women in whom we did caesarean sections. The women with an unripe cervix did not have a high level of oxytocin receptors and the women with a ripe cervix did.

Nathanielsz: Were these decidual or myometrial oxytocin receptors?

Husslein: There was very good correlation: whenever we found oxytocin receptors in the myometrium we also found decidua. We did not find any situation where there was a discrepancy.

MacKenzie: I would agree that there are women whom we cannot get into labour with oxytocin unless they have some PGs, but the reverse also applies. There are women to whom we give prostaglandins to get them into labour and we fail, but if we then add oxytocin we can stimulate them.

I think it inappropriate to make a distinction between cervical ripening and induction of labour. I think that is an artificial distinction. I think we are talking about induction of labour and then taking into account the state of the cervix and that determines how we should try to induce labour. Cervical ripening is not an entity on its own.

Husslein: I fully agree that there is this other group of women where we start with prostaglandins and on the final round we have not put them into labour. We have apparently changed something but we do not understand what it is. It may be responsiveness towards oxytocin. It may because prostaglandins induce oxytocin receptors, but that is difficult to prove, but in theory that would make a lot of sense.

On the other aspect, I fully agree. I am a little unhappy that apparently I did not get my message across. The distinction between ripening and induction is an artificial one. The point I wanted to make is that induction of an unripe cervix is a totally different situation from induction with a ripe cervix. I agree that in physiology the two things go together, and if we try to distinguish them, then this is a little artificial.

Rådestad: What should we do if the third prostaglandin application has failed to ripen the cervix and we still think that there is a strong indication to induce labour? Should we section that woman or what?

Greer: It depends on the ripeness of the cervix. If it is extremely unripe and it has not been possible to effect ripening, then probably I would do a section – if I had reasonable indications for induction in the first place. If I was having some success with ripening then I would do what Mr MacKenzie was suggesting, rupture the membranes, give her some oxytocin, see if she responds, and if not do a section. If it was very unripe one can rupture the membranes: that is probably a lost cause, but I would make an attempt with oxytocin if possible.

Coming back to Mr MacKenzie's point about the distinction. I agree entirely that it is an artificial one, but it is a very important one to conceptualise for the practising obstetrician. Traditionally we think of induction as forewater amniotomy followed by intermittent oxytocin, and that is often inappropriate if the cervix is unripe. We have to think, does labour need to be induced: yes or no? And then, does the process start with trying to prepare the cervix for labour as opposed to the traditional induction techniques? It is artificial, but it is important for clinical practice.

Husslein: I want to reinforce the point that if PGs have been applied a number of times – whether it is two or three may be open to debate – then even if the cervix is ripe, there is a group of women who cannot be put into labour with two, or even three, prostaglandin applications. It is important to put this over to the public. In such women either the indications for induction should be considered, or if the obstetrician really believes that they should be delivered, then probably they should be sectioned. But first the indications should be considered because sometimes the indications are not that strict and a couple more days could be allowed to pass.

Amy: Referring to the use of oxytocin following PGs, it is clear that PGs have one property that oxytocin lacks, namely that PGs induce the formation of gap junctions and that the stimulation of myometrial activity can be much more effective once there is a sufficient level of gap junction, so that the stimulus can be generalised through the entire myometrium.

I am always very surprised that those who write and talk about vaginal administration of prostaglandins seem to forget that it is a systemic method of administering PGs, not a local method. The PGs have to be absorbed via the vaginal wall into the systemic circulation to reach the end organ. I am always surprised when I see data which mention that the vaginal administration of PGs does not give rise to any side effects. I saw some of the worst side effects when we were experimenting with some of the analogues and used them via the vaginal route. It was always difficult to control them, and I am not talking solely about hypotonus.

Husslein: It is an old debate and probably in theory Professor Amy is right. In clinical practice if we use those doses that are used to induce labour around term, 3 mg in a vaginal tablet or 2 ml in gel form, we virtually never see a systemic reaction. If the levels reached with this type of application are compared to intravenous PGs in a group in whom labour is induced, the intravenous levels are extremely high until the contractions begin, compared to the vaginal tablet levels which are not that high at all.

In theory I agree. I do not see how it gets to the uterus without getting into the circulation, but the fact is that the contractions are induced with very low systemic levels.

Rådestad: I suppose that when side effects are seen with endocervical application of prostaglandins, the gel has probably been applied in the lower uterine segment. How would one know that the gel has been applied strictly intracervically?

Greer: It is a good question. We do not.

Husslein: It is a good, and old, and difficult question. The answer is: by experience. The problem is that if it is inserted too high there is too much resorption with side effects, but if it is too low there is not enough resorption with not enough efficacy. We have to understand that the closer we are to the uterus, the more resorption we have, and so it is a difficult problem. It is an argument that has always been brought against the use of endocervical gel.

Another argument, but on the same lines, is how can one put 3 ml of a gel into a completely closed cervix? The cervix will not take the 3 ml, so part of it will run into the retroamniotic space and part of it will run into the vagina.

Mackenzie: There is another answer to that, that the dose that is placed endocervically is the same dose that is placed extra-amniotically. Any gastrointestinal side effects from that dose (PGE$_2$ 0.5 mg) are very infrequent.

It is a legitimate question. Who knows whether or not it is in the cervical canal? But it does not matter: even if it goes into the lower uterine pool it achieves the same result in the myometrium.

Nathanielsz: I should like to get back to the debate between Mr MacKenzie and Professor Greer. Should one look at the individual portion of the process of parturition, cervical ripening, as being at fault, or should we look at the whole of the labour process?

It is clear that labour is an interlocked series of events which have to take place in a particular time sequence. There are the fetal membranes, the decidua, the myometrium and the cervix. Perhaps one of the problems that the clinicians have is that, when they ask which is the organ at fault, and name the cervix inadequately ripened, they then try to treat that, whereas they should perhaps go further back in the whole process. In normal term delivery I believe that it is the fetus that starts this all off, through the mechanisms that I discussed earlier. There is one paper in the English literature, written by a Japanese group who used dihydroepiandrosterone (DHEA) sulphate to treat post-term labour, and by trying to put PGs locally the situation is similar to what I referred to earlier, as to why we give androgens rather than oestrogens. The list of things for ripening the cervix had oestrogens in it. I do not think we can ripen the cervix by giving exogenous oestrogens. If the oestrogens work, they do not get there by the same route as if they were synthesised by the organisms themselves.

We should be looking at the whole parturition process. We have been discussing two- and three-phase regimens, PGs first and oxytocin later. Could somebody try to give some androgen. DHEA sulphate? It is a totally physiological molecule: one can measure its concentration and reassure oneself that one is not doing something nasty and pharmacological. Then perhaps one would be going back further up the pathway.

Smith: To develop that idea, has anybody tried, in those cases where they have been giving oxytocin and have failed to get a rise in prostaglandins, giving low-dose PGs to those women who are already in labour with oxytocin? If one gives PGs and they fail, one gives oxytocin. In those women who are given oxytocin who are not establishing in labour and in whom the PG levels do not rise, why not give them PGs secondarily? Has it been tried, and if not, why not?

Husslein: In theory that is a very good point. But in practice if both are given at the same time one will run into tremendous hyperstimulation problems. It is difficult to explain because from a physiological point of view, normal labour probably has a bit of oxytocin and a lot of prostaglandins. But the clinical fact is that if they are added at the same time there is a high risk of hyperstimulation.

Keirse: I think it was done in the early 1970s, and the main problem was hyperstimulation.

Smith: So the failure of other actions of the PGs cannot be that important.

Keirse: But that was not looking specifically at those who were receiving oxytocin and who were not doing anything. It was routinely combining oxytocin with prostaglandins.

Smith: In these women who are being given oxytocin and there is no progress, why does someone not try a trial with low-dose prostaglandin?

Preterm Labour

Chapter 14

Cellular Endocrinology

A. López Bernal and S. P. Watson

Introduction

The importance of preterm birth as a cause of perinatal mortality and morbidity cannot be overemphasised. Rush et al. [1] concluded that preterm birth (deliveries before 37 weeks' gestation) was responsible for 85% of early neonatal deaths not due to lethal congenital deformities. This figure was derived from deliveries at the John Radcliffe Maternity Hospital in Oxford during 1973–74. The highest neonatal mortality occurred when preterm labour was spontaneous rather than elective. A review of the deliveries during 1978–88 in the same hospital (P. Yudkin and A. López Bernal, Oxford Data System) revealed that preterm deliveries accounted for 84% of early neonatal deaths, excluding congenital malformations. Thus over the last decades, despite considerable advances in obstetric and neonatal care, the impact of preterm birth on perinatal mortality remains virtually unchanged. A more detailed analysis of the 1978–88 figures from the John Radcliffe Hospital (Fig. 14.1) shows that early preterm births (less than 32 weeks' gestation) accounted for only 1.2% of births, yet they accounted for a disproportionately high percentage (45%) of perinatal deaths (comprising stillbirths and early neonatal deaths). Consequently the perinatal mortality rate in this group was enormous: 211 per thousand births; compared to 29 per thousand at 32–36 weeks; and two per thousand after 37 weeks' gestation. Moreover, Fig. 14.2 shows that spontaneous preterm deliveries accounted for more than half the total neonatal deaths. Hence it is likely that prevention of spontaneous preterm labour, especially before 32 weeks' gestation, would considerably reduce neonatal mortality. These figures can generally be applied to other communities in the UK [2] and in other Western countries [3].

The prevention of preterm labour is a major goal in modern obstetrics, not only to decrease neonatal deaths but also to prevent the wide range of short- and long-

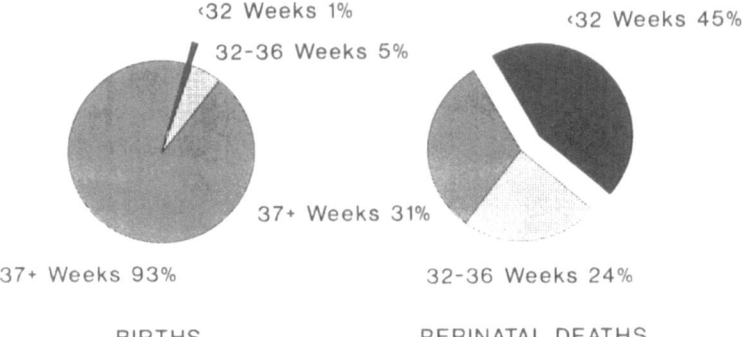

Fig. 14.1. Distribution of perinatal mortality by gestational age at delivery. The number of births (excluding congenital malformations) at the John Radcliffe Maternity Hospital during 1978–88 was 63 067 and the number of perinatal deaths was 362.

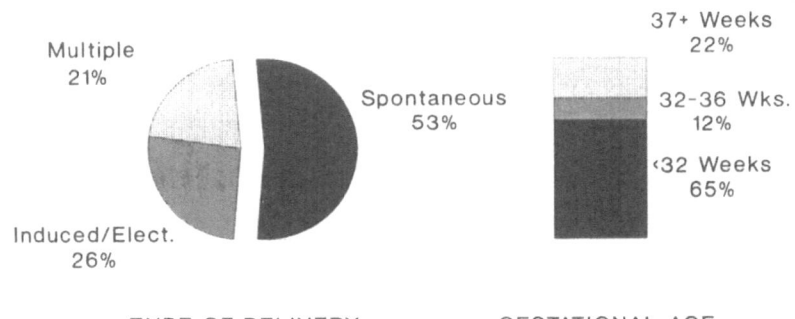

Fig. 14.2. Distribution of early neonatal deaths by type of delivery and gestational age. The number of early neonatal deaths (excluding congenital malformations) during 1978–88 was 154.

term infant morbidity associated with prematurity. Public awareness of the need to deal with this problem is illustrated by the fact that in the USA more than a $100 m per year is given to "birth defects"-related charities, a figure only surpassed by cancer and heart-related charities [4]. Because we know so little about the physiological control of the onset of labour it is very difficult to provide adequate management to prevent preterm labour and delivery. This chapter will focus on the role of prostaglandins and the involvement of second messenger pathways in the control of myometrial contractility.

Role of Prostaglandins

Parturition is associated with increased intrauterine prostaglandin (PG) release as shown by the rising levels of PGE, $PGF_{2\alpha}$, and their metabolites in utero-ovarian veins [5], amniotic fluid [6–9], maternal circulation [10,11] and urine [12] during progressing labour. It is believed that the increased PG output during labour originates in intrauterine tissues (placenta, fetal membranes, decidua), because following placental separation in the third stage of labour there is a precipitous fall in PG metabolites in the maternal circulation [13,14]. There are many publications concerned with PG production by intrauterine tissues [15–21] and this chapter will concentrate on the role of fetal lung phospholipids (surfactant) in PG synthesis, and the identification of PG-producing cell types in decidua by flow cytometry.

Availability of Substrate

Arachidonic acid is the obligatory precursor for PGs of the 2 series (containing two unsaturated double bonds, e.g. PGE_2, $PGF_{2\alpha}$, PGD_2). Since only a few cells in the body can synthesise arachidonic acid (from the essential fatty acid linoleic acid) it is itself considered to be an essential fatty acid. During the third trimester of pregnancy arachidonic acid is present in relatively high concentrations in fetal membranes (amnion and chorion) incorporated mostly into phospholipids and cholesterol esters [22–25]. Quantitatively the most important phospholipids in fetal membranes are phosphatidylcholine (PC), phosphatidylethanolamine (PE) and phosphatidylinositol (PI). At the onset of labour arachidonic acid is released from PE (by phospholipase A_2) and PI (by phospholipase C, diacyl- and monoacylglycerol lipases) [23,26,27]. Once liberated arachidonic acid can be rapidly converted into prostaglandins and lipo-oxygenase products. Because the fetal membranes are not vascularised the question arises as to the source of arachidonate for these tissues. By measuring arachidonate distribution in diamniotic–dichorionic twin membranes (where it is possible to obtain samples of amnion/chorion without any decidual contamination) Okita et al. [28] concluded that arachidonic acid in amnion cells is derived primarily from essential fatty acids in the amniotic fluid, and in chorion cells it is derived partly from the amniotic fluid and partly from the underlying decidua.

Surfactant constitutes a major source of lipid in amniotic fluid and may supply arachidonate to the fetal membranes. Surfactant is a complex lipid–protein mixture and appears in the fetal lung secretions which are intermittently discharged into the amniotic fluid from the beginning of the third trimester [29]. It consists of about 85% phospholipid, 5% non-polar lipids including cholesterol, glycerides and fatty acids, and about 10% protein. Lecithin (phosphatidylcholine) constitutes about 80% of surfactant phospholipids and of this about 60% is dipalmitoyl phosphatidylcholine. The next most important phospholipid is phosphatidylglycerol (5%–10%). The apoproteins specifically associated with pulmonary surfactant have been classified into four main groups designated SP–A, B, C [30,31] and, more recently, D [32]. When the fatty acid content of surfactant lecithin was estimated by gas chromatography palmitate was found to be most abundant (87%); however, arachidonate accounted for more than 2% [33]; hence surfactant represents an important source of arachidonate for the fetal membranes.

Moreover, surfactant has a direct stimulatory effect on PGE_2 production by amnion and choriodecidua which requires both the lipid and protein components for full expression [34]. The mechanism of stimulation has not been fully elucidated. During labour, platelet activating factor (PAF) is secreted in association with surfactant [35]. PAF stimulates PG production in human amnion and endometrial tissue [36,37]. Lecithin itself at high concentrations can stimulate PG production by human amnion, probably by enhancing phospholipase A_2 activity on the cell membranes [38]. However these effects are unlikely to account for the full stimulatory effect of whole surfactant at physiological concentrations [34].

It is possible that amnion cells have a mechanism for recognising surfactant and selectively incorporating arachidonic acid which can be used for PG synthesis. By using a monoclonal antibody against human SP-B it is possible to localise surfactant apoprotein material on the amniotic epithelium in vivo and on cells incubated with surfactant in vitro [39]. Furthermore, cells incubated in the presence of surfactant containing PC labelled at position 2 with [^{14}C]arachidonic acid can readily transfer the label to other phospholipids (PE, PI). When these cells are challenged with calcium ionophore or phorbol esters (to stimulate phospholipase activity and prostaglandin synthesis) they release free [^{14}C]arachidonic acid and ^{14}C-labelled PGE_2. It is clear from these experiments that surfactant phospholipid arachidonate provides a precursor for PG synthesis.

Although these findings provide a potential link between the process of menstruation of the fetus in preparation for birth (surfactant synthesis and secretion) and the activation of PG production in the fetal membranes at the onset of labour, the precise nature of the stimulus that initiates parturition in women is not known.

Chorioamnionitis-Associated Preterm Labour

However, if it is assumed that increased PG production is important for parturition, the question arises as to whether PG release is prematurely activated in preterm labour. Studies in Oxford and in Capetown [40,41] have shown that, in idiopathic or uncomplicated preterm labour, PGE and PGF production by placenta, fetal membranes and decidua is relatively low compared to spontaneous labour at term. However, in chorioamnionitis-associated preterm labour (with histological evidence of placental inflammation, including chorioamnionitis, funisitis, intervillositis, deciduitis) PG output is greatly increased. Moreover tissues with inflammatory infiltration have a large output of leukotriene B_4 (LTB_4), a potent chemotactic agent. Since chorioamnionitis is often the result of bacterial infection these findings provide an explanation for the high levels of prostanoids and lipo-oxygenase products in the amniotic fluid of women with intrauterine infection [42,43], and it has been shown that bacterial products increase arachidonic acid metabolism in the fetal membranes [44]. Another finding in these and other studies [45,46] is the difference in gestational age between chorioamnionitis-associated preterm labour, which tends to occur before 30 weeks' gestation and therefore has a very poor neonatal outcome, and uncomplicated-preterm labour which occurs, on average, 4 weeks later. Hence, chorioamnionitis can be an important cause of early preterm labour by provoking a premature activation of prostaglandin release.

Inflammation is a complex process involving several cell types and chemical mediators. Some of the mediators, including PGs, PAF, bradykinin, histamine, serotonin can provoke uterine contractions by stimulating myometrial cells directly. Other agents, such as LTB_4 and a number of cytokines, amplify the inflammatory reaction. The prevention of chorioamnionitis-associated preterm labour will require methods to decrease the incidence of vaginal infection [47,48] and the use of potent and safe antibiotics and anti-inflammatory drugs, including perhaps prostanoid- and LTB$_4$-receptor antagonists. The effectiveness of such an approach will need to be tested by controlled clinical trials. There is also an urgent need to develop tests for the rapid and accurate diagnosis of chorioamnionitis.

Identification of Prostaglandin-Producing Cell Populations in Human Term Decidua

The decidua is a major intrauterine source of PGs at term [16,18,19,49,50]; however, this tissue comprises several different cell populations and it is therefore important to determine which cell type(s) are responsible for PG production. Using monoclonal antibodies to label specific cell surface antigens in combination with histochemistry and flow cytometry it has been possible to determine that in the third trimester 47% of decidual cells are of bone-marrow origin. Of these 18% are tissue macrophages and the rest comprise T cells, large granular lymphocytes, B cells and granulocytes [51]. The remaining cells include stromal cells and residual glandular elements [52,53].

Flow cytometry allows the preparation of highly homogeneous (>95% pure) cell suspensions and this technique has been used to separate decidual cells obtained from the maternal surface of the fetal membranes following spontaneous vaginal deliveries at term [54]. Fragments of decidual tissue were digested with a mixture of collagenase/hyaluronidase/DNAse and the resulting cell suspensions were prepurified on Percoll density gradients. The cells were labelled with mouse monoclonal antibodies: F10/89/4 [55] which labels the leukocyte common antigen, CD45, found exclusively on cells of bone-marrow origin, or L243 [56] which binds to MHC class II HLA-DR and is specific for macrophages in human decidual tissue [57,58]. The cells were then labelled with a second (goat-antimouse) fluorescein-conjugated antibody and sorted in a flow cytometer by virtue of their fluorescence. After sorting, the cells were incubated in a defined medium and their PG output was measured by radioimmunoassay. The results showed that bone-marrow derived (CD45-positive) cells had higher PGF$_{2\alpha}$ and PGE$_2$ production rates than CD45-negative cells (Fig. 14.3). Moreover cells labelled with anti HLA-DR (macrophages) had a higher PG output than non-macrophages (Fig. 14.3). Bone-marrow derived cells, and specifically the macrophage population have the highest PG output among decidual cells. Further experiments using gas chromatography/mass spectrometry identified PGD$_2$ as a major prostanoid produced by CD45-positive decidual cells (E.R. Norwitz, J. Yerguei and A. López Bernal, unpublished observations).

It is tempting to speculate that bone-marrow derived cells may play a role in the spontaneous onset of labour at term, although PG production rates of decidual macrophages obtained before and after labour have not as yet been compared. Moreover, in chorioamnionitis there is a large increase in PG release by decidua and fetal membranes and this is probably associated with increased cytokine release by decidual macrophages [59]. Interleukin-1 [60], interleukin-6 [61–63] and tumour necrosis factor-α [64,65] levels are increased in the amniotic fluid of

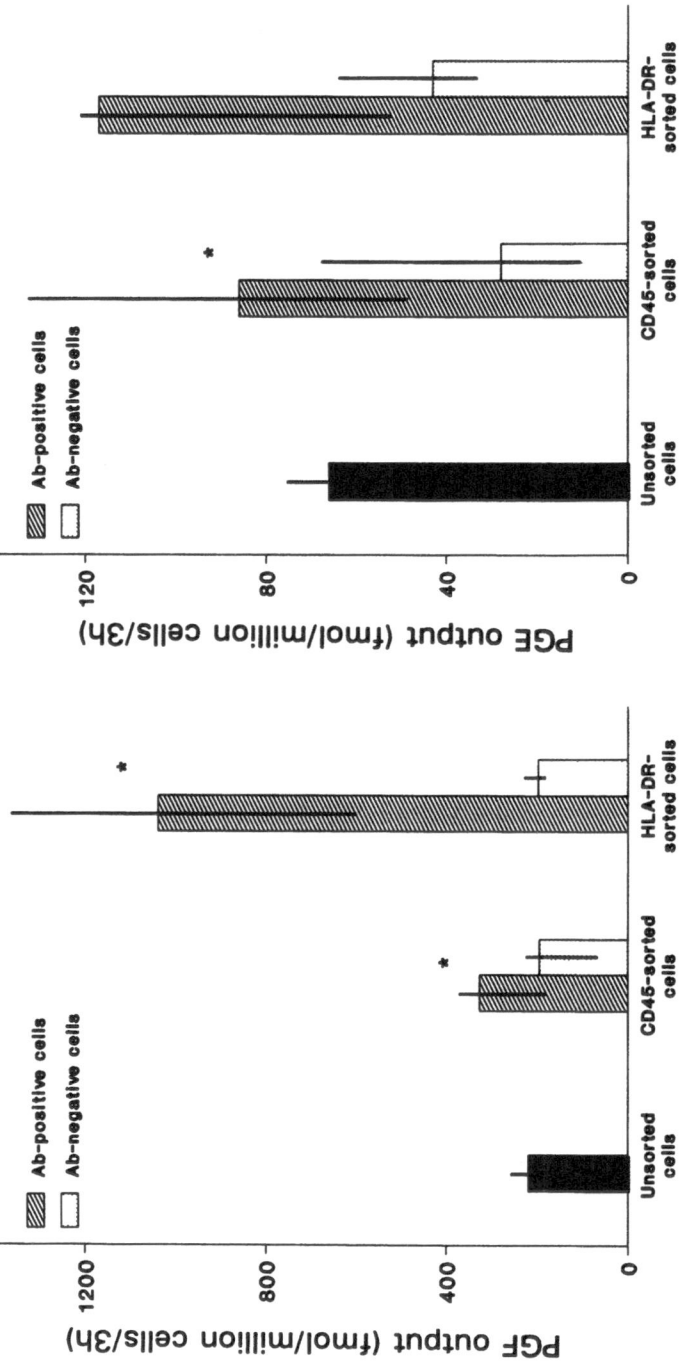

Fig. 14.3. Prostaglandin production by human term decidual cells sorted by flow cytometry. CD45-positive cells were of bone-marrow origin; HLA-DR-positive cells were macrophages. The results are given as the median range from nine experiments. The asterisks indicate significant ($P<0.01$) differences between antibody-positive and -negative cell populations. Adapted from Norwitz et al. [54].

women with chorioamnionitis. These cytokines stimulate PG production by decidual cells and may be involved in the pathogenesis of infection-associated preterm labour.

Role of Second Messengers in Myometrial Contractility

Although there is evidence for a role of PGs in the regulation of myometrial activity and of their involvement in chorioamnionitis-associated preterm labour, the trigger for the onset of idiopathic preterm labour is unknown. There are no apparent changes in the levels of circulating hormones at the initiation of preterm labour and the possibility should be considered that there may be increased sensitivity of the myometrium. This may also be the case for the onset of labour at term. A change in myometrial sensitivity may be brought about by a number of mechanisms such as an upregulation of stimulatory receptors or a downregulation of inhibitory ones. There may also be a change in their signal transduction pathways and evidence in favour of this is beginning to emerge. Therefore the second half of this chapter deals with the cellular endocrinology of uterine contractility and the possible changes that might occur during pregnancy. The discussion will focus on second messengers, with little reference to electrophysiological mechanisms which remain outside the scope of this chapter.

Many hormones have strong effects on myometrial activation and relaxation. Their action depends on the binding to specific receptors on the cell membrane and the transmission of information to an effector system within the cell usually via a G protein. There are at least two major second messenger pathways operating in human myometrium, adenylyl cyclase and phospholipase C (Figs. 14.4 and 14.5). It is noteworthy that each hormone–receptor complex can interact with several G proteins providing a signal amplification system. The number of second messenger molecules generated depends not so much on the number of

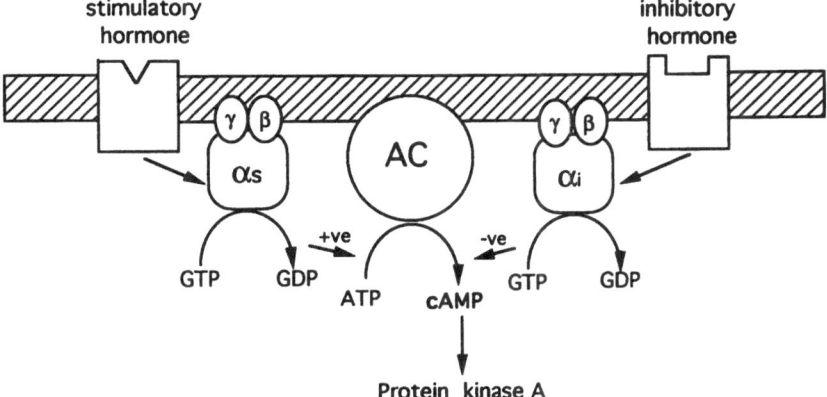

Fig. 14.4. Adenylyl cyclase (AC) can be stimulated or inhibited by a hormone–receptor complex coupled to α_s (left) or to α_i (right) leading to increased/decreased synthesis of cAMP.

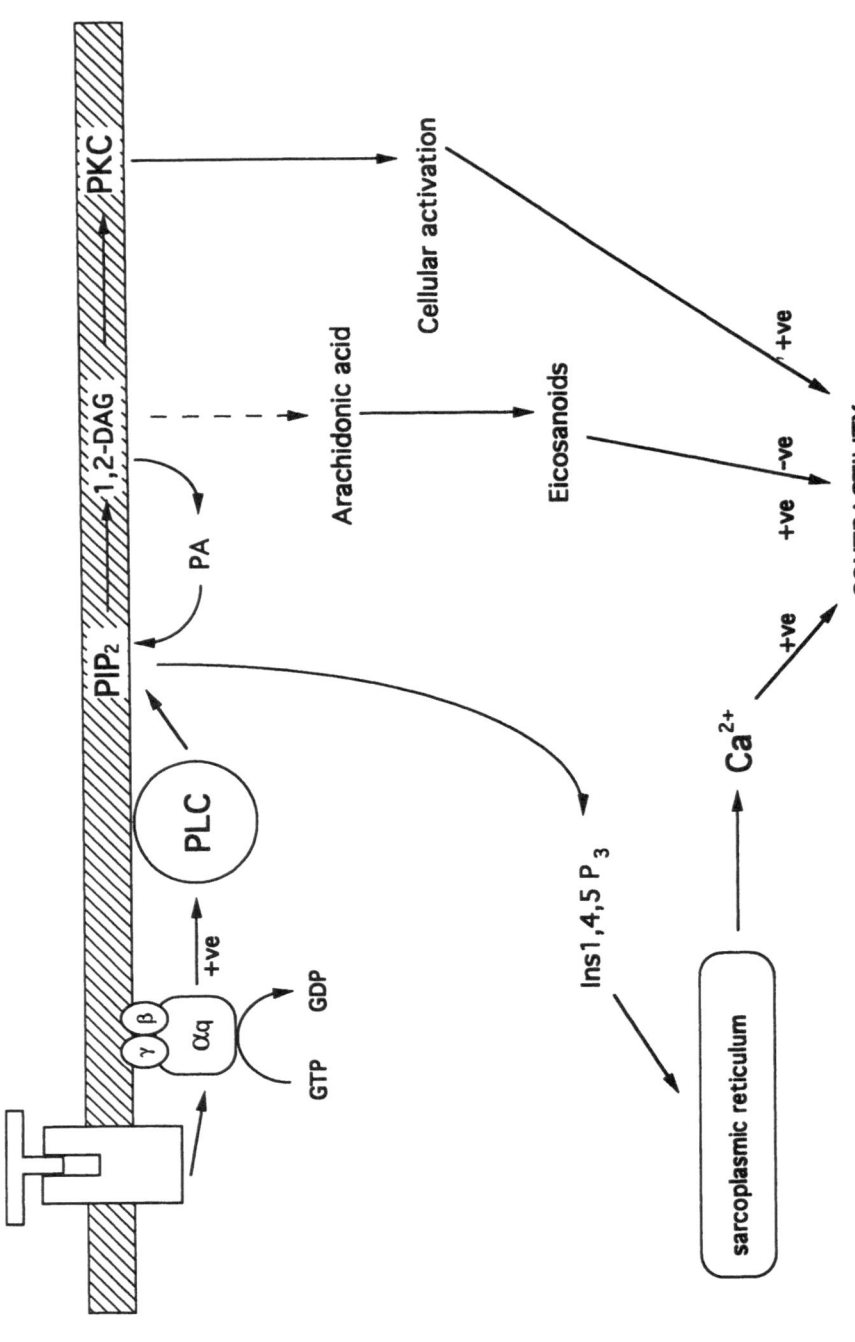

Fig. 14.5. The inositol phospholipid pathway. The binding of a hormone to its receptor stimulates GTP/GDP exchange by α_q and this activates phospholipase C (PLC), leading to the hydrolysis of phosphatidylinositol 4,5-bisphosphate (PIP_2). This generates two second messengers: inositol 1,4,5-trisphosphate (Ins 1,4,5 P_3) which mobilises calcium from the sarcoplasmic reticulum, and 1,2-diacylglycerol (1,2-DAG) which activates protein kinase C (PKC). These two pathways can stimulate smooth muscle contractility. DAG can be converted into phosphatidic acid (PA) and reincorporated into PIP_2 or it can be metabolised to release arachidonic acid. Arachidonic acid can have a second messenger role itself, probably by mobilising calcium, or it can be converted into prostaglandins and other eicosanoids which further regulate contractility.

occupied hormone binding sites on the cell membrane, but on the level of interaction or "coupling" between the hormone–receptor complex and the G protein, and between the G protein and its effector enzyme.

Involvement of G Proteins

Regulatory GTP-binding proteins (G proteins) constitute a family of proteins involved in signal transduction across the plasma membrane [66–70]. They consist of three different subunits α, β and γ. G proteins are classified according to their α subunits, some of which are substrates for ADP-ribosylating bacterial exotoxins, such as pertussis toxin (the toxin uncouples the G protein from its receptor thus blocking signal transduction) (Table 14.1). Sixteen G protein α subunits encoded by different genes are known. Three types of β and four types of γ subunits have also been identified but are thought to be functionally identical. G proteins transduce signals from membrane receptors to effectors such as enzymes (for example, adenylyl cyclase and phospholipase C) and ion channels (for example, the voltage-sensitive calcium or potassium channels) and they are likely to play a major role in myometrial activation and relaxation.

Table 14.1. Examples of G proteins involved in signal transduction. To date the best characterised pathways are those for G_s, the stimulatory G protein of adenylyl cyclase, for the retinal G proteins or transducins, which mediate between activated photoreceptors and a cyclic GMP phosphodiesterase, and for G_o which mediate calcium channel inhibition.

Family	Subtypes	Transduction-pathways	Pertussis sensitive
G_s	$G_{\alpha s}$	Adenylyl cyclase	No
Transducin	$G_{\alpha t}$	cGMP phosphodiesterase	Yes
G_i	$G_{\alpha i1}$, $G_{\alpha i2}$, $G_{\alpha i3}$	Adenylyl cyclase inhibition K^+ channel stimulation Ca^{2+} channel inhibition (?)	Yes
G_o	$G_{\alpha o1}$, $G_{\alpha o2}$	Ca^{2+} channel inhibition	Yes
G_q	$G_{\alpha q}$, $G_{\alpha 11-16}$	Phospholipase C	No

The Adenylyl Cyclase Pathway

The adenylyl cyclase pathway is initiated by the binding of a hormone or agonist to its receptor (Fig. 14.4). The receptor so activated interacts with either a G protein which stimulates (G_s) or inhibits (G_i) the catalytic subunit of adenylyl cyclase thus increasing or inhibiting agonist-stimulated synthesis of adenosine 3',5'-monophosphate (cAMP). The second messenger action of cAMP results from its activation of protein kinase A which, by phosphorylating selected target proteins, provokes a cellular response. In myometrium, calcium binds to calmodulin and this complex activates the enzyme myosin light chain kinase (MLCK) which phosphorylates myosin, thus promoting the interaction between actin and myosin that results in contraction. Protein kinase A phosphorylates MLCK and decreases the affinity of this enzyme for the calcium–calmodulin complex; phosphorylation of myosin is blocked and relaxation occurs (Fig. 14.6).

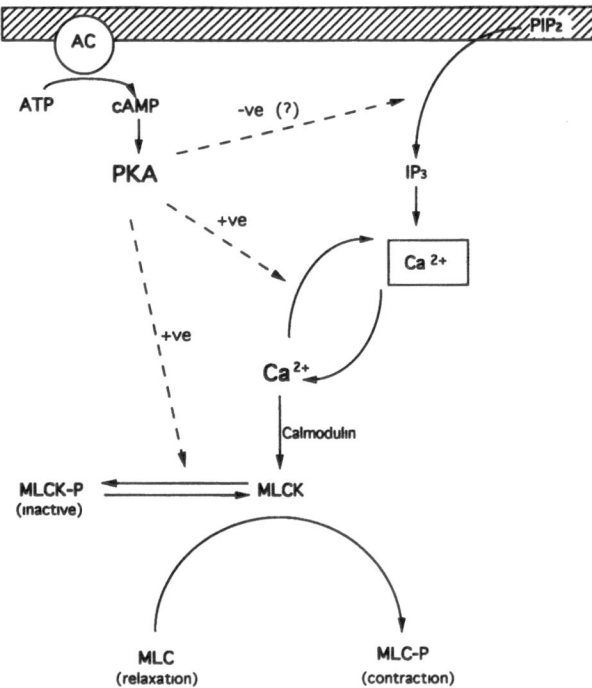

Fig. 14.6. Myosin light chain kinase (MLCK) is activated by the Ca^{2+}–calmodulin complex and phosphorylates myosin (MLC) leading to contraction. This reaction can be inhibited by cAMP-dependent protein kinase (PKA) which by phosphorylating MLCK renders it inactive. PKA can also lower intracellular calcium by promoting Ca^{2+} uptake by the sarcoplasmic reticulum or by inhibiting the formation of IP_3. By these mechanisms cAMP provokes smooth muscle relaxation.

Moreover, cAMP-dependent protein kinase A may promote relaxation of smooth muscle by lowering intracellular calcium; this can be achieved by promoting calcium uptake by the sarcoplasmic reticulum or by inhibiting formation of IP_3 (Fig. 14.6). Hence hormones that raise cAMP relax the uterus and hormones that decrease cAMP enhance contractility. Other cyclic nucleotides, for example cGMP, may have second-messenger roles in human myometrium and activators of guanylyl cyclase are known to relax myometrial cells in vitro [71], although the role of cGMP remains controversial [72].

The Inositol Phospholipid Pathway

The role of receptor-stimulated inositol phospholipid hydrolysis in many systems has become increasingly clear [73–75], however the steps in this pathway are not so well characterised as those linking receptors to adenylyl cyclase. Hokin and Hokin [76] made the initial observation that cholinergic stimulation of pancreatic cells stimulated the incorporation of radiolabelled phosphate into phosphatidyl-inositol (PI) and phosphatidic acid. The presence of this type of "PI" response was later established in many tissues, but it was only with the discovery of inositol trisphosphate and its ability to mobilise intracellular calcium that the PI cycle became established as a major cell signalling pathway [74]. This pathway is intimately associated with smooth muscle contractility and is summarised in Fig. 14.5. The binding of a hormone or agonist to its cell surface receptor stimulates a G-protein which in turn activates phospholipase C. The hydrolysis of phosphatidylinositol 4,5-bisphosphate (PIP_2) by phospholipase C generates two molecules both of which have second messenger roles: inositol 1,4,5-trisphosphate (IP_3) which mobilises calcium from the sarcoplasmic reticulum, and 1,2-diacylglycerol which activates protein kinase C, leading to the phosphorylation of several cellular proteins. There is considerable amplification of the signal in this pathway because each hormone–receptor complex can activate several G-proteins and each phospholipase C molecule can hydrolyse many molecules of PIP_2; so, as with the adenylyl cyclase pathway, the extent of coupling between receptor and G-protein and between G-protein and phospholipase C is probably more important for cellular responsiveness than the number of hormone receptors on the cell surface.

The action of IP_3 is terminated by its rapid metabolism to inositol bis- and monophosphates and finally to inositol which can be reincorporated into PI. IP_3 can also be converted into inositol 1,3,4,5-tetrakisphosphate (IP_4), which may be a second messenger in its own right [77,78] but whose role in myometrium is not clear. Diacylglycerol can be converted into phosphatidic acid and reutilised for PI synthesis or it can be hydrolysed by diacylglycerol and monoacylglycerol lipases. The latter pathway is of great interest because the fatty acid in position 2 of the 1,2-diacylglyercol molecule derived from PI is usually arachidonate which, once released, becomes available for prostaglandin synthesis. Hence, prostaglandins and other eicosanoids modulate further the response of the cell to the original agonist.

It must be emphasised that this description of the inositol phospholipid pathway is probably oversimplified. Phosphoinositides other than PIP_2 may be hydrolysed following hormone stimulation; assignment of G-protein types to specific myometrial receptors has not been achieved; there are several phospholipase C isozymes in smooth muscle and it is not known which are involved in the transmission of contractile stimuli; the role of protein kinase C and the identification of the relevant phosphorylation substrates in myometrium remain to be investigated. Moreover phospholipases A_2 and D activities may also be involved in cell signalling [79–82] but their role in myometrium is not known. Despite these uncertainties the inositol phospholipid pathway is now thought to have a major influence on myometrial function.

Role of IP_3 in Human Myometrium

Oxytocin and other stimulatory peptides cause a rapid increase in endogenous IP_3 levels in human myometrium (Fig. 14.7). Moreover IP_3 releases calcium from the sarcoplasmic reticulum of myometrial cells [83–85]. While this evidence is consistent with the second messenger role of IP_3 in myometrium, the identification of specific IP_3 binding sites in this tissue has further strengthened the role of IP_3. Rivera et al. [86] demonstrated the presence of binding sites in membrane preparation of human myometrium with the characteristics of IP_3 receptors, i.e. very fast association and dissociation rates, high affinity (saturation in the low

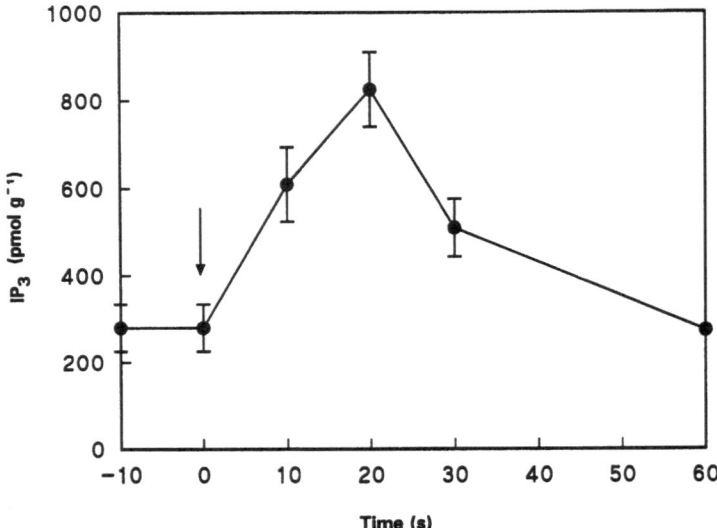

Fig. 14.7. Mass IP$_3$ levels estimated by radioreceptor assay in slices of term human myometrium exposed to 1 μM-oxytocin (*arrow*). Means ± SEM from three experiments.

nanomolar range) and specificity. The sites distinguished between IP$_3$ and other inositol-polyphosphates (IP$_1$, IP$_2$, IP$_4$, IP$_5$, IP$_6$) and showed excellent discrimination between inositol 1,4,5-trisphosphate and the substantially less active inositol 2,4,5-trisphosphate and inositol 1,3,4-trisphosphate isomers. The myometrial IP$_3$ receptor is similar to that present in other tissues (cerebellum, adrenal cortex, platelets) [87] although small differences in binding affinity between tissues exist. Calcium inhibits the binding of IP$_3$ to its myometrial receptor, probably due to an allosteric effect mediated by the calcium binding protein calmedin loosely associated with the receptor [86]. This may provide a regulatory mechanism by which increased intracellular calcium following receptor-stimulated IP$_3$ generation may lead to attenuation of the IP$_3$ response by inhibition of its binding.

Prostaglandins and Uterine Contractility

Prostaglandins have stimulatory and inhibitory effects on myometrial contractility and are well suited to participate in the balance between uterine quiescence and the transition into labour. Binding sites for PGE$_1$/PGE$_2$ and for PGF$_{2\alpha}$ have been described in human myometrium by several groups [88–95]. These sites have high affinity for PGE$_2$ (K_d 1 nM) and poorer affinity (K_d 30 nM) for PGF$_{2\alpha}$ [95]. A link between PG binding to these sites and second messenger generation is suggested by the fact that drugs that inhibit PGE$_2$ binding (i.e. sodium meclofenamate) also inhibit cAMP formation [96]. Pharmacological studies

Table 14.2. Prostanoid receptors

	Receptors				
	DP	EP_1, EP_2, EP_3	FP	IP	TP
Potency order	D>E,F,I,T	E>F,I>D,T	F>D>E>LT	I>D,E,F,>T	T=H>>D,E,F,I
Example agonists	BW245C ZK110841	EP_1: 17-phenyl-ω-trinor-PGE_2 EP_2:butaprost EP_3: enprostil; GR63799	fluprostenol	cicaprost	U46619 STA_2
Example antagonists	BWA868C	EP_1: SC19220 AH6809	–	–	GR32191 SQ29548
Effector pathways	cAMP↑	EP_1: IP_3/DG EP_2: cAMP↑ EP_3: IP_3/DG;cAMP↓	IP_3/DG	cAMP↑	IP_3/DG

Prostanoids: PGD_2 (D), PGE_2 (E), $PGF_{2\alpha}$ (F), PGH_2 (H), PGI_2 (I), TXA_2 (T) reveal a complex pattern of responses [97]: PGs of the E and D type and their analogues tend to relax the uterus acting on "EP_2" and "DP" receptors linked to cAMP generation; $PGF_{2\alpha}$ analogues stimulate contractility through "FP" receptors [98–100]. The effector pathway for FP receptors in the uterus is not known although in other tissues they are linked to IP_3 generation. PGE_2 and its analogues are potent stimulatory drugs in vivo and have been used successfully for the treatment of postpartum haemorrhage. However, in vitro PGE_2 is stimulatory at low doses (nM) whereas at high (μM) doses it has a biphasic effect with an initial contraction followed by profound relaxation [101,102]. Coleman et al. [98–100] have suggested the presence of three functional EP receptor subtypes in myometrium: EP_2 relaxatory, linked to cAMP generation, and EP_1 and EP_3, stimulatory, linked to the inositol phospholipid pathway (Table 14.2). These putative receptors can be distinguished pharmacologically with a variety of specific PG agonists and antagonists.

PGE_2 inhibits calcium uptake and enhances calcium release from myometrial sarcoplasmic reticulum vesicles [103–105] thus leading to a net increase in available intracellular calcium. By contrast, $PGF_{2\alpha}$ promotes calcium entry into myometrial cells from the extracellular medium [106]. It is not clear whether these effects of PGs on intracellular calcium are mediated by second messengers. Much of the uncertainty about the mechanism of action of PGs on the uterus will be dispelled when the structure of PG receptors is known. It will be necessary to identify the receptors present in the uterus using molecular biology techniques and selective agonists and antagonists. Unfortunately, the receptors have not yet been cloned and the latter compounds are poor discriminators.

Prostacyclin receptors linked to adenylyl cyclase by G_s [107] and the recently cloned thromboxane A_2 receptor [108] linked to phospholipase C by G_q may also be involved in the complex regulation of uterine contractility by eicosanoids.

Other Uterine Stimulants

Oxytocin has long been associated with human parturition. Caldeyro-Barcia and Poseiro [109] documented the increased sensitivity of the uterus to oxytocin in vivo with advancing gestation, and it has been suggested that women who go into preterm labour have higher sensitivity to oxytocin than women who deliver at term [110]. The mechanism of action of oxytocin on human myometrial cells has recently been investigated. Oxytocin stimulates the inositol phospholipid pathway [111] and increases intracellular calcium via an IP_3 dependent mechanism [106]. Oxytocin causes very rapid increases in mass levels of IP_3 (Fig. 14.7) and the time course correlates well with the calcium fluxes visualised in isolated myometrial cells [112], i.e. peak levels of IP_3 and calcium are obtained within 10–20 s after oxytocin stimulation, and with the stimulation of contractions. High affinity (K_d 1 nM) oxytocin binding sites are present in human myometrium and increase during pregnancy [86,113]. These sites cross-react with vasopressin. Similar binding sites are present in sheep myometrium and endometrium [114,115] and experiments with specific oxytocin antagonists suggest that these sites represent oxytocin receptors [116–118]. Because oxytocin receptors are relatively specific for myometrial cells, the use of oxytocin antagonists which block oxytocin binding and IP$_3$ formation [119] represents an interesting approach to inhibit preterm labour with no side effects [120]. The nature of the G protein mediating the action of oxytocin is not known, although it is partially sensitive to pertussis toxin in human and rat [106,121,122], but not guinea-pig [123] myometrium. It is likely that the pertussis-insensitive G protein belongs to the G$_q$ class which has recently been shown to activate phospholipase C [124,125].

Other peptide hormones which stimulate uterine contractility include vasopressin, angiotensin and endothelin, and the action of the latter has been studied in some detail. Endothelin is a potent vasoconstrictor related to the sarafotoxins from snake venom. The name is derived from its production by vascular endothelial cells [126]. Endothelin is present in plasma and amniotic fluid of pregnant women near term [127] and stimulates the contractility of human myometrium in vitro [104,128,129], hence, like oxytocin it may be an endogenous modulator of uterine activity. Endothelin binds to high affinity receptors in human myometrial cells which are distinct from the oxytocin receptor, and increases intracellular calcium by a mechanism involving mobilisation from intracellular stores and calcium entry through cell membrane channels [129]. The rise in intracellular calcium is accompanied by increased phosphorylation of MLCK [128]. Although it seems clear that the action of endothelin involves inositol phospholipid hydrolysis, the nature of the G protein involved is unknown, although it is resistant to pertussis toxin [121].

The existence of α and β-adrenergic responses which mediate uterine contraction and relaxation, respectively, has been known for many years [130]. Further studies with various pharmacological agonists/antagonists and binding experiments with selective radioligands has demonstrated the presence of α_1, α_2 and β_2 receptor subtypes in uterine tissue from many species including human [131–134]. Recent experiments using membrane preparations from human pregnant myometrium indicate that α_1 adrenergic receptors are linked to the inositol phospholipid pathway by an uncharacterised G protein [135] and α_2 receptors are linked to adenylyl cyclase inhibition via G$_i$ [136]. In contrast, β-adrenergic receptors stimulate cAMP formation via G$_s$ [137]. Thus the uterine stimulatory effect of catecholamines is exerted primarily through α_1, and, possibly, through α_2 receptors whereas the relaxant effect of these compounds is mediated by β_2 receptors.

Because of the extensive use of β-agonists in preterm labour β-adrenergic mechanisms have been studied by several groups. It is believed that cAMP mediates the relaxant effect of these drugs and it is of interest that the adenylyl cyclase activity of human myometrium in response to the β_2 agonist isoproterenol was found to decrease towards term [137]. cAMP generation in response to GTP-analogues also decreased after 35 weeks' gestation whereas the response to forskolin (which activates adenylyl cyclase directly) remained intact [137]. Thus it seems that in human term myometrium there is uncoupling of β_2 receptors to adenylyl cyclase via G$_s$ and the relaxant effect of these drugs is diminished; in other words there should be enhanced responsiveness to tocolytic drugs mediated by cAMP before 35 weeks compared to term. A loss of PGE-induced cAMP responses in human myometrium at term has also been described [138]. Tocolytics are effective in suppressing preterm labour for some time and postponing delivery, but it has been suggested that their main benefit is to provide time for other therapeutic measures, e.g. to administer glucocorticoids to promote fetal lung maturation or to transfer the mother to a centre with adequate facilities for preterm delivery [139].

In many species, including human, the uterus contracts in response to acetylcholine and to carbachol. This system has been studied in some detail in the rat [122] and the evidence suggests that carbachol attenuates cAMP production by stimulating a calcium-dependent phosphodiesterase, but it also stimulates phospholipase C and IP_3 formation. In guinea-pig uterus carbachol inhibits the rise in cAMP in response to prostacyclin; the effect of carbachol is blocked by pertusis toxin thus suggesting that in this species muscarinic receptors are linked to adenylyl cyclase via G_i [122,140].

Are There Changes in G Protein Function in Myometrium During Pregnancy?

The hypothesis that changes in signal transduction pathways in the uterus may be involved in parturition is attractive, because it could explain the increase in contractility without a need for changes in circulating hormone levels or myometrial receptor concentrations. Evidence that changes in the content and/or function of G proteins in myometrium may be responsible for uterine quiescence during pregnancy and for increased contractility at the onset of labour, is beginning to accumulate from studies on animal and human tissue. For example, in the guinea pig the establishment and maintenance of pregnancy is associated with a significant decrease in GTP-stimulated phosphoinositide hydrolysis, with little change in phospholipase C activity [141]. This suggests that the coupling of G proteins to phospholipase C is impaired during pregnancy, and the uterus is therefore less sensitive to hormones that stimulate the inositol phospholipid pathway, i.e. it becomes quiescent. Also in the guinea pig pregnancy provoked a significant increase in myometrial GTP-dependent adenylyl cyclase activity, without changes in enzyme concentration, suggesting an increased coupling of G_s to adenylyl cyclase [142]. This would contribute to uterine quiescence by increasing uterine sensitivity to relaxants. In human myometrium the activation of adenylyl cyclase by β-adrenergic drugs and PGE_2 disappears at the end of pregnancy with no change in receptor levels [137,138], so that cAMP-mediated relaxation is attenuated. In the rat there are quantitative changes in the levels of myometrial G protein subunits linked to adenylyl cyclase: G_{i2} α and β subunits increase at midgestation and return to normal values at term, whereas $G_{i3\alpha}$ decreases with advancing gestation [143]. Interestingly, some of these changes may be hormone-dependent: in rabbits, progesterone treatment desensitises myometrial α_2-adrenergic receptors [144,145]. Since these receptors are coupled to adenylyl cyclase inhibition through G_i, the effect of progesterone is to favour cAMP formation and uterine relaxation. In guinea pigs progesterone and oestradiol have opposing effects on G-protein coupling to adenylyl cyclase. Further evidence from studies on small rodents suggests a complex "cross-talk" between the adenylyl cyclase and inositol phospholipid pathways. In rats, isoproterenol and relaxin (which acts as a uterine relaxant by increasing cAMP), inhibit oxytocin-stimulated inositol phosphate formation and intracellular calcium release [146,147], and prostaglandins and carbachol, which stimulate contractility, attenuate cAMP formation by relaxatory agonists [148]. This inhibitory effect of the prostaglandins (PGE_2 and $PGF_{2\alpha}$) on cAMP generation was blocked by pertussis toxin thus suggesting the involvement of G_i [148].

It is possible that changes in G protein coupling and content modify the sensitivity of the myometrium to hormones and agonists during pregnancy by altering the balance of IP_3 and cAMP formation. In addition G proteins regulate calcium and potassium channels providing alternative mechanisms for contraction and relaxation. The identification and quantitation of G proteins linked to contractility pathways in human myometrium and their assignment to specific receptors is obviously of paramount importance. The onset of term and preterm labour may depend not so much on changes in the levels of hormones reaching the myometrium, but on changes in their signal transduction pathways mediated at the level of the G proteins.

Conclusions

Normal parturition is associated with increased intrauterine PG release but the control of PG production at the onset of labour is not well understood. Fetal surfactant is an important source of arachidonate and may play a part in the events that initiate parturition at term by stimulating arachidonate turnover and PG production in the fetal membranes. Chorioamnionitis can cause early preterm labour by provoking a premature release of PGs and other inflammatory mediators in the decidua/fetal membranes area. Bone marrow-derived cells and, specifically, decidual macrophages have a relatively high PG output compared to other decidual cells making them potential candidates for the increase in PG production. The role of bone marrow-derived decidual cells in normal and chorioamnionitis-associated labour needs to be defined. However, idiopathic preterm labour is probably due to increased sensitivity of the myometrium to endogenous agonists.

Our failure to deal effectively with preterm labour is related to the difficulty in anticipating or even diagnosing this condition. However, it also stems from our ignorance about the control of uterine contractility. Recent progress in cell signalling pathways, the characterisation of regulatory G-proteins, and the ability to clone and sequence cell surface receptors has provided the tools to study the mechanism of action of hormones in fine detail. When these tools are applied to the human myometrium the role of PGs, oxytocin, adrenergic agonists and other hormones known to influence myometrial contractility should become clearer. From a therapeutic point of view, knowledge of the dominant stimulatory/inhibitory pathways should facilitate the design of better drugs to control uterine activity in a safe and specific manner. This approach should improve the management of both preterm and term labour.

Acknowledgement. We are grateful to Dr P. J. R. Phizackerley for valuable comments.

References

1. Rush RW, Keirse MJ, Howat P, Baum JD, Anderson AB, Turnbull AC. Contribution of preterm delivery to perinatal mortality. Br Med J 1976; 2:965–8.
2. Collaborative Survey of Perinatal and late Neonatal Mortality. Newcastle upon Tyne: Northern Regional Health Authority, 1986; 3–42.
3. National Institutes of Health. Infant mortality. 1988 Research Accomplishments. US Department of Health and Human Services 1989; 1–26.
4. Max B. This and that: error, observation and education in pharmacology. TiPS 1991; 12:176–80.
5. Davidson BJ, Murray RD, Challis JR, Valenzuela GJ. Estrogen, progesterone, prolactin, prostaglandin E_2, prostaglandin F_2 alpha, 13,14-dihydro-15-keto-prostaglandin $F_{2\ alpha}$, and 6-keto-prostaglandin $F_{1\ alpha}$ gradients across the uterus in women in labor and not in labor. Am J Obstet Gynecol 1987; 157:54–8.
6. Keirse MJNC, Turnbull AC. E prostaglandins in amniotic fluid during late pregnancy and labour. Br J Obstet Gynaecol 1973; 80:970–3.
7. Keirse MJNC, Flint APF, Turnbull AC. F prostaglandins in amniotic fluid during pregnancy and labour. Br J Obstet Gynaecol 1974; 81:131–5.
8. Dray F, Frydman R. Primary prostaglandins in amniotic fluid in pregnancy and spontaneous labor. Am J Obstet Gynecol 1976; 126:13–19.
9. Keirse MJNC, Mitchell MD, Turnbull AC. Changes in prostaglandin F and 13,14-dihydro-15-keto-prostaglandin F concentrations in amniotic fluid at the onset of and during labour. Br J Obstet Gynaecol 1977; 84:743–6.
10. Gréen K, Bygdeman M, Toppozada M, Wiqvist N. The role of prostaglandin F_{2alpha} in human parturition. Endogenous plasma levels of 15-keto-13,14-dihydro-prostaglandin F_{2alpha} during labor. Am J Obstet Gynecol 1974; 120:25–31.
11. Sellers SM, Mitchell MD, Bibby JG, Anderson AB, Turnbull AC. A comparison of plasma prostaglandin levels in term and preterm labour. Br J Obstet Gynecol 1981; 88:362–6.
12. Granström E, Kindahl H. Radioimmunoassay for urinary metabolites of prostaglandin F_{2alpha}. Prostaglandins 1976; 12:759–83.
13. Sellers SM, Hodgson HT, Mitchell MD, Anderson AB, Turnbull AC. Raised prostaglandin levels in the third stage of labor. Am J Obstet Gynecol 1982; 144:209–12.
14. Noort WA, van Bulck B, Vereecken A, de Zwart FA, Keirse MJ. Changes in plasma levels of $PGF_{2\ alpha}$ and PGI_2 metabolites at and after delivery at term. Prostaglandins 1989; 37:3–12.
15. Liggins GC, Forster CS, Grieves SA, Schwartz AL. Control of parturition in man. Biol Reprod 1977; 16:39–56.
16. Keirse MJNC. Endogenous prostaglandins in human parturition. In: Keirse MJNC, Anderson ABM, Bennebroek Gravenhorst J, eds. Human parturition. Leiden: Leiden University Press, 1979; 101–42.
17. Kinoshita K, Satoh K, Yasumizu T, Sakamoto S, Green K. Bioconversion of arachidonic acid in human amnion during pregnancy and labor. Adv Prostaglandin Thromboxane Leukotriene Res 1980; 8:1419–22.
18. Okazaki T, Casey ML, Okita JR, MacDonald PC, Johnston JM. Initiation of human parturition. XII. Biosynthesis and metabolism of prostaglandins in human fetal membranes and uterine decidua. Am J Obstet Gynecol 1981; 139:373–81.
19. Mitchell MD. Pathways of arachidonic acid metabolism with specific application to the fetus and mother. Semin Perinatol 1986; 10:242–54.
20. Liggins GC. Initiation of labour. Biol Neonate 1989; 55:366–75.
21. Lundin Schiller S, Mitchell MD. The role of prostaglandins in human parturition. Prostaglandins Leukotrienes Essent Fatty Acids 1990; 39:1–10.
22. Schwartz AL, Forster CS, Smith PA, Liggins GC. Human amnion metabolism. II. Incorporation of fatty acids into tissue phospholipids in vitro. Am J Obstet Gynecol 1977; 127:475–81.
23. Okita JR, MacDonald PC, Johnston JM. Mobilization of arachidonic acid from specific glycerophospholipids of human fetal membranes during early labor. J Biol Chem 1982; 257:14029–34.
24. Foster HWJ, Das SK. Study of lipids in human amnion and chorion. Am J Obstet Gynecol 1984; 149:670–3.
25. Olson DM, Smieja Z. Arachidonic acid incorporation into lipids of term human amnion. Am J Obstet Gynecol 1988; 159:995–1001.
26. Okazaki T, Sagawa N, Bleasdale JE, Okita JR, MacDonald PC, Johnston JM. Initiation of

human parturition: XIII. Phospholipase C, phospholipase A_2, and diacylglycerol lipase activities in fetal membranes and decidua vera tissues from early and late gestation. Biol Reprod 1981; 25:103–9.

27. Okazaki T, Sagawa N, Okita JR, Bleasdale JE, MacDonald PC, Johnston JM. Diacylglycerol metabolism and arachidonic acid release in human fetal membranes and decidua vera. J Biol Chem 1981; 256:7316–21.

28. Okita JR, Johnston JM, MacDonald PC. Source of prostaglandin precursor in human fetal membranes: arachidonic acid content of amnion and chorion laeve in diamnionic-dichorionic twin placentas. Am J Obstet Gynecol 1983; 147:477–82.

29. Gluck L. Biochemical development of the lung: clinical aspects of surfactant development, RDS and the intrauterine assessment of lung maturity. Clin Obstet Gynecol 1971; 14:710–21.

30. Metcalfe IL, Enhorning G, Possmayer F. Pulmonary surfactant-associated proteins: their role in the expression of surface activity. J Appl Physiol 1980; 49:34–41.

31. Possmayer F. A proposed nomenclature for pulmonary surfactant-associated proteins. Am Rev Respir Dis 1988; 138:990–8.

32. Persson A, Chang D, Rust K, Moxley M, Longmore W, Crouch E. Purification and biochemical characterization of CP4 (SP-D), a collagenous surfactant associated protein. Biochemistry 1989; 28:6362–7.

33. López Bernal A, Newman GE, Phizackerley PJ, Turnbull AC. Surfactant stimulates prostaglandin E production in human amnion. Br J Obstet Gynaecol 1988; 95:1013–17.

34. López Bernal A, Newman GE, Phizackerley PJ, Turnbull AC. Effect of lipid and protein fractions from fetal pulmonary surfactant on prostaglandin E production by a human amnion cell line. Eicosanoids 1989; 2:29–32.

35. Billah MM, Johnston JM. Identification of phospholipid platelet-activating factor (1-O-alkyl-2-acetyl-sn-glycero-3-phosphocholine) in human amniotic fluid and urine. Biochem Biophys Res Commun 1983; 113:51–8.

36. Billah MM, Di Renzo GC, Ban C et al. Platelet-activating factor metabolism in human amnion and the responses of this tissue to extracellular platelet-activating factor. Prostaglandins 1985; 30:841–50.

37. Smith SK, Kelly RW. Effect of platelet-activating factor on the release of PGF-2 alpha and PGE-2 by separated cells of human endometrium. J Reprod Fertil 1988; 82:271–6.

38. Ohtsuka T, Lee HC, Yamaguchi M, Mori N. Dipalmitoylphosphatidylcholine (L-alpha-lecithin) stimulates prostaglandin E production in human amnion. Br J Obstet Gynaecol 1990; 97:843–6.

39. Newman GE, Phizackerley PJR, Lopez Bernal A, Noble GR, Willis AC. Adsorption of fetal surfactant protein SP-B on the human amnion at term and on amniocytes incubated with fetal surfactant in vitro. Reprod Fertil Dev 1991; 3:421–30.

40. López Bernal A, Hansell DJ, Khong TY, Keeling JW, Turnbull AC. Prostaglandin E production by the fetal membranes in unexplained preterm labour and preterm labour associated with chorioamnionitis. Br J Obstet Gynaecol 1989; 96:1133–9.

41. van der Elst CW, López Bernal A, Sinclair Smith CC. The role of chorioamnionitis and prostaglandins in preterm labor. Obstet Gynecol 1991; 77:672–6.

42. Romero R, Emamian M, Wan M, Quintero R, Hobbins JC, Mitchell MD. Prostaglandin concentrations in amniotic fluid of women with intra-amniotic infection and preterm labor. Am J Obstet Gynecol 1987; 157:1461–7.

43. Romero R, Quintero R, Emamian M et al. Arachidonate lipoxygenase metabolites in amniotic fluid of women with intra-amniotic infection and preterm labor. Am J Obstet Gynecol 1987; 157:1454–60.

44. Bennett PR, Rose MP, Myatt L, Elder MG. Preterm labor: stimulation of arachidonic acid metabolism in human amnion cells by bacterial products. Am J Obstet Gynecol 1987; 156:649–55.

45. Lamont RF, Taylor Robinson D, Newman M, Wigglesworth J, Elder MG. Spontaneous early preterm labour associated with abnormal genital bacterial colonization. Br J Obstet Gynaecol 1986; 93:804–10.

46. Hillier SL, Martius J, Krohn M, Kiviat N, Holmes KK, Eschenbach DA. A case-control study of chorioamnionic infection and histologic chorioamnionitis in prematurity. N Engl J Med 1988; 319:972–8.

47. McGregor JA, French JI, Richter R et al. Antenatal microbiologic and maternal risk factors associated with prematurity. Am J Obstet Gynecol 1990; 163:1465–73.

48. McDonald HM, O'Loughlin JA, Jolley P, Vigneswaran R, McDonald PJ. Vaginal infection and preterm labour. Br J Obstet Gynaecol 1991; 98:427–35.

49. López Bernal A, Hansell DJ, Alexander S, Turnbull AC. Steroid conversion and prostaglandin production by chorionic and decidual cells in relation to term and preterm labour. Br J Obstet Gynaecol 1987; 94:1052–8.

50. Olson DM, Skinner K, Challis JR. Prostaglandin output in relation to parturition by cells dispersed from human intrauterine tissues. J Clin Endocrinol Metab 1983; 57:694–9.

51. Vince GS, Starkey PM, Jackson MC, Sargent IL, Redman CW. Flow cytometric characterisation of cell populations in human pregnancy decidua and isolation of decidual macrophages. J Immunol Methods 1990; 132:181–9.

52. Bulmer JN, Wells M, Bhabra K, Johnson PM. Immunohistological characterization of endometrial gland epithelium and extravillous fetal trophoblast in third trimester human placental bed tissues. Br J Obstet Gynaecol 1986; 93:823–32.

53. Bulmer JN, Smith J, Morrison L, Wells M. Maternal and fetal cellular relationships in the human placental basal plate. Placenta 1988; 9:237–46.

54. Norwitz ER, Starkey PM, Lopez Bernal A, Turnbull AC. Identification by flow cytometry of the prostaglandin-producing cell populations of term human decidua. J Endocrinol 1991; 131:327–9.

55. Dalchau R, Kirkley J, Fabre JW. Monoclonal antibody to a human leukocyte-specific membrane glycoprotein probably homologous to the leukocyte-common (L-C) antigen of the rat. Eur J Immunol 1980; 10:737–44.

56. Lampson LA, Levy R. Two populations of Ia-like molecules on a human B cell line. J Immunol 1980; 125:293–9.

57. Sutton L, Mason DY, Redman CW. HLA-DR positive cells in the human placenta. Immunology 1983; 49:103–12.

58. Bulmer JN, Morrison L, Smith JC. Expression of class II MHC gene products by macrophages in human uteroplacental tissue. Immunology 1988; 63:707–14.

59. Vince CS, Shorter SC, Starkey PM et al. Localisation of tumor necrosis factor production in cells at the materno/fetal interface in human pregnancy. Clin Exp Immunol 1991; 87:in press.

60. Romero R, Brody DT, Oyarzun E et al. Infection and labor. III. Interleukin-1: a signal for the onset of parturition. Am J Obstet Gynecol 1989; 160:1117–23.

61. Romero R, Avila C, Santhanam U, Sehgal PB. Amniotic fluid interleukin 6 in preterm labor. Association with infection. J Clin Invest 1990; 85:1392–400.

62. Liechty KW, Koenig JM, Mitchell MD, Romero R, Christensen RD. Production of interleukin-6 by fetal and maternal cells in vivo during intraamniotic infection and in vitro after stimulation with interleukin-1. Pediatr Res 1991; 29:1–4.

63. Mitchell MD, Dudley DJ, Edwin SS, Schiller SL. Interleukin-6 stimulates prostaglandin production by human amnion and decidual cells. Eur J Pharmacol 1991; 192:189–91.

64. Romero R, Manogue KR, Mitchell MD et al. Infection and labor. IV. Cachetin-tumor necrosis factor in the amniotic fluid of women with intraamniotic infection and preterm labor. Am J Obstet Gynecol 1989; 161:336–41.

65. Casey ML, Cox SM, Beutler B, Milewich L, MacDonald PC. Cachectin/tumor necrosis factor-alpha formation in human decidua. Potential role of cytokines in infection-induced preterm labor. J Clin Invest 1989; 83:430–6.

66. Gilman AG. G proteins: transducers of receptor-generated signals. Annu Rev Biochem 1987; 56:615–49.

67. Bourne HR, Sanders DA, McCormick F. The GTPase superfamily: conserved structure and molecular mechanism. Nature 1991; 349:117–27.

68. Birnbaumer L, Pérez Reyes E, Bertrand P et al. Molecular diversity and function of G proteins and calcium channels. Biol Reprod 1991; 44:207–24.

69. Simon MI, Strathmann MP, Gautam N. Diversity of G proteins in signal transduction. Science 1991; 252:802–8.

70. Kaziro Y, Itoh H, Kozasa T, Nakafuku M, Satoh T. Structure and function of signal-transducing GTP-binding proteins. Annu Rev Biochem 1991; 60:349–400.

71. Word RA, Casey ML, Kamm KE, Stull JT. Effects of cGMP on myosin light chain phosphorylation, and contraction in human myometrium. Am J Physiol 1991; 260:C861–C867.

72. Diamond J. Beta-adrenoceptors, cyclic AMP and cyclic GMP in control of uterine motility. In: Carsten ME, Miller JD, eds. Uterine function. Molecular and cellular aspects. New York: Plenum Press, 1990; 249–75.

73. Michell RH. Inositol phospholipids and cell surface receptor function. Biochim Biophys Acta 1975; 415:81–47.

74. Berridge MJ, Irvine RF. Inositol trisphosphate, a novel second messenger in cellular signal transduction. Nature 1984; 312:315–21.

75. Hokin LE. Receptors and phosphoinositide-generated second messengers. Annu Rev Biochem 1985; 54:205–35.
76. Hokin LE, Hokin MR. Effects of acetylcholine on the turnover of phosphonyl units in individual phospholipids of pancreas slices and brain cortex slices. Biochim Biophys Acta 1955; 18:102–110.
77. Irvine RF, Moor RM. Micro-injection of inositol 1,3,4,5-tetrakisphosphate activates sea urchin eggs by a mechanism dependent on external Ca^{2+}. Biochem J 1986; 240:917–20.
78. Cullen PJ, Irvine RF, Dawson AP. Synergistic control of Ca^{2+} mobilization in permeabilized mouse L1210 lymphoma cells by inositol 2,4,5-trisphosphate and inositol 1,3,4,5-tetrakisphosphate. Biochem J 1990; 271:549–53.
79. Burgoyne RD, Morgan A. The control of free arachidonic acid levels. TiBS 1990; 15:365–6.
80. Billah MM, Anthes JC, Mullmann TJ, Receptor-coupled phospholipase D: regulation and functional significance. Biochem Soc Trans 1991; 19:324–9.
81. Ferguson JE, Hanley MR. The role of phospholipases and phospholipid-derived signals in cell activation. Curr Opinion Cell Biol 1991; 3:206–12.
82. Shukla SD, Halenda SP. Phospholipase D in cell signalling and its relationship to phospholipase C. Life Sci 1991; 48:851–66.
83. Carsten ME, Miller JD. Ca^{2+} release by inositol trisphosphate from Ca^{2+}-transporting microsomes derived from uterine sarcoplasmic reticulum. Biochem Biophys Res Commun 1985; 130:1027–31.
84. Carsten ME, Miller JD. Calcium control mechanisms in the myometrial cell and the role of the phosphoinositide cycle. In: Carsten ME, Miller JD, eds. Uterine function. Molecular and cellular aspects. New York: Plenum Press, 1990; 121–67.
85. Ver A, Mullner N, Szollar L, Somogyi J. Oxytocin regulates Ca^{2+} level in myometrium by influencing phosphoinositide metabolism. Acta Physiol Hung 1989; 74:189–94.
86. Rivera J, López Bernal A, Varney M, Watson SP. Inositol 1,4,5-trisphosphate and oxytocin binding in human myometrium. Endocrinology 1990; 127:155–62.
87. Varney MA, Rivera J, Lopez Bernal A, Watson SP. Are there subtypes of the inositol 1,4,5-trisphosphate receptor? Biochem J 1990; 269:211–16.
88. Wakeling AE, Wyngarden LJ. Prostaglandin receptors in the human, monkey and hamster uterus. Endocrinology 1974; 95:55–64.
89. Schillinger E, Prior G. Characteristics of prostaglandin receptor sites in human uterine tissue. Adv Prostaglandin Thromboxane Res 1976; 1:259–63.
90. Crankshaw DJ, Crankshaw J, Branda LA, Daniel EE. Receptors for E type prostaglandins in the plasma membrane of nonpregnant human myometrium. Arch Biochem Biophys 1979; 198:70–7.
91. Bauknecht T, Krahe B, Rechenbach U, Zahradnik HP, Breckwoldt M. Distribution of prostaglandin E2 and prostaglandin F2 alpha receptors in human myometrium. Acta Endocrinol (Copenh) 1981; 98:446–50.
92. Carsten ME, Miller JD. Prostaglandin E_2 receptor in the myometrium: distribution in subcellular fractions. Arch Biochem Biophys 1981; 212:700–4.
93. Hofmann GE, Rao CV, Barrows GH, Sanfilippo JS. Topography of human uterine prostaglandin E and F2 alpha receptors and their profiles during pathological states. J Clin Endocrinol Metab 1983; 57:360–6.
94. Chegnini N, Rao CV. Wakim N, Sanfilippo J. Prostaglandin binding to different cell types of human uterus: quantitative light microsocope autoradiographic study. Prostaglandins Leukotrienes Med 1986; 22:129–38.
95. Adelantado JM, López Bernal A, Turnbull AC. Topographical distribution of prostaglandin E receptors in human myometrium. Br J Obstet Gynaecol 1988; 95:348–53.
96. López Bernal A, Buckley S, Rees CM, Marshall JM. Meclofenamate inhibits prostaglandin E binding and adenylyl cyclase activation in human myometrium. J Endocrinol 1991; 129:439–45.
97. Pickles VR. The myometrial action of six prostaglandins: consideration of a receptor hypothesis. In: Bergstrom S, Samuelsson B, eds. Nobel Symposium 2: Prostaglandins. Stockholm: Almqvist and Wiksell, 1967; 79–83.
98. Kennedy I, Coleman RA, Humphrey PP, Levy GP, Lumley P. Studies on the characterisation of prostanoid receptors: a proposed classification. Prostaglandins 1982; 24:667–89.
99. Coleman RA. Prostanoid receptors and their significance in myometrial contractility. In: Keirse MJNC, Noort WA, eds. Prostaglandins in reproduction. The Hague: 2nd ECPR, 1991; 83–4.
100. Coleman RA, Kennedy I, Humphrey PPA, Levy GP, Lumley P. Prostanoids and their receptors. In: Hansch C, Sammes PG, Taylor JB, eds. Comprehensive medical chemistry. Oxford: Pergamon Press, 1990; 643–714.

101. Wikland M, Lindblom B, Wilhelmsson L, Wiqvist N. Oxytocin, prostaglandins, and contractility of the human uterus at term pregnancy. Acta Obstet Gynecol Scand 1982; 61:467–72.
102. Cañete Soler R, López Bernal A. A comparison of leukotriene and prostaglandin binding to human myometrium. Eicosanoids 1988; 1:79–84.
103. Carsten ME, Miller JD. A new look at uterine muscle contraction. Am J Obstet Gynecol 1987; 157:1303–15.
104. Word RA, Kamm KE, Stull JT, Casey ML. Endothelin increases cytoplasmic calcium and myosin phosphorylation in human myometrium. Am J Obstet Gynecol 1990; 162:1103–8.
105. Mackenzie LW, Word RA, Casey ML, Stull JT. Myosin light chain phosphorylation in human myometrial smooth muscle cells. Am J Physiol 1990; 258:C92–C98.
106. Molnar M, Hertelendy F. Regulation of intracellular free calcium in human myometrial cells by prostaglandin F2 alpha: comparison with oxytocin. J Clin Endocrinol Metab 1990; 71:1243–50.
107. Tanfin Z, Harbon S. Heterologous regulations of cAMP responses in pregnant rat myometrium. Evolution from a stimulatory to an inhibitory prostaglandin E_2 and prostacyclin effect. Mol Pharmacol 1987; 32:249–57.
108. Hirata M, Hayashi Y, Ushikubi F et al. Cloning and expression of cDNA for a human thromboxane A2 receptor. Nature 1991; 349:617–20.
109. Caldeyro-Barcia R, Poseiro JJ. Oxytocin and contractility of the pregnant human uterus. Ann NY Acad Sci 1959; 75:813–30.
110. Takahashi K, Diamond F, Bieniarz J, Yen H, Burd L, Uterine contractility and oxytocin sensitivity in preterm, term, and postterm pregnancy. Am J Obstet Gynecol 1980; 136:774–9.
111. Schrey MP, Cornford PA, Read AM, Steer PJ. A role for phosphoinositide hydrolysis in human uterine smooth muscle during parturition. Am J Obstet Gynecol 1988; 159:964–70.
112. Tasaka K, Masumoto N, Miyake A, Tanizawa O. Direct measurement of intracellular free calcium in cultured human puerperal myometrial cells stimulated by oxytocin: effects of extracellular calcium and calcium channel blockers. Obstet Gynecol 1991; 77:101–6.
113. Fuchs AR, Fuchs F, Husslein P, Soloff MS. Oxytocin receptors in the human uterus during pregnancy and parturition. Am J Obstet Gynecol 1984; 150:734–41.
114. Sheldrick EL, Flint AP. Endocrine control of uterine oxytocin receptors in the ewe. J Endocrinol 1985; 106:249–58.
115. Ayad VJ, Wathes DC. Characterization of endometrial and myometrial oxytocin receptors in the non-pregnant ewe. J Endocrinol 1989; 123:11–18.
116. Antoni FA, Chadio SE. Essential role of magnesium in oxytocin-receptor affinity and ligand specificity. Biochem J 1989; 257:611–14.
117. Tence M, Guillon G, Bottari S, Jard S. Labelling of vasopressin and oxytocin receptors from the human uterus. Eur J Pharmacol 1990; 191:427–36.
118. Ayad VJ, Guldenaar SE, Wathes DC. Characterization and localization of oxytocin receptors in the uterus and oviduct of the non-pregnant ewe using an iodinated receptor antagonist. J Endocrinol 1991; 128:187–95.
119. López Bernal A, Phipps SL, Rosevear SK, Turnbull AC. Mechanism of action of the oxytocin antagonist 1-deamino-2-D-Tyr-(OEt)-4-Thr-8-Orn-oxytocin. Br J Obstet Gynaecol 1989; 96:1108–10.
120. Åkerlund M, Stromberg P, Hauksson A et al. Inhibition of uterine contractions of premature labour with an oxytocin analogue. Results from a pilot study. Br J Obstet Gynaecol 1987; 94:1040–4.
121. Hertelendy F, Molnar M. Mode of action of endothelin in rat myometrial cells: comparison with oxytocin and prostaglandin F2alpha. SGI 1991; Abs 218.
122. Harbon S, Marc S, Goureau O et al. Multiple regulation of the generation of inositol phosphates and cAMP in myometrium. In: Garfield RE, ed. Uterine contractility. Norwell, MA: Serono Symposia, USA, 1990:123–40.
123. Marc S, Leiber D, Harbon S. Fluoroaluminates mimic muscarinic- and oxytocin-receptor-mediated generation of inositol phosphates and contraction in the intact guinea-pig myometrium. Role for a pertussis/cholera-toxin-insensitive G protein. Biochem J 1988; 255:705–13.
124. Taylor SJ, Chae HZ, Rhee SG, Exton JH. Activation of the beta 1 isozyme of phospholipase C by alpha subunits of the Gq class of G proteins. Nature 1991; 350:516–18.
125. Smrcka AV, Hepler JR, Brown KO, Sternweis PC. Regulation of polyphosphoinositide-specific phospholipase C activity by purified Gq. Science 1991; 251:804–7.
126. Yanagisawa M. A novel potent vasoconstrictor peptide produced by vascular endothelial cells. Nature 1988; 332:411–15.
127. Casey ML, Word RA, MacDonald PC. Endothelin-1 gene expression and regulation of

endothelin mRNA and protein biosynthesis in avascular human amnion. Potential source of amniotic fluid endothelin. J Biol Chem 1991; 266:5762–68.

128. Word RA, Kamm KE, Stull JT, Casey ML. Endothelin increases cytoplasmic calcium and myosin phosphorylation in human myometrium. Am J Obstet Gynecol 1990; 162:1103–8.

129. Maher E, Bardequez A, Gardner JP, et al. Endothelin- and oxytocin-induced calcium signaling in cultured human myometrial cells. J Clin Invest 1991; 87:1251–8.

130. Ahlquist RP. The adrenergic receptor. J Pharm Sci 1966; 55:359–67.

131. Wansbrough H, Nakanishi H, Wood C. Effect of epinephrine on human uterine activity in vitro and in vivo. Obstet Gynecol 1967; 30:779–89.

132. Bottari SP, Vokaer A, Kaivez E, Lescrainier JP, Vauquelin G. Identification and characterization of alpha 2-adrenergic receptors in human myometrium by rauwolscine binding. Am J Obstet Gynecol 1983; 146:639–43.

133. Bottari SP, Vauquelin G, Lescrainier JP, Kaivez E, Vokaer A. Identification and characterization of alpha 1-adrenergic receptors in human myometrium by prazosin binding. Biochem Pharmacol 1983; 32:925–8.

134. Falkay G, Kovacs L. Characterization of beta-adrenergic receptors in human myometrium and placenta. Acta Physiol Hung 1985; 65:491–5.

135. Breuiller-Fouche M, Doualla-Bell Kotto Maka F, Geny B, Ferre F. Alpha-1 adrenergic receptor: binding and phosphoinositide breakdown in human myometrium. J Pharmacol Exp Ther 1991; 258:82–7.

136. Breuiller M, Rouot B, Litime MH, Leroy MJ, Ferre F. Functional coupling of the alpha 2-adrenergic receptor-adenylate cyclase complex in the pregnant human myometrium. J Clin Endocrinol Metab 1990; 70:1299–304.

137. Litime MH, Pointis G, Breuiller M, Cabrol D, Ferre F. Disappearance of beta-adrenergic response of human myometrial adenylate cyclase at the end of pregnancy. J Clin Endocrinol Metab 1989; 69:1–6.

138. Breuiller M, Doulla Bell F, Litime MH, Leroy MJ, Ferre F. Disappearance of human myometrial adenylate cyclase activation by prostaglandins at the end of pregnancy. Comparison with beta-adrenergic response. Adv Prostaglandin Thromboxane Leukotriene Res 1991; 21B: 811–14.

139. Keirse MJNC, Grant A, King JF. Preterm labour. In: Chalmers I, Enkin M, Keirse MJNC, eds. Effective care in pregnancy and childbirth. Oxford: Oxford University Press, 1989:694–745.

140. Leiber D, Marc S, Harbon S. Pharmacological evidence for distinct muscarinic receptor subtypes coupled to the inhibition of adenylate cyclase and to the increased generation of inositol phosphates in the guinea pig myometrium. J Pharmacol Exp Ther 1990; 252:800–9.

141. Arkinstall SJ, Jones CT. Pregnancy suppresses G protein coupling to phosphoinositide hydrolysis in guinea pig myometrium. Am J Physiol 1990; 259:E57–E65.

142. Arkinstall SJ, Jones CT. Influence of pregnancy on G-protein coupling to adenylate cyclase activation in guinea-pig myometrium. J Endocrinol 1990; 127:15–21.

143. Tanfin Z, Goureau O, Milligan G, Harbon S. Characterization of G proteins in rat myometrium. A differential modulation of Gi2 alpha and Gi3 alpha during gestation. FEBS Lett 1991; 278:4–8.

144. Wu YY, Riemer RK, Goldfien A, Roberts JM. Progesterone prevents linkage of rabbit myometrial alpha 2-adrenergic receptors to inhibition of adenylate cyclase. Am J Obstet Gynecol 1989; 160:838–43.

145. Roberts JM, Riemer RK, Bottari SP, Wu YY, Goldfien A. Hormonal regulation of myometrial adrenergic responses: the receptor and beyond. J Dev Physiol 1989; 11:125–34.

146. Anwer K, Hovington JA, Sanborn BM. Antagonism of contractants and relaxants at the level of intracellular calcium and phosphoinositide turnover in the rat uterus. Endocrinology 1989; 124:2995–3002.

147. Anwer K, Hovington JA, Sanborn BM. Involvement of protein kinase A in the regulation of intracellular free calcium and phosphoinositide turnover in rat myometrium. Biol Reprod 1990; 43:851–9.

148. Goureau O, Tanfin Z, Harbon S. Prostaglandins and muscarinic agonists induce cyclic AMP attenuation by two distinct mechanisms in the pregnant-rat myometrium. Interaction between cyclic AMP and Ca^{2+} signals. Biochem J 1990; 271:667–73.

Chapter 15

Infection and Preterm Labour

M. G. Elder

Introduction

The physiological and biochemical mechanisms which take place in preterm and term labour are similar. An understanding of the process by which preterm labour might be induced by infection could provide valuable clues as to the mechanisms of spontaneous term labour. The understanding of those mechanisms involved in spontaneous labour is increasing very rapidly, but the interaction is not clear and more information is needed. Prostaglandins (PG) are uterotonic compounds and there is substantial evidence that they are essential in the onset and maintenance of human labour. Whether they are the final common pathway or important facilitators of some other mechanism is not known. The concentrations of $PGF_{2\alpha}$ and PGE_2 increase in the amniotic fluid during the last few weeks of pregnancy [1] and in association with dilatation of the cervix [2]. A coincidental increase in maternal urinary PG metabolites supports the contention that there is increased production of these substances during late pregnancy. In amniotic fluid, the concentration of 6-keto-$PGF_{1\alpha}$, the hydrolytic breakdown product of prostacyclin (PGI_2), does not change during labour [3]. Studies in the human and in the sheep suggest that prostacyclin may inhibit myometrial contractility. This combination results in an increase in the output of stimulatory prostaglandins but the synthesis is also directed away from the formation of inhibitory eicosanoids [4]. This pattern of PG output, which increases PGE_2 and $PGF_{2\alpha}$ relative to the concentration of 6-keto-$PGF_{1\alpha}$, can be reproduced in vitro by treating decidual tissue with oestrogen.

In contrast to oxytocin, prostaglandins induce uterine contractions at all stages of pregnancy. This suggests that they play a central role and are not too dependent on the uterus being prepared by endocrine events. Uterotrophins such as oestrogens are also important and act by increasing myometrial gap junctions

[5] and oxytocin receptors in myometrium [6]. Preterm labour may be a normal signal occurring too early in pregnancy, but is more likely to be due to an abnormal signal and there is increasing evidence to implicate infection as this signal.

Before considering the potential role of infection in the aetiology of preterm labour it is important to consider the difficulties in defining normal vaginal flora.

Vaginal Flora

The portal of entry for infection to the intrauterine tissue is the vagina and cervix. The skin, the mouth, the upper respiratory tract and the gastrointestinal tract have characteristic and unique patterns of microbial colonisation. Although there is a superficial similarity between the vaginal and faecal flora, there are essential differences in prevalence and concentration. It is reasonable to assume that faecal organisms may be introduced into the vagina from perineal sources but it is not known whether these organisms are transient colonisers or whether they persist in some women. When a single culture is taken from an individual at one point in time it is difficult to ascertain whether any given organism is a permanent member of the endogenous flora.

Although species occurring in the vagina may overlap with those of the oral cavity, both of these sites appear to be unique in terms of the prevalence and relative concentrations of particular species. It was initially assumed that the microbiology of saliva reflected that of the oral cavity as a whole. It is now known that the microbial populations that reside on the various tooth surfaces are very different from those which colonise the tongue [7]. Similarly to the oral cavity there may be specific ecological niches in the lower genital tract [8]. The anatomy of the cervix, with the presence or absence of an ectropion influenced by age, oral contraception, the stage of the menstrual cycle or pregnancy, as well as the extent of the ectropion or patulous nature of the cervical os influenced by parity, will all have significant influence on "endocervical" flora.

The mechanisms which control the microflora of the vagina are poorly understood. The question of whether the host determines the vaginal milieu, which in turn dictates the specific mirco-organisms that can thrive under those conditions, or alternatively whether the microflora themselves determine the vaginal milieu by virtue of their metabolic activity, or both, is still controversial. The most popular theory for control of the vaginal flora in the premenopausal population has been that the host's production of oestrogen increases glycogen in the vaginal epithelium which in turn is metabolised to lactic acid by the microbial flora, consisting mainly of lactorbacilli. The production of lactic acid in the vagina selectively favours its colonisation by acidophilic species such as lactobacilli. This hypothesis is supported by the relatively higher frequency and abundance of lactobacilli in premenopausal and pregnant women than in prepubertal girls and postmenopausal women. However, the factors regulating pH are not well defined and further studies are needed to assess the longitudinal relationship of endogenous vaginal flora from juvenile, prepubertal, pregnant, premenopausal and postmenopausal subjects using modern bacteriological techniques.

It is likely that the endogenous flora in healthy asymptomatic, premenopausal women contains not only one or more species of lactobacilli but includes mixed species of aerobes and/or anaerobes [9].

Clearly, for the majority of women, these organisms are commensal in that they co-exist with each other and with the host, which may be more important. However, subtle changes in these relationships could alter the proportion of one bacterial species to another and their relationship to the host, thereby upsetting a delicate balance.

Abnormal vaginal colonisation was defined by Lamont et al. using very strict criteria [10]. In the presence of polymorphonuclear leucocytes, *Neisseria gonorrhoeae or Haemophilus influenzae* at any concentration, or other organisms such as *Escherischia coli or Bacteroides fragilis* if they were isolated in large numbers, were considered to be abnormal [10]. Using these criteria, abnormal colonisation was associated with preterm labour in 47% of study patients compared with 15% of control patients. The presence of organisms (in study v. control group) such as *Mycoplasma hominis* (80% versus 46%) or *Ureaplasma urealyticum* (24% versus 8%) has also been shown to be associated with a greater incidence of preterm labour [10,11]. Whether or not individual organisms are important is unclear but preterm labour is much more likely to be the effect of an inflammatory response induced by the abnormal flora rather than the specific effects of any one organism.

Local Defence Mechanisms

The acidophilic lactobacilli which keep the vaginal pH at between 3.5 and 4.5 produce a reduction in bacterial growth [12]. A pH of greater than 4.4 has been shown to be associated with a greater presence of organisms such as *Mycoplasma hominis and Ureaplasma urealyticum* [13]. Pilot data suggest that women in preterm labour with intact membranes have a significantly higher vaginal pH than women in early labour at term (pH 5.4 versus 4.1) [12]. This suggests that the role of vaginal acidity may be to restrain excessive growth of organisms that could induce an inflammatory response. More data are needed on the changes of vaginal pH seen in preterm labour. Whether or not changes occur beforehand and so could predict the condition needs to be determined.

Subtle changes in host resistance could be reflected in small but significant changes in bacterial flora. In a large longitudinal study, 800 women were screened in early second trimester. Abnormal colonisation was detected by the diagnosis of bacterial vaginosis (BV) using Gram stain. In those women who were BV-positive the subsequent incidence of pregnancy loss (second trimester miscarriage or preterm labour) was 15% compared to 2.7% in the BV-negative women ($P<0.00001$). For delivery between 18 and 37 weeks the odds ratio was greater than 5 and the relative risk was 3.5:1 (R.F. Lamont; Hay and D. Taylor-Robinson, personal communication). This is in keeping with a recent study from Adelaide, Australia, where two distinct bacterial groupings were commonly found in women in preterm labour, especially when this was at less than 34 weeks gestation. One group of women were found to have BV and the other group were vaginally colonised with enteropharyngeal bacteria [13].

The local immune response, of vaginal secretion of IgA to protect mucus membranes, may also play a part in maintaining the balance between vaginal bacterial flora and the host. A reduction in immune response may be a factor in initiating preterm labour. Many bacterial species produce proteases that degrade IgA and possibly IgG [14]. The amounts of IgA present in vaginal and cervical secretions in cases of preterm labour, normal pregnancy and normal labour need to be assessed and this work is currently in progress.

If there is an abnormal vaginal flora with organisms present which have the capacity to stimulate an inflammatory response, they still need to gain access to the appropriate tissues within the uterus where this response may have some effect. The ability of bacteria to gain access to the uterus through the cervical mucus plug would be an important element of the interaction between the organisms and the host. The ability of various bacteria to secrete mucinase may be critical to their ability to gain access through the cervical canal but nothing is known of this in the context of preterm labour. Again much work needs to be done to identify the factors that influence the passage of bacteria within the cervical canal. Proteolytic enzymes in the seminal fluid increase the permeability of cervical mucus [15], and bacteria can facilitate their penetration through the cervical mucus plug by attaching themselves to mobile spermatozoa [16].

Cervical Flora

Both aerobic and anaerobic species are found in the endocervix. The commonest aerobes are diphtheroides, streptococci, staphylococci, *E. coli* and aerobic species of lactobacilli. The commonest anaerobes are *Bacteroides* and peptostreptococci. In non-pregnant women, 70% were found to have both aerobic and anaerobic species present in the endocervix whereas 27% had only aerobes, and 3% were sterile [17]. A fairly large study assessing the flora quantitatively in non-pregnant and pregnant subjects showed that in pregnancy there were more pure cultures of a single organism than in the non-pregnant state and that on average there were 1.5 types of organism present. The incidence of anaerobic species declined as pregnancy progressed. It was shown that the number of lactobacilli in the cervix increased in pregnancy compared with non-pregnancy from 10^7ml^{-1} to 10^9ml^{-1} [9]. Despite this large number of acidophilic organisms, the pH in the cervical canal is considerably higher than in the vagina. This is thought to be due to the lack of glycogen, which acts as a substrate for the lactobacilli to convert into lactic acid in the vagina. As a result of this more neutral pH organisms within the cervix have a greater ability to multiply and to induce an inflammatory response.

Goplerud et al. [18] reported on the endocervical flora of pregnant women during the first, second and third trimesters of pregnancy, the third postpartum day and the sixth postpartum week. The prevalence of significant organisms varied between the groups but some general trends appeared. Groups of micro-organisms, such as anaerobic cocci and Gram-negative rods, decreased during pregnancy. The most substantial decrease during pregnancy was in the anaerobic portion of the flora.

Further work confirmed the reduction in anaerobic organisms from early pregnancy to labour, whereas aerobic organisms remained relatively constant [19]. Aerobic lactobacilli and yeasts appeared to increase as pregnancy progressed [18].

Once through the cervix, the bacteria will encounter the decidua and the fetal membranes. Placentitis, funicitis and amnionitis are found most frequently in association with preterm birth [20]. Whereas in the past, chorioamnionitis was thought to be induced by non-infectious agents or factors such as changes in pH, anoxia or meconium [21], it is now accepted that inflammatory lesions of the chorion and amnion and umbilial cord are due to infection. Bacteria have been recovered from 82% of placentae of women with clinical and histological evidence of chorioamnionitis [22]. This confusion probably arose because many organisms, such as mycoplasmas, which would not have been cultured in the past with routine techniques, are now isolated through more sophisticated culture methods. In addition, the fragility of some bacteria, like gonococci and chlamydiae and the administration of antibiotics to the mother, may have influenced the lack of success of cultures. Finally, many positive cultures were classified as irrelevant in the past because the organisms grown were considered to be non-pathogenic. It is now established that organisms of low virulence may be pathogenic to the fetus and newborn [23] and may enhance the pathogenicity of other bacteria [24], as well as inducing a low grade inflammatory response.

Bacteria from the vagina reach the fetal membranes through the cervix and can reach the amniotic cavity through either ruptured or intact membranes. Many studies have shown positive amniotic fluid cultures within a short time of membrane rupture and no correlation between duration of rupture and incidence of positive culture [25]. An early peak in neonatal cord immunoglobulin levels has been found immediately after rupture of the membranes, suggesting that some infants were infected before the membranes ruptured [26].

Bacterial Enzymes and Premature Rupture of the Membranes

The ability of certain strains of bacteria to secrete enzymes such as mucinase or collagenase may facilitate their passage through the cervical canal and access to the fetal membranes. Bacterial proteases could weaken the membranes, causing rupture. Studies in vitro using membranes and protease-producing bacteria have shown that the membranes are weakened, that human neutrophils and their constituent enzymes can enhance this effect and that antibiotics can reduce this effect [27,28]. Three parameters of membrane integrity (bursting tension, elasticity and work required to rupture) were decreased by contact with preparations of group B streptococci or *Staphylococcus aureus* in the presence or absence of neutrophils. Elastase released from neutrophils seemed to enhance the effect of bacterial proteases. Erythromycin and clindamycin given in subinhibitory doses did not alter bacterial growth but inhibited protease release and subsequent membrane damage.

Prostaglandin Production by Fetal Membranes

The fetal membranes and the decidua are known to be able to produce prostaglandins in response to a variety of stimuli and it is from these tissues that the prostaglandins responsible for labour are produced. In addition, arachidonic acid metabolism via the lipoxygenase and epoxygenase pathways can take place and has been shown to have a direct but weak stimulatory effect on myometrium. The synthetic pathways have been described [29]. It is less clear which tissue is responsible for the production and what stimulates this response. Much work in the past has been done on single cell types in monolayer culture or in explants of a single tissue. This ignores the fact that the fetal membranes consist of distinct tissues, namely amnion and chorion and the adjacent maternal decidua, each of which will synthesise and metabolise prostaglandins differently.

Amnion

There is no doubt that in vitro the amnion will produce PGE_2 whether stimulated or not. Output of PGE_2 by amnion cells obtained from women following spontaneous labour is significantly higher than from tissues obtained after elective caesarean section [30]. We have demonstrated that the addition of conditioned media in which various pathogens had been cultured gave a dose-dependent increase of the folowing:

1. Arachidonic acid metabolism
2. Increase in cyclo-oxygenase compared to lipoxgenase activity
3. PGE_2 production.

The organisms studied were group B haemolytic streptococcus, *Bacteroides fragilis and E. coli.*

Lactobacilli did not produce an alteration in any of these three parameters [30]. Subsequent to this study, a wide range of micro-organisms found in association with chorioamnionitis and preterm delivery produced a significant increase in PGE_2 production by amnion cells [31]. This demonstrates that the amnion is capable of producing prostaglandins in response to a bacterial stimulus.

Chorion

The amnion lies in opposition to the chorion, which produces low concentractions of eicosanoids but contains high levels of prostaglandin dehydrogenase enzyme activity. Prostaglandins produced in the amnion would have to cross the chorion before gaining access to the myometrium. Nakla et al. [32] showed that both arachidonic acid and PGE_2 crossed from the amnion to the chorio-decidua in vitro. They used a short-term incubation (6 h) which may have rendered the membranes permeable. Similar short-term incubations have shown passage of small amounts of PGE_2 across the membranes at a similar rate of sucrose. This is suggestive of an extracellular transfer [33]. There is further evidence to suggest that prostaglandins are synthesised in the amnion and then cross the chorion and decidua to activate the myometrium. This comes from the suggestion that, although the chorion is a major site of prostaglandin dehydrogenase (PGDH) activity, this activity is not uniform throughout the chorion. Finally, a relative deficiency of PGDH in the chorion may account for preterm labour in a small number of women [34].

Full Thickness Membranes

Our own recent work has used full thickness membranes in a different in vitro culture system. The period of culture was much longer and experiments only started after 24 h to give the membranes time to recover from the trauma of labour, delivery and the tissue culture process. The membranes produce large amounts of PGE_2, virtually all of which is recovered on either side of the membrane in the form of PGE metabolites [35]. Using the same system we have shown that very little PGE_2 added to fetal side crosses from amnion to chorion in the unmetabolised form [36] and this has been confirmed by others [37]. Both platelet activating factor (PAF) [38] and interleukin-1-beta (unpublished data) caused a short-term increase in PGE_2 metabolites recovered from the maternal side of the membranes.

Decidua

Decidual tissue was scraped off the membranes and the cells were separated using a two-stage enzyme incubation [39]. The cell suspension was separated into various cell populations using a percoll density gradient method. The largest band of cells was found in the 20% percoll fraction at sp. gr. 1.033 and a smaller band of cells was located in the 40% percoll fraction (sp. gr. 1.056). The number of cells obtained was approximately 8×10^6 cells g^{-1} of tissue. The cells in the 20% percoll fraction were not LCA positive and therefore not bone marrow derived. They produced large quantities of prolactin and did not produce human placental lactogen, suggesting that they were decidual stromal cells with no significant contamination from trophoblast. The cells in the 40% percoll fraction were positive for LCA and most were macrophages (EMB-11 positive) with a few T lymphocytes. Most cells in this band were expressing cyclo-oxygenase enzyme [40].

The biochemical interplay between these two cell types and their role in preterm and term labour warrants study. PGE_2 production by decidual stromal cells obtained before the onset of labour was in the range $0.1–1.0$ ng/10^6 cells/ 24 h. Substantially increased amounts of both PGE_2 and $PGF_{2\alpha}$ were produced by decidual stromal cells obtained after the onset of labour (Table 15.1). The values in Table 15.1 are after 24 h in culture, and were maintained at similar levels for up to 72 h of culture in the absence of added stimuli. This suggests that some form of decidual activation had occurred involving a major change in stromal cell function. By contrast, PGE_2 production by decidual bone marrow-derived cells was the same before labour (3.4 ± 0.9 mg/10^6 cells/24 h) and after the onset of labour (3.1 ± 0.3) (mean $\pm$ SD, $n = 4$). Studies in our department have suggested that prostaglandin production by decidual stromal cells is dependent on extracellular arachidonic acid [41] and that changes in the levels of cyclo-oxygenase

Table 15.1. Production of prostaglandins by decidual stromal
cells obtained before or after onset of labour

	PGE_2 (ng/10^6 cells/24 h)	$PGF_{2\alpha}$
Not in labour	1.6±1.2	1.8±0.2
In labour	18.4±1.1	32.8±4.3

Values are mean±SD, $n=4$.

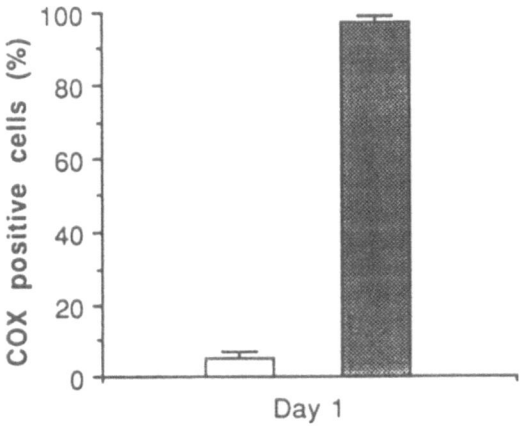

Fig. 15.1. Numbers of cyclo-oxygenase-positive decidual stromal cells before (□) and after (▇)
normal term labour. Data are mean ± SEM (n = 3 experiments).

enzyme may be important in the regulation of prostaglandin production by these
cells. Immunocytochemistry was used to assess changes in cyclo-oxygenase levels
in decidual stromal cells obtained before and after labour. Of these cells, 3 ± 2%
stained positively for cyclo-oxygenase before labour, compared with 95 ± 3% of
cells obtained after labour (Fig. 15.1).

This work suggests that decidual stromal cells are a major source of prostaglandins in labour and that this increase in production may be important in normal
labour. It is consistent with studies implicating decidual activation in preterm
labour associated with intrauterine infection [42,43].

Bacterial Effects on Decidual Cells

It has been suggested that bacterial phospholipase A_2 (PLA_2) may be a major
determinant of increased prostaglandin production by fetal membranes [44,45].
Recent studies indicate that this is unlikely to be the case since several organisms
associated with preterm labour have very low levels of PLA_2 [46]. Bacterial
components such as lipopolysaccarides (LPS) are associated with preterm labour
[47] and may have a direct stimulatory effect on prostaglandin production by

decidual cells. This has been shown to be the case for both stromal cells and macrophages (Table 15.2). The mechanism for this increased production is not known but it is thought to be independent of IL-1-beta as there was no significant increase in the production of IL-1-beta by either stromal cells or macrophages.

Table 15.2. Effect of LPS on PGE_2 production by decidual stromal or bone marrow-derived cells

	Stromal cells	Bone marrow derived cells
	PGE2 (ng/10^6 cells/24 h)	
Control	0.97±0.47	3.06±0.33
LPS	5.53±1.0	7.2 ±0.8

Values are mean±SD, $n=4$.

Cytokines such as interleukins, tumour necrosis factors (TNF) and PAF have been demonstrated in the amniotic fluid in cases of preterm labour due to infection [48–50]. Their source is not yet known but they are probably fetal in origin.

Given that bacteria can reach the decidua, which contains large numbers of macrophages, it is reasonable to postulate that they could be derived from activated decidual macrophages and that they would then affect the stromal cells. We have shown that IL-1-beta increased PGE_2 production by decidual stromal cells in culture in a time- and dose-dependent manner and that the increase in cyclo-oxygenase preceded the production of PGE_2. The optimum conditions were 24 h in culture and a concentration of 100 pg ml^{-1} of IL-1-beta (Fig. 15.2).

An increase in cyclo-oxygenase enzyme synthesis (45% of cells positive) accompanied the increase in prostaglandin production. This was inhibited by the protein synthesis inhibitor cycloheximide. This implicates protein synthesis in the stimulatory effects of IL-1-beta, which may be mediated through the increase in cyclo-oxygenase. Interleukin-6 increased the numbers of stromal cells staining for cyclo-oxygenase to 95% but had no significant effect on prostaglandin synthesis (Fig. 15.3). The combination of IL-6 and IL-1-beta therefore produces the same changes in decidual stromal cells as those seen after the onset of spontaneous labour. However, the increase in PGE_2 production was not seen until day 3 of culture despite an increase in cyclo-oxygenase activity on day 1 (Fig. 15.4), suggesting the presence during the first 48 h of an inhibitory factor produced by decidua.

Oxytocin has been clearly implicated in the process of term labour by its clinical usefulness in the induction of labour. One study [51] suggested that oxytocin may also be involved in preterm labour, since an oxytocin antagonist decreased the frequency of uterine contractions in women with preterm labour. Non-purified decidual cells have been shown to produce 2–3-fold more $PGF_{2\alpha}$ in the presence of 200 pM-oxytocin [52]. Purified decidual stromal cells showed only limited (less than twofold) increases in prostaglandin production in response to physiological concentrations of oxytocin (100 pM) at all time points examined (2 h–24 h) (unpublished data). Co-addition of IL-1-beta resulted in an increase in PGE_2 production (control 0.6 ± 0.2, IL-1-beta 1.0 ± 0.4, oxytocin 0.6 ± 0.3, IL-1-beta + oxytocin 5.9 ± 3.1 ng/10^6 cells/ 2 h), but this was observed only over short incubation times (2 h–4 h). This suggests that IL-1-beta and oxytocin have

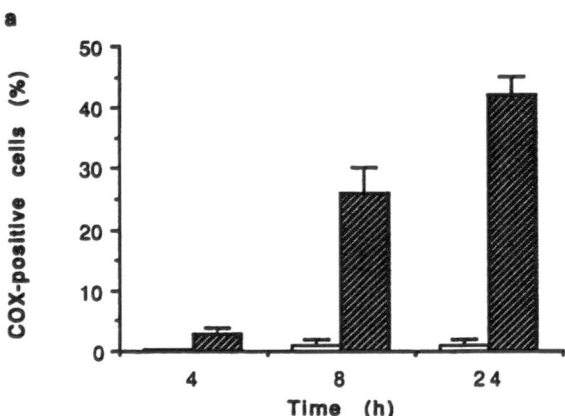

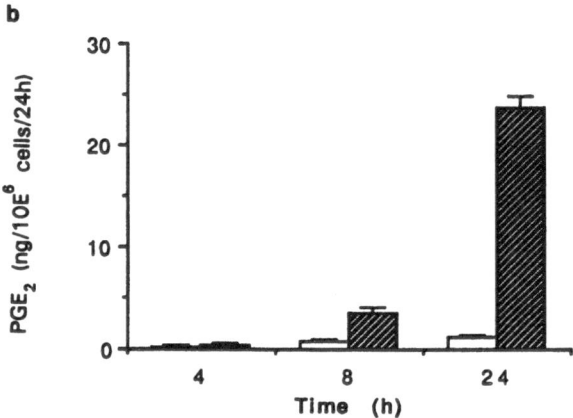

Fig. 15.2. Time response of (**a**) numbers of cyclo-oxygenase positive cells or (**b**) PGE$_2$ production by the same cells in the presence (▨) or absence (□) of IL-1 beta (100 pg ml^{-1}). All data are means ± SEM (n = 4), and are typical of three replicate experiments.

synergistic actions on prostaglandin production by decidual stromal cells, but further studies are needed to identify the mechanism of this effect.

Inhibitory Protein and Decidua

If there is a natural autocrine drive to prostaglandin synthesis by decidual stromal cells stimulated by activated macrophages releasing cytokines within the decidua, it is likely that there is a brake on this system to prevent inappropriate stimulation of the myometrium. It is known that decidua produces a compound which inhibits

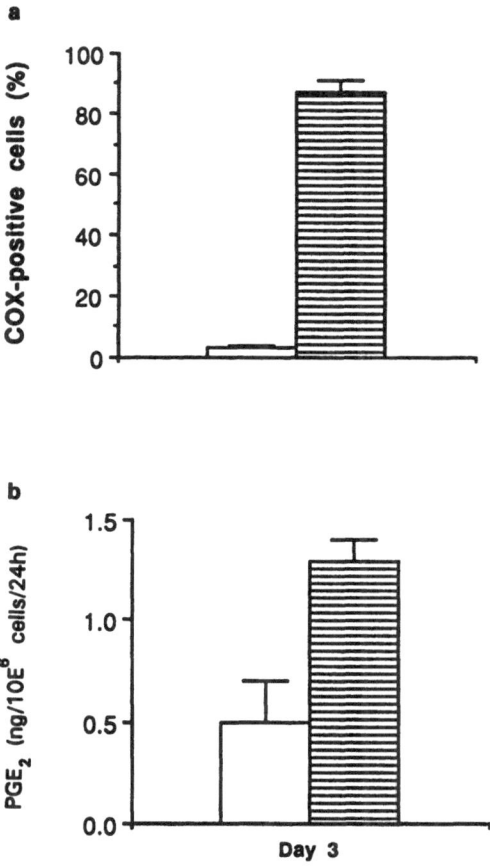

Fig. 15.3. Effects of IL-6 (100 pg ml^{-1}) (▤) added on day 3 of culture on (**a**) numbers of cyclo-oxygenase positive decidual stromal cells or (**b**) PGE$_2$ production by the same cells. All data are mean ± SEM ($n = 3$), and are typical of three replicate experiments.

prostaglandin production [53,54]. This factor is acidic, has a molecular weight of approximately 60 kD [53] and inhibits prostaglandin production by interaction with the cyclo-oxygenase enzyme [55].

Basal production of PGE$_2$ by decidual stromal cells is increased during the first 48 h of culture by the addition of cycloheximide, an inhibitor of protein synthesis (Table 15.3). This again suggests the production of a protein which inhibits prostaglandin synthesis.

We have carried out some preliminary investigations as to whether progesterone, which is known to regulate prostaglandin production, might exert its effects through regulating the production of this protein. Cycloheximide was used to inhibit the synthesis of the presumptive inhibitor, leading to increased PGE$_2$ production. Progesterone alone (10^{-7}M) had a small inhibitory effect on basal PGE$_2$ synthesis by decidual stromal cells and opposed the effects of cycloheximide on PGE$_2$ synthesis (Table 15.4). We interpret these results as showing that

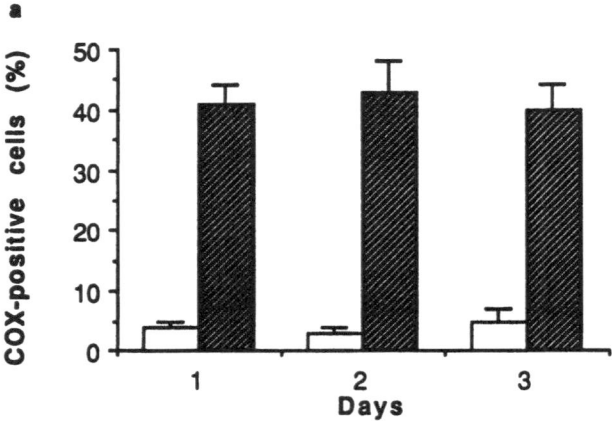

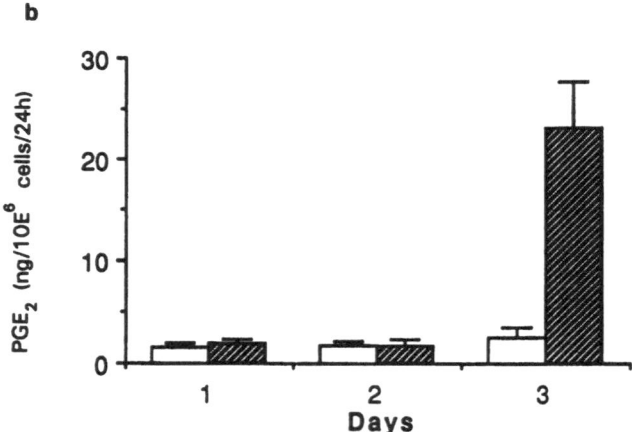

Fig. 15.4. Effects of IL-1-beta (100 pg ml^{-1}) (▨) added on day 1, day 2 or day 3 of culture on (**a**) numbers of cyclo-oxygenase positive decidual stromal cells or (**b**) PGE$_2$ production by the same cells. All data are means ± SEM (n = 3), and are typical of four replicate experiments.

Table 15.3. Basal production of PGE$_2$ by decidual stromal cells

	PGE$_2$ (ng/10^6 cells/24 h)		
	Day 1	Day 2	Day 3
Control	1.6±0.4	2.5±0.3	3.7±0.6
Cycloheximide (0.5 μg ml^{-1})	15.6±8.2	12.9±2.4	4.1±0.5

Values are mean ± SD, N = 4.

progesterone increased production of the inhibitory protein, thus opposing the effects of cycloheximide in decreasing protein synthesis. Further studies are required to confirm this finding, but this suggests that progesterone may be an inhibitor of prostaglandin production by increasing synthesis of the 60 kDa protein which inhibits decidual prostaglandin production.

Table 15.4. Effects of progesterone on PGE_2 synthesis by decidual stromal cells

	PGE_2 (ng/10^6 cells/24 h)	
	No progesterone	Progesterone (10^{-7}M)
Basal synthesis	1.3±0.2	0.9±0.2
Cycloheximide (0.5 μg ml^{-1})	4.2±0.6	1.4±0.4

Values are mean ± SD, $n = 4$.

Determination of this protein and the factors controlling its expression is likely to be very important in understanding the mechanism of uterine quiescence as well as activation.

It is postulated that the mechanism of preterm and term labour may be the same and that they involve an inflammatory response. This could be induced by bacteria but there could be other signals which trigger a non-infective inflammatory response.

PAF and IL-1-beta are known to increase in the liquor prior to labour [48,56] and these cytokines could act as fetal signals activating the decidua. PAF may come from the maturing fetal lung or from activated decidual macrophages.

Our results show that in the intact fetal membrane, PAF stimulated a small increase in production of PGE_2 by amnion (10–20 ng/ml/24 h) and a similar increase by choriodecidua. Membranes obtained after labour showed higher basal production of PGE_2. PAF added to the amnion did not increase this further but when added on the decidual side there was a 6–10-fold increase [35]. These results suggest that PAF may be a factor in the maintenance of raised prostaglandin production integral to the process of labour. PAF secretion into the liquor does not cross the membranes but is concentrated in the chorion and is metabolised there. Fetal PAF does not seem to be a likely initiator of increased prostaglandin synthesis in maternal decidua.

In conclusion there is good evidence that the decidua is the main site of increased synthesis of prostaglandins. A cytokine-mediated mechanism may be responsible for this process. This can be initiated by bacteria in cases of clinically obvious infection but also in the form of a low-grade inflammatory response triggering the biochemical amplification that can lead after several days or weeks to normal labour. Fetal cytokines may be involved in similar mechanisms leading to term labour.

Acknowledgement. I am grateful to Drs M. Sullivan, O. Ishihara and H. Khan for carrying out the experimental work, and to Action Research, The Aga Khan Foundation, Ono Pharmaceuticals UK, the British Council and the Institute Trust Fund who supported the work.

References

1. Dray F, Frydman R. Primary prostaglandins in amniotic fluid in pregnancy and spontaneous labour. Am J Obstet Gynecol 1976; 126:13–19.
2. Keirse MJNC, Flint APC, Turnbull AC. Prostaglandins in amniotic fluid during pregnancy and labour. J Obstet Gynaecol Br Cwlth 1974; 81:131–6.
3. Mitchell MD. Pathways of arachidonic acid metabolism with specific application to the fetus and mother. Semin Perinatol 1986; 10:242–54.
4. Lye SJ, Challis JRG. Inhibition by PGI_2 of myometrial activity in vivo in non pregnant ovariectomised sheep. J Reprod Fertil 1982; 66:311–15.
5. Garfield RE, Kannan MS, Daniel EE. Gap junction formation in myometrium: control by oestrogens, progesterone and prostaglandins. Am J Physiol 1980; 238:81–9.
6. Soloff MS. Uterine receptors for oxytocin: effects of estrogen. Biochem Biophys Res Commun 1975; 56:205–12.
7. Bowden GHW, Ellwood DC, Hamilton IR. In: Alexander M, ed. Microbial ecology of the oral cavity. Advances in Microbial Ecology. New York: Plenum Press, 1979; 135–217.
8. Bartlett JG, Moon NE, Goldstein PR, Goren B, Onderdonk AB, Polk BF. Cervical and vaginal bacterial flora: ecologic niches in the female lower genital tract. Am J Obstet Gynecol 1978; 130:658–61.
9. Lindner JGEM, Plantema FHF, Hoogkamp-Korstanje JAA. Quantitative studies of the vaginal flora of healthy women and of obstetrics and gynaecological patients. J Med Microbiol 1978; 11:233–41.
10. Lamont RF, Taylor-Robinson D, Newman M, Wigglesworth J, Elder MG. Spontaneous early preterm labour associated with abnormal genital bacterial colonisation. Br J Obstet Gynaecol 1986; 93:804–10.
11. Minkoff H, Grunebaum AN, Schwarz RH et al. Risk factor for prematurity and premature rupture of membranes: a prospective study of the vaginal flora in pregnancy. Am J Obstet Gynecol 1984; 150:965–72.
12. Gleeson RP, Elder AM, Turner MJ, Rutherford AJ, Elder MG. Vaginal pH in pregnancy in women delivered at and before term. Br J Obstet Gynaecol 1989; 96:183–7.
13. McDonald HM, O'Loughlin JA, Jolley P, Vigneswaran R, McDonald PJ. Vaginal infection and preterm labour. Br J Obstet Gynaecol 1991; 98:427–35.
14. McGregor JA, Lawellin D, Franco-Buff A, Todd JK, Makowski E. Protease production of micro-organisms associated with reproductive tract infection. Am J Obstet Gynecol 1986; 154:109–14.
15. Moghissi KS. Sperm migration through cervical mucous. In: Sherman AI, ed. Pathways of conception. The role of the cervix and oviduct in reproduction. Springfield, IL: CC Thomas, 1971; 214–36.
16. Gnarpe H, Friberg J. T-mycoplasmas on spermatozoa and infertility. Nature 1973; 254:97–8.
17. Gorbach SL, Menda KB, Thadepalli H, Keith L. Anaerobic mocroflora of the cervix in healthy women. Am J Obstet Gynecol 1973; 177:1053–5.
18. Goplerud CP, Ohm MJ, Galask RP. Aerobic and anaerobic flora of the cervix during pregnancy and the puerperium. Am J Obstet Gynecol 1976; 126:858–65.
19. Moberg P, Eneroth P, Harlin J, Ljung-Wastrom A, Nord CE. Cervical bacterial flora in infertile and pregnant women. Med Microbiol Immunol 1978; 165:139–45.
20. Bobitt JR, Ledger WR. Amniotic fluid analysis, its role in maternal and neonatal infection. Obstet Gynecol 1978; 51:56–62.
21. Lauweryns J, Bernat R, Lerut A, Detourney G. Intra-uterine pneumonia. An experimental study. Biol Neonate 1973; 22:301–18.
22. Pankuch GA, Applebaum PC, Lorenz RP, Botti JJ, Schachter J, Naeye RL. Placental microbiology and histology and the pathogenesis of chorioamnionitis. Obstet Gynecol 1984; 64:802–6.
23. Miller JM, Hill GB, Welt SI, Pupkin MJ. Bacterial colonisation of amniotic fluid in the presence of ruptured membranes. Am J Obstet Gynecol 1980; 137:451–8.
24. Cooperman NR, Kasim M, Rajachekaraiah KR. Clinical significance of amniotic fluid, amniotic membranes and endometrial biopsy cultures at the time of caesarean section. Am J Obstet Gynecol 1980; 137:536–41.
25. Garite TJ, Freeman RK. Chorioamnionitis in the preterm gestation. Obstet Gynecol 1982; 54:539–45

26. Cederquist LL, Ewool LC, Bousness RL, Litwin SD. Detectability and patterns of immunoglobulins in normal amniotic fluid throughout gestation. Am J Obstet Gynecol 1978; 130:220–6.

27. Schoonmaker JN, Lawellin DW, Lunt B, McGregor JA. Bacteria and inflammatory cells reduce chorioamniotic membrane integrity and tensile strength. Obstet Gynecol 1989; 74:590–6.

28. McGregor JA, Schoonmaker JN, Lunt BD, Lawellin DW. Antibiotic inhibition of bacterially induced fetal membrane weakening. Obstet Gynecol 1990; 76:124–8.

29. Bennett PR, Elder MG, Myatt L. The effects of lipoxygenase metabolites of arachidonic acid on human myometrial contractility. Prostaglandins 1987; 33:837–44.

30. Bennett PR, Rose MP, Myatt L, Elder MG. Preterm labour: stimulation of arachidonic acid metabolism in human amnion cells by bacterial products. Am J Obstet Gynecol 1987; 156:649–55.

31. Lamont RF, Anthony R, Myatt L, Booth L, Furr PM, Taylor-Robinson D. Production of PGE$_2$ by human amnion in vitro in response to addition of media conditioned by microorganisms associated with chorioamnionitis and preterm labour. Am J Obstet Gynecol 1990; 162:819–25.

32. Nakla S, Skinner K, Mitchell BF, Chalis JRG. Changes in prostaglandin transfer across human fetal membranes obtained after spontaneous labour. Am J Obstet Gynecol 1986; 155:1337–41.

33. Bennett PR, Chamberlain GVP, Patel L, Elder MG, Myatt L. Mechanisms of parturition. The transfer of prostaglandin E$_2$ and 5-hydroxy-eicosatetraenoic acid across fetal membranes. Am J Obstet Gynecol 1990; 162:683–7.

34. Cheung PYC, Walton JC, Tal HH, Riley SC, Challis JRG. Immunocytochemical distribution and localisation of 15-hydroxy prostaglandin dehydrogenase in human fetal membranes, decidua and placenta. Am J Obstet Gynecol 1990; 163:1445–9.

35. Khan H, Sullivan MHF, Helmig R, Roseblade CK, Uldbjerg N, Elder MG. Quantitative production of prostaglandin E$_2$ and its metabolites by human fetal membranes. Br J Obstet Gynaecol 1991; 98:712–15.

36. Roseblade CK, Sullivan MHF, Khan H, Lumb MR, Elder MG. Limited transfer of prostaglandin E$_2$ across the fetal membranes before and after labour. Acta Obstet Gynecol Scand 1990; 69:399–403.

37. McCoshen JA, Hoffman DR, Kredentser JV, Arenda C, Johnston JM. The role of fetal membranes in regulating production transport and metabolism of PGE$_2$ during labour. Am J Obstet Gynecol 1990; 163:1632–40.

38. Morris C, Khan H, Sullivan MHF, Elder MG. Effects of platelet activating factor on PGE$_2$ production by intact fetal membranes. Am J Obstet Gynecol 1992; in press.

39. Vince GS, Starkey PM, Jackson ML, Sargent IL, Redman CG. Flow cytometric characterisation of cell populations in human pregnancy decidua and isolation of decidual macrophages. J Immunol Methods 1990; 132:181–9.

40. Khan H, Ishihara O, Elder MG, Sullivan MHF. A comparison of two populations of decidual cells by immunocytochemistry and prostaglandin production. Histochemistry 1991; 96:149–52.

41. Ishihara O, Khan H, Sullivan MHF, Elder MG. Differential metabolism of intracellular and extracellular arachidonic acid by decidual stromal cells and macrophages. Eicosanoids 1991; 4:143.

42. Casey ML, MacDonald PC. Biomolecular processes in the initiation of parturition: decidual activation. Clin Obstet Gynecol 1988; 31:533–52.

43. Romero R, Mazor M, Wu YK, Sirtori M, Oyarzun E, Mitchell MD, Hobbins JC. Infection in the pathogenesis of preterm labour. Semin Perinatol 1988; 12:262–79.

44. Bejar P, Curbeol V, Davis C, Gluck L. Premature labour II: bacterial sources of phospholipase. Obstet Gynecol 1981; 57:479–82.

45. Lamont RF, Rose MP, Elder MG. Effect of bacterial products on prostaglandin E production by amnion cells. Lancet 1985; ii:1331–3.

46. Lumb MR, Roseblade CK, Helmig R, Uldbjerg N, Sullivan MHF, Elder MG. Use of a new simplified assay for PLA$_2$ to measure bacterial enzyme levels. Clin Chim Acta 1990; 189:39–46.

47. Romero R, Roslansky P, Oyarzun E et al. Labor and infection. Bacterial endotoxin in amniotic fluid and its relationship to the onset of preterm labor. Am J Obstet Gynecol 1988; 158:1044–9.

48. Romero R, Brody DT, Oyarzun E, Mazor M, Wu YK, Hobbins JC, Durum SK. Infection and labor III: Interleukin-1 a signal for the onset of parturition. Am J Obstet Gynecol 1089; 160:1117–21.

49. Romero R, Manogue KR, Mitchell MD, Wu YK, Oyarzun E, Hobbins JC, Cerami A. Infection and labor IV: Cachetin – tumor necrosis factor in the amniotic fluid of women with intra-amniotic infection and preterm labor. Am J Obstet Gynecol 1990; 161:336–41.

50. Romero R, Avila C, Santhanam U, Segal PB. Amniotic fluid interleukin 6 in preterm labor – association with infection. J Clin Invest 85:1392–400.

51. Akerhind M, Stromberg P, Hanksson A, Andersen LF, Lyndrup J, Trojnar J, Melin P. Inhibition

of uterine contractions of premature labour with an oxytocin analogue. Results from a pilot study. Br J Obstet Gynaecol 1987; 94:1040–4.

52. Wilson T, Liggins GC, Whittaker DJ. Oxytocin stimulates the release of arachidonic acid from human decidual cells. Prostaglandins 1988; 35:771–80.
53. Ishihara O, Kinoshita K, Satoh K, Mizuno M. The inhibitory effect of cytosolic fraction of human decidua on prostaglandin synthesis. Endocrinol Jpn 1987; 34:793–6.
54. Romero R, Lafreniere D, Hobbins JC, Mitchell MD. A product from human decidua inhibits prostaglandin production by human amnion. Prostaglandin Leukotriene Med 1987; 30:29–35.
55. Ishihara O, Kinoshita K, Satoh K, Mizuno M, Shimuzu T. An inhibitor of prostaglandin biosynthesis from human decidua: partial purification and properties. Prostaglandin Leukotriene Essent Fatty Acids 1990; 40:223–6.
56. Hoffman DR, Romero R, Johnston JM. Detection of platelet activating factor in amniotic fluid of complicated pregnancies. Am J Obstet Gynecol 1990; 162:525–8.

Discussion

Lumsden: Would Dr Lopez-Bernal amplify on his comment that receptor numbers were not important, and it was the coupling with the G-proteins that was important? Does that imply that, for example, there might be another receptor that will influence this coupling, or is it just a matter of receptor occupancy?

López Bernal: That is a fundamental question. I did not say that receptor numbers are not important. The receptors have to be there as otherwise the tissue does not respond. But what happens is that ultimately the response will depend on the number of second messenger molecules generated. So in a coupling situation where one receptor activates 10 G-proteins, and then each G-protein activates 10 units of PLC, for example, there is 100-fold amplification. In a situation where the coupling has been lost and one receptor can only activate, say, half a G-protein, and then only 5 units of enzyme, it is a 100 to five situation, and doubling or tripling or even multiplying the receptors by 20 will not make a lot of difference. The tissue is not responsive because it is uncoupled and it can be uncoupled by a variety of mechanisms. Other receptors can certainly influence that.

For example, in myometrium there is a classic situation in the rat where increases in cyclic AMP decrease the production of IP_3 by other agonists. If we give, say, a beta-mimetic to a rat and then try to increase IP_3 with oxytocin, because cyclic AMP production has been increased, the coupling is lost. And so whether there are 10 receptors for oxytocin or 100 becomes in some ways irrelevant.

But the sheep is the classical model where receptor numbers are important in the endometrium. They must be there at certain times in the cycle, and that is an important point of regulation. But then the coupling also becomes important and that could be a good place for pharmacological intervention.

Nathanielsz: In relation to infection and the host bacterium response there were a couple of papers that I found very exciting in a recent issue of *Science*, about differential responses to leprosy, in which they looked at the lepromatous form of the disease and the tuberculous form of the disease and found that the white cell populations in the lesions in the patients that responded in these different ways were different and their cytokine productions were different. The concept that the patient can be responding differently to the same infection put it in a very nice way for me.

The issue of the heterogeneity of the receptor populations and the fact that PGE_2 can do totally opposite things if the receptor is there suggests to me that we should not be trying to treat these deficiency diseases, if that is what we consider failure of cervical dilatation, with the agonist, but trying to manipulate the receptor populations by again going further up the pathway and producing the right milieu into which to put whatever pharmacology we wish to place.

López Bernal: I did not say this but some of the coupling and uncoupling changes are steroid-dependent – in rabbits, for example.

Nathanielsz: And in Roberts's study with the catecholamines. Catecholamines have not featured very much in this discussion about prostaglandins, but with the catecholamines the heterologous regulation of receptors by steroids has been very nicely worked out. And I think the same will apply with prostaglandins eventually.

López Bernal: I agree.

Keirse: I had forgotten about the decidual supernatant inhibiting seminal vesicle PGE production but I remember having seen it. Would boiled supernatant do the same thing?

Elder: We do not know.

Keirse: There are some data on boiled cytosols which, particularly in placenta, interfered with PGH synthase.

Kelly: Is the inhibitor similar in character to the gravidin of Teresa Wilson?

Elder: No. I was interested in the earlier comments on gravidin. We are hoping to start that work in the next few months and try and characterise it.

Husslein: I was interested in the result with oxytocin receptors. In our first study we found lower receptor values for oxytocin when we took the samples from women who were in labour. We tried to explain it on the basis of another observation that we made when we looked at a whole uterus removed at a caesarean hysterectomy. We measured oxytocin receptors at different points of that uterus and we found a very dramatic gradient from the fundus down to the cervix. We argued that in women who are in labour we make the incision much further down compared to women who are not in labour and who have no stretching of the lower uterine segment. Is that a reasonable explanation? What is the explanation for finding lower receptors in women in labour?

López Bernal: I am very aware of that study. I keep asking if the lower uterine segment changes so dramatically.

I have done a similar study, not yet published, and I find (in rough numbers) that if the concentration of oxytocin receptors in the fundus is 1000 fmol per ml of protein, then in the corpus it is 400. But I find that it only begins to decrease close to the cervix. Only when we get collagen rather than smooth muscles, is there a dramatic decrease when the values are expressed per ml of protein.

The other thing that puzzles me is why in preterm labour, with an average cervical dilatation of only 2 cm, there is a drop in receptors. I think it may be downregulation. If the oxytocin halves once labour is established, maybe the receptor number decreases or is internalised and the system works well because of the second messenger pathway so the number of receptors may not be as important.

It is possible that there is an anatomical explanation, but it may not be the complete explanation.

Olson: Is there any evidence to suggest that PGs induce oxytocin receptors?

López Bernal: I do not know of any evidence. I know that Linda Sheldrick can induce the oxytocin receptor with steroids in uterine explants.

With the samples that I took, I tried to subclassify the women. Those who had had an induction seemed to have intermediate receptor levels. Their levels are not as low as in women after spontaneous preterm labour or as high as in women having elective caesarean section. I tried to correlate that to the use of prostaglandins and the previous number of sections and so on, and I could not find any clear correlation. So I do not think that there is evidence that the receptor number is altered by prostaglandins.

Nathanielsz: Not even in primates, which we use as experimental animals for postmaturity, as far as I know. Certainly in none of our animals do we ever see it. I was intrigued with gravidin and these inhibitors – whether the disease of postmaturity might be an excess production of them.

Elder: That is an obvious possibility. First we need to be sure what they are and that they exist.

Olson: Those of us who do experiments on preterm labour want to differentiate those women who are infected and those who are not infected. How rigorous do we need to be in our examination of those women and their tissues? For instance, is the obvious lack of sepsis plus no histology, or no infiltration of neutrophils into the fetal membranes, adequate enough?

Elder: I am not sure. Romero, who has probably done the most work in this field, takes amniotic fluid samples from amniocentesis in all these women before delivery and looks for the presence of organisms in culture.

Olson: Is that the ultimate test?

Elder: I would have thought so. It is the ultimate in invasiveness as well, I suppose. But why is it so important to know?

Olson: That is the issue. Are there two groups of women who deliver with preterm labour – those who are infected and those who are not? Do we look for different aetiologies in those women?

Elder: To take the comments I made on interleukin-6: high levels were found in women in whom there was a positive amniotic fluid culture, but levels were also found to be significantly increased over normal in women who did not have any positive cultures – the so-called uncomplicated labours. Then a potent cytokine that is associated with inflammatory responses is present in the amniotic fluid. What is it doing there?

Olson: But a number of studies have also shown that women who have no indication of chorioamnionitis have low levels of prostaglandins. We have looked at amnion tissue levels of the cyclo-oxygenase enzyme activity and find that the V_{max} is elevated in some women – these are all without infection by our criteria – and it is very very low in others. I wonder if we are coming to the point where we might have to look for other mediators as activators of cervical dilatation and uterine contractility in that group of women who did not present with any infection and yet have delivered preterm. It raises the issue that prostaglandins might not be the trigger.

López Bernal: In the cases where there is a controlled infiltration, I believe there is increasing cyclo-oxygenase activity. The evidence is indirect. If we add exogenous arachidonic acid, the prostaglandin output becomes colossal. If we add a lot of arachidonic acid to tissue that is normal, we can never bring the prostaglandins up to anywhere near the level that we see with infection.

I believe there is a time course here, and this is relevant to something that was said earlier about not having evidence of infection. Paradoxically, the early stages of inflammation are when the PG release is highest. Women can have no clinical symptoms whatsoever with an initial inflammatory reaction, whereas the prostaglandins, especially PGE, may be recruiting cells. And those are the worst cases. In a very florid inflammatory reaction with cell necrosis, prostaglandin production goes down.

But I do think that it is a pathological situation and I think we need to start doing some sort of controlled trial, treating women between, say, 25 and 30 weeks, with some sort of antibiotic and anti-inflammatory regimen. I know it is difficult to predict who will go into labour, but people are now measuring fibronectin in vaginal fluid and that is apparently a quite good predictor. That, plus one or two other tests, and some of the classical broad-spectrum antibiotics and a leucotriene B-receptor antagonist or meclofenamate could be used. Why do we not do it?

Nathanielsz: I think NIH has a trial right now.

Olson: Professor Elder presented data showing the unlikelihood of PGE crossing the fetal membranes to the maternal side. What is the source of $PGF_{2\alpha}$ found in the amniotic fluid with labour, as published by Keirse and by Amy many years ago? If it is not from the fetus, it has to be from the fetal membranes and decidua; it is most probably not the amnion. And it has to cross the chorion to get there.

Elder: I do not know. It does not fit. It does not fit with the data that I have shown.

Chapter 16

Prevention of Preterm Labour

J.-J. Amy and H. Cammu

Introduction

Preterm birth has been defined by the World Health Organization as a birth occurring at a gestational age of less than 37 completed weeks (<259 days). The duration of gestation is measured from the first day of the last menstrual period and expressed in days or completed weeks. Preterm labour may be defined as labour ensuing before the 37th completed week of pregnancy.

Preterm birth of otherwise normal babies is a universal problem affecting both developed and developing countries, and a cause of considerable expenditure of health care resources. It is responsible for more than one-half and possibly three-quarters of the mortality among neonates without congenital anomalies [1,2]. With the decrease of perinatal morbidity and mortality due to other causes, the relative magnitude of the problem of preterm delivery has grown.

Various intervention programmes have claimed success in reducing the number of preterm deliveries, but the results have been difficult to reproduce or sustain. Despite many efforts in various fields encompassing governmental funding of medical care, improved antenatal care, earlier diagnosis of multiple gestation, large-scale use of tocolytics, the frequency of preterm births has not been markedly lessened in the past decades. The most important challenge of contemporary obstetrics will consist in elucidating the pathophysiology of preterm birth, in defining the relevant risk factors, and in applying rational and effective prevention and intervention policies. As stated by Eastman [3], "only when the factors causing prematurity are clearly understood, can any intelligent attempt at prevention be made".

Factors Predisposing to Preterm Labour

The principal risk factors that have been identified [4–6] are listed in Table 16.1.

Table 16.1. Principal risk factors of preterm birth

Demographic risks
Age <17 or >35
Nulliparity
Non-white race
Low socioeconomic and educational level

Behavioural risks
Deficient nutrition before and during pregnancy
Grossly excessive physical activity
Inadequate prenatal care

Pre-existent medical and obstetric risks
Prior preterm delivery
Prior second trimester loss
Uterine or cervical defect

Current pregnancy risks
Overdistension of the uterus (multiple pregnancy, hydramnios)
Bleeding from the uterus
Injury
Abdominal surgery
Pyrexial illness
Genital tract infection
Excessive myometrial activity
Cervical dilatation >2 cm
PPROM

Adapted from Iams et al. [6]

It must be realised that about half of all preterm births affect women not thought to be at risk. Conversely, except in cases of multiple gestation, most women in whom risk factors have been detected do not go into labour before term. With the sole exception of multiple pregnancy, the predictive value of each of the individual risk factors is less than 30% [6]. This, and the knowledge that preterm birth is often related to an unfavourable social background, beyond the practioner's control, have caused resignation and apathy among obstetricians, in the past. Papiernik and his team [7–11] should be credited for having stressed that, on the contrary, it was the obstetrician's task to thoroughly investigate this important problem, to identify patients at risk, to institute preventive measures prenatally, and to spread information among patients and authorities alike.

Biological and Social Characteristics

Age

There is an association between preterm birth and extremes of maternal age. In Aberdeen, between 1976 and 1980, the frequency of preterm delivery after spontaneous onset of labour in teenagers was nearly twice that in women aged 20–29 [12] (Table 16.2). However, as emphasised by Hall and Carr-Hill [12], youth is associated with factors such as minimum education, low social class and illegitimacy. Moreover, teenagers also have a higher incidence of prolonged pregnancy, which almost certainly rules out a biological effect.

Table 16.2. Spontaneous preterm delivery rate by maternal age (Aberdeen 1976–1980; $n = 11\,454$)

Age (years)	Preterm delivery rate (%)
14–19	7.8
20–29	3.8
30+	4.3

Adapted from Hall [4].

Parity

Preterm labour is more common in first pregnancies, and then less frequent with successive pregnancies up to the fourth [13] (Table 16.3).

Table 16.3. Spontaneous preterm delivery rate by parity (Aberdeen 1976–1980; $n = 11\,454$)

Parity	Preterm delivery rate (%)
0	5.0
1–2	3.6
3+	6.5

Adapted from Hall [4].

Ethnic Group

Race also has a major bearing on the prevalence of preterm births at each income, occupational and educational level considered. In the USA, both in black women (comparable in body size to white women) and in Puerto-Rican women (of shorter stature), the proportion of preterm deliveries is higher than in white women [14].

Maternal Height and Weight

Short stature, low prepregnancy weight, and suboptimal weight gain in pregnancy possibly increase the risk of preterm delivery although, particularly in these matters it is not clear whether the associations described are with low birth weight, spontaneous preterm birth, the obstetrician's active interference, or some combination of these [5].

Uterine and Cervical Defects

Congenital malformations of the uterus are associated with miscarriage in the first and second trimesters and, later in pregnancy, with preterm premature rupture of membranes (PPROM). Likewise, Asherman's syndrome carries an increased incidence of both miscarriage and preterm delivery, if the patient becomes pregnant [5].

A congenital or traumatically acquired weakness of the cervix may render the uterus incapable of containing a gestation normally. Belief in such "incompetence" of the cervix is the basis for performing cerclage. The condition is not a common one and tends to be overdiagnosed.

Socioeconomic Class

Social class, defined by the husband's occupation, is an indicator of the woman's behaviour, education, professional activity, nutrition, alcohol intake and smoking habits during pregnancy, as well as previous social and medical exposure. The lower socioeconomic groups are more at risk [14].

Occupation and Working Conditions of the Gravida

Gestation is not shortened in women working during pregnancy, even if they remain active well into the third trimester [15]. Saurel-Cubizolles et al. [16] have even reported a lower risk of preterm birth, in comparison with women without a professional occupation.

Various factors explain why women engaged in a professional activity are at a lower risk of delivering preterm: they are better educated and belong to a higher socioeconomic class, they are of lesser parity, they take better care of their health, and they attend the prenatal clinic and antenatal classes with greater regularity [16].

Dissimilar findings relating to this topic can be explained by failure to control for confounding factors. For instance, maternal age unquestionably varies between working and non-working women, among categories of employment, and even among women doing the same job [16,17]. Nevertheless, certain occupations and working conditions appear to carry a higher risk of preterm delivery. This applies to standing for extended periods of time, work on a production line, cumulation of strenuous tasks, and carrying of heavy loads [16,18]. Klebanoff et al. [19] found only a modestly increased risk of preterm delivery in women exposed to prolonged periods of standing, and no increase at all in association with heavy work or exercise. Yet the same group of investigators reported the same year that female resident doctors working more than 100 h per week were twice as likely to deliver preterm as residents working fewer hours [20]. A 50% higher risk of preterm delivery has been described in women working with electrical, metal or leather goods, when compared with other female manual workers [21].

Urinary catecholamine excretion, which reflects the total endogenous production of these substances, is augmented by nearly 60% during work periods that are physically, emotionally and intellectually very demanding [22], and it is possible that the deleterious effect of certain occupations and working conditions is mediated by an increased production of these hormones.

Travelling daily to and from work for more than 1.5 h would also increase the risk of preterm delivery, according to certain authors [8].

Stress

A significant association has been found between the experience of major life-events in pregnancy and preterm delivery. It appeared that the effects of stress might be additive, that is the more life-events encountered during pregnancy, the higher the risk of preterm delivery [23].

Nutrition

Deficiencies in the quality of nutrition are only of borderline importance in the aetiology of preterm birth [24].

Coitus

Theoretically, a variety of stimuli may elicit uterine contractions during or following coitus, and, in predisposed women, initiate the train of events leading to preterm labour. These stimuli include:

1. The excitation of sensory nerves in the cervix and the upper part of the vagina;
2. The release in the vagina of the prostanoates contained in the ejaculate;
3. The female orgasm, which is frequently associated with contractions of the uterus;
4. The release of oxytocin following stimulation of the nipples.

Several authors have postulated a correlation between coitus, orgasm, uterine contractions and preterm labour. From a review of the literature [25], it can only be concluded that although it is possible that intercourse and/or orgasm can precipitate preterm labour, the clinical studies give conflicting answers. One of the reasons is that most studies are retrospective, based on interviews at delivery. Such studies compare the sexual behaviour of women at term with that of women before term, which differs regardless of outcome, sexual activity declining with advancing gestation [25].

Uncertain Gestation

Uncertain gestation relates more closely to preterm delivery than the majority of other maternal indices, and is quite independent of these latter [4] (Table 16.4).

Table 16.4. Spontaneous preterm delivery rate by certainty of gestation (Aberdeen 1976–1980; $n = 11\,454$)

Certainty of gestation	Preterm delivery rate (%)
Certain	3.7
Approximative	5.3
Uncertain	8.7

Adapted from Hall [4].

Past Obstetric History

A multiparous woman's reproductive history may give important prognostic clues. The risk for preterm delivery is trebled after one previous preterm birth and increased sixfold after two (Table 16.5).

Table 16.5. Risk of repetition of preterm birth in two consecutive births (Aberdeen; $n = 6072$)

First birth	Second birth preterm (%)
Preterm	15.4
Term	4.7

Adapted from Carr-Hill and Hall [26].

It is not clear whether the association of short interpregnancy intervals with preterm labour is due predominantly to the tendency to "replace" without delay an unsuccessful pregnancy [4].

Fetal Factors

Preterm labour is more frequent when the fetus is male [12] (Table 16.6).

Table 16.6. Risk of preterm birth by fetal sex in singletons (spontaneous onset of labour) in Aberdeen 1961–1979

	Number	Preterm birth rate (%)
Male fetus	18 591	6.8
Female fetus	17 699	5.7

Adapted from Hall and Carr-Hill [12].

Multiple Pregnancy

Multiple pregnancy is a strong marker of preterm labour. The median gestational length in twin pregnancy is 37 weeks; that is 50% of twins are born preterm. The median gestations for triplets and quadruplets are 33 and 31 weeks, respectively [27] (Table 14.7).

Table 16.7. Preterm delivery in multiple pregnancy

	Median gestational length (weeks)	Percentage preterm infants
Twins	37	50
Triplets	33	95
Quadruplets	31	97

Preterm labour in twins is related to zygosity and placentation: it is most frequent in monozygotic monochorionic twins, next most frequent in monozygotic dichorionic twins, and least frequent in dizygotic twins [4].

Women with monozygotic monochorionic twins are more prone to suffer PPROM, whereas those with dizygotic twins will more often present with contractions. There is a high male to female sex ratio in preterm twins, and it is highest in monozygotic twins [28].

Other Complications of Pregnancy

Hydramnios

Polyhydramnios is another condition causing "uterine stretch", leading to an untimely increase in prostaglandin production and the onset of uterine activity before term. Preterm labour is particularly frequent when hydramnios has developed acutely, as can be the case with monochorionic twins.

Bleeding in Pregnancy

Bleeding from the uterus, irrespective of the stage of pregnancy and the cause of the bleeding, predisposes to preterm birth. Threatened abortion, accidental haemorrhage, placenta praevia and non-specific antepartum haemorrhage are all associated with a high preterm delivery rate [5].

Abdominal Surgery

The surgical treatment of appendicitis or of a complication of an ovarian cyst carry an increased incidence of both miscarriage and preterm delivery.

Genital Tract Infection

Many epidemiological, microbiological and histological data indicate that microbial infestation of the genital tract is linked to the occurrence of preterm labour and that of PPROM. However, descriptive, prospective and retrospective cohort studies have failed to identify with any consistency specific micro-organisms or associations thereof. Germs incriminated have included *Neisseria gonorrhoeae*, group B streptococci, *C. trachomatis*, *Mycoplasma hominis*, *Ureaplasma urealyticum*, *Trichomonas vaginalis*, and microorganisms found in bacterial vaginosis [29]. Numerous microbial species present in the genital tract are capable of releasing phospholipases A_2 and C, and of activating the arachidonic acid cascade. The ensuing increase in the local production of prostaglandins E_2 and $F_{2\alpha}$ may result in the ripening of the cervix and, ultimately, in the stimulation of uterine activity. Some of these germs produce collagenases, mucinases, and proteases, capable of facilitating microbial invasion of the uterine cavity, weakening the fetal membranes, and causing preterm labour or premature rupture of the membranes.

It is likely that in many cases chorioamnionitis antedates labour and/or rupture of the membranes. The frequency of positive amniotic fluid cultures in women in preterm labour with intact membranes varied from 0 to 61% in 16 studies published between 1980 and 1990. This extreme variability seems to be the result of differences in patient populations, definitions of preterm labour, and microbiological techniques [30].

Findings of micro-organisms within the membranes in over half of preterm deliveries suggest that germs present in the lower genital tract can ascend and exert effects on the cervix, lower uterine segment decidua, and membranes, without necessarily causing infection of the fetus or the amniotic fluid [29]. Be that as it may, preterm birth is associated with a significant increase in the incidence of puerperal endometritis, which indicates clearly a relationship between genital tract infection and prematurity [31].

Bacteriuria

There is no clear relationship between bacteriuria and preterm birth [31–33]. In studies that have reported a statistically significant increase in the rate of preterm births in bacteriuric patients, it is possible that bacteriuria simply acted as a confounding variable or marker of increased risk. Bacteriuria and preterm birth share the common risk factor of lower socioeconomic status, and of young age at first pregnancy. Further, the efficacy of antimicrobial therapy in reducing the risk of preterm birth in bacteriuric women may result from its action on germs in the vagina and in the cervix, that are causally associated with preterm labour [33].

Miscellaneous Infections

Protozoal infections (toxoplasmosis, malaria), bacterial infections (syphilis, tuberculosis, leprosy, typhoid fever, listeriosis, infections due to *Campylobacter*) and viral infections (hepatitis, measles, smallpox) have been associated with preterm labour [33].

Preterm Premature Rupture of the Membranes

Rupture of the membranes precedes the onset of labour in many patients delivering preterm. The overwhelming majority of women in preterm labour and with ruptured membranes, will deliver before term, in contrast to women thought to be in preterm labour, but with intact membranes, most of whom will deliver at term [5].

Other Maternal and Fetal Complications

Isoimmunisation, proteinuric hypertension, intrauterine growth retardation and other complications may require the obstetrician to terminate pregnancy before term.

Prediction of Preterm Labour

The concept of allocating individual women to certain "risk categories" in early pregnancy is appealing. Theoretically, this approach should allow the obstetrician to make rational decisions during antenatal care. With proper knowledge of the earliest signs of departure from normality, one should also be able to intervene in a beneficial way [34].

Several scoring systems, based on established risk factors for preterm labour, have been devised [7,35]. Papiernik [7] was the first to devise such a system, considering factors in all areas nowadays thought to be important: general and social factors, unfavourable medical or obstetric antecedents, danger signals at examination, and factors of fatigue. Later, systems of predicting spontaneous preterm delivery have been described, that take into acount not only characteristics ascertainable at the initial evaluation, but also assessment at later stages of pregnancy, with reassignment of the risk [8,9,36,37]. The predictive power of the system was improved by this rescoring later in pregnancy.

Since many components of these scores are based on factors related to past pregnancy performance, prediction of preterm birth is more reliable in parous than in nulliparous women [5,31,34], yet these latter account for an increasing proportion of the total obstetric population [34]. Overall, however, all these risk scoring systems have low sensitivities and they carry a high rate of false prediction of preterm delivery [5,38]. Furthermore, a given scoring system is devised for a given population: it takes into account the risk factors prevailing in that population [39] and, hence, cannot be extrapolated unaltered to other populations [40].

Savitz et al. [39] emphasised that if preterm birth is to be prevented, a detailed study of each separate cause of preterm birth is required. If this is not done, a specific exposure resulting in a specific cause of preterm birth will be attenuated when projected on the whole incidence of preterm delivery. If for instance, a prevention programme is based on intervention in early preterm labour, its success will in part depend on the contribution of preterm labour to all preterm deliveries.

There are methodological concerns with the use of a risk scoring system. A woman may be assigned to the high-risk group because of the rigid definition of the risk markers, whereas an experienced clinician might have assessed the situation more sensitively by applying implicit, but sound, clinical judgement [41]. Furthermore, Alexander and Keirse [41] correctly stated that scoring systems perform better in assessing the risk, if they are implemented late in pregnancy, or if they allow for readjustment during pregnancy. However, this leads to the paradoxical situation that the most accurate prediction is made at a moment when there is less need for this information, whereas the much needed early identification is grossly imprecise.

Yet, despite these shortcomings, formalised risk assessment has provided methods which can be tested for the prevention of preterm birth [31]. The greatest accomplishment of scoring systems has consisted in making clinicians more conscious of the need to prevent preterm labour [42].

Dynamic Assessment of the Risk, During Pregnancy

Cervical Scoring

Many obstetricians perform a vaginal examination (VE) routinely, at each prenatal visit. In the practitioner's mind, the VE aims at determining the status of the cervix and, on the basis of this and previous examinations, at defining whether there is a greater than normal chance that the woman might go spontaneously into labour, within a short interval of time. If such is the purpose, the VE is particularly important before term, so that measures can be implemented to delay the onset of labour, if deemed necessary [43].

Doubts have been raised regarding the predictability of the onset of labour, based on the subjective interpretation of changes in the cervix, should they occur [44]. These latter changes do indeed take place very gradually in the course of a normal pregnancy, particularly during the third trimester. Detractors of the routine VE have even claimed that it could be harmful, by accelerating cervical maturation and/or stimulating myometrial activity, as well as by increasing the risk of PPROM [45]. Despite the fact that VE may cause a very short-lived release of prostanoates locally, there are no hard data substantiating the detrimental effects [43,46]. O'Donovan et al. [44], to our mind wrongly, consider that preterm labour in patients with cervical changes, is unlikely to be prevented by modification of life-style, and that the costs of the implementation of such a policy are unwarranted.

After reviewing the literature, Heringa and Huisjes [47] concluded that dilatation of the internal cervical os to 2 cm, early in the third trimester, could not be interpreted as necessarily abnormal, in the absence of effacement. However, they felt that dilatation exceeding 2 cm, with simultaneous effacement of the cervix, was abnormal.

Newman et al. [48] calculated the cervical score of patients with multiple pregnancy, by subtracting cervical dilatation in centimetres from cervical length in centimetres. Cervical scores declined progressively with advancing gestation and subsequent preterm delivery. A cervical score ≤0 before 34 weeks' gestation was strongly predictive of preterm delivery (75%). Only 2 of 78 women (2.6%) with a score >0 delivered within a week of the examination. The earlier in pregnancy a cervical score ≤0 was found, the greater the positive predictive value that could be ascribed to it (e.g. 92% at 20–28 weeks' gestation). The first appearance of a score ≤0 had the best correlation with gestational length at delivery and provided the best sensitivity, specificity, and predictive values for preterm birth. Used in this way, cervical scoring proved to be simple, quantifiable, reproducible, and safe, in the evaluation of the risk of preterm delivery [48].

Myometrial Activity Monitoring at Home

Portable tocodynamometers allowing transmission of digitised tracings by telephone for interpretation, have been used for monitoring women at high risk of preterm labour, at home. A number of small, randomised trials were carried out to determine the effectiveness of myometrial activity monitoring at home, in preventing preterm delivery. Preterm labour was diagnosed at an earlier stage, amenable to tocolysis, and preterm birth was less frequent in women monitored than in control patients submitted to routine care. These trials left unanswered the question whether the observed beneficial effect was due to the monitoring per se, or whether it was achieved by the accompanying nursing support, or the extra periods of limited physical activity during monitoring. Trials that compared women who were monitored, with others who received equivalent nursing support but no monitoring, did not show a clearly positive effect of monitoring, suggesting that nursing support alone might be sufficient to reduce the frequency of preterm delivery in women at risk [49].

Nipple Stimulation Test

Eden et al. [38] hypothesised that a provocative test of myometrial contractility at the beginning of the third trimester could identify women destined to deliver prematurely. They studied a standard protocol of nipple stimulation, under cardiotocographic control, at about 28 weeks' gestation. Uterine activity was elicited twice as frequently among women who delivered preterm, as among those who delivered at term. A positive nipple stimulation test correctly identified 16 of the 19 patients who delivered preterm (sensitivity: 84%). In addition, a negative test preceded term delivery in 44 of 47 patients (negative predictive value: 94%).

Fetal Fibronectin as a Marker for Preterm Delivery

Lockwood et al. [50] postulated that separation of the chorion from the decidua might release fibronectin into the cervix and the vagina, which could serve as a biochemical marker for preterm delivery. Identification of this substance in the lower genital tract had a positive predictive value for preterm delivery of 83%, when used in a group of patients with excessive uterine activity and intact membranes; the sensitivity of the test was 82%. The test may serve to diagnose preterm labour in women with preterm contractions, allowing for an earlier and more satisfactory selection of subjects requiring tocolysis. For the finding to be really useful, however, future studies should confirm that the presence of fetal fibronectin in the cervical and vaginal secretions can identify asymptomatic patients at risk for preterm delivery while they are still amenable to therapy.

Intervention to Reduce the Risk of Preterm Delivery

Papiernik [7–9] developed the first model of intervention. This latter begins with education and counselling regarding risk factors and danger signs associated with pre-term delivery. Early in pregnancy, intervention consists of risk assessment, psychological support, rest and supplementation of nutrition. Leaves of absence are granted, particularly to women with strenuous occupations and with long distances to travel to and from work. Risk assessment continues as a dynamic process throughout pregnancy. VE to assess cervical status and station of the presenting part is regularly performed. Liberal use is made of pharmacological interventions, such as progestins (at one point, 25% of all patients, 100% of patients at risk) and tocolysis, and surgical procedures, such as cervical cerclage (at one point, 50% of patients at risk).

Application of this model of intervention at the Béclère Maternity Hospital in Clamart, France, was associated with a stepwise reduction in preterm births from 10.1% to 3.4%, between 1973 and 1979. In the city of Haguenau, France, a reduction in preterm deliveries was observed over a 12-year period, following implementation of this intervention model. In Haguenau, the observed reduction was more important for early preterm births (50% reduction of births before 34 weeks) than for total preterm births (30% reduction). The birthweight distribution showed similar trends, with a reduction of very low birthweights and of birthweights below 2000 g. The reduction of preterm deliveries was observed in low and medium risk women, but not in women considered to be at high risk (previous preterm delivery; less than 22 or more than 35 years of age; bleeding during pregnancy). The incidence of the "classical" risk factors declined in the observed population over the 12-year period [10].

The components of the prevention programme applied in Haguenau were basically the same as those implemented nationally in France, in 1971, and a similar reduction in preterm births was also observed in many other centres in France.

Papiernik et al. [10] attributed the improvement in the preterm birth rate observed in Haguenau to two different mechanisms: (a) a reduction in the short term (during pregnancy itself), affecting women without strong predisposing factors; (b) a reduction in the long term, due to the decrease in the prevalence of strong predisposing risk factors in the whole population.

In San Francisco, the implementation of a prevention programme was associated with a decrease in the preterm delivery rate from 6.7% to 2.4% between 1978 and 1979 [37].

The real impact of models of intervention such as that implemented in Haguenau [10,11] is difficult to define. These studies did not include a control group of women at similar risk, in whom intervention was withheld, which could have established a causal relation between the measures being taken and the changes that were witnessed [17,51]. Instead, the conclusions of the investigators rested on the comparison of preterm birth rates before and after implementation of a given programme, or on comparisons of trends in the population under study, with those in populations not taking part in a similar programme [51]. It is clear that the introduction of a prevention programme nationwide in France in 1971, has made assessment of the impact of the Haguenau study more arduous still.

Intervention models have been criticised for having caused obstetricians to intervene unnecessarily and far too often with aggressive prevention measures, such as the administration of tocolytic drugs, or the performance of cervical cerclage [5, 41, 52].

In conclusion, whether application of scoring systems and implementation of interventions actually reduce the rate of preterm delivery is not proven. But the endeavour of Papiernik et al. is an illustration of how the change over time in care-seeking behaviour of the better educated has spread to less educated groups in the population [17].

Specific Interventions

With respect to preterm births, there are at least two kinds of intervention to be considered: (a) those that prevent conception and/or completion of pregnancy in women at higher risk, and (b) those that alter the condition of the pregnant woman in such a way that a normal pregacy outcome is enhanced [52].

It is almost certain that procedures or processes that prevent births in populations of high risk women, also reduce the frequency of abnormalities in babies being born [52]. Liberalised abortion has been shown to improve pregnancy outcome.

In the following paragraphs, we discuss a number of specific interventions. One should keep in mind the multivariate character of preterm birth. Elimination of one risk factor is not very helpful, and intervention schemes based on only one risk factor are bound to fail.

Social Support

Social support systems have been shown to be of value in improving pregnancy outcome. However, the real problem is how to deliver support to women who do not establish contact with health care providers, and who usually present the greatest risk with regard to pregnancy outcome. For these women, a system of community-based social support may prove to be beneficial, cost effective, and more humane than existing hospital based services [23].

Nutritional Supplementation

Programmes have often been instituted to supplement the nutrition of low-income pregnant women to promote a favourable outcome of pregnancy. One large-scale programme instituted in the USA was associated with an increase in mean birthweight. This was ascribed partly to an average of 5 days' increase in the duration of gestation, and, to a lesser degree, to an increase in fetal growth [24].

A randomised controlled study of antenatal nutritional supplementation in New York City yielded ambiguous results: balanced protein-calorie supplements increased the length of gestation (with borderline significance), whereas high-protein supplementation, on the contrary, seemed to increase the number of very early preterm births [53].

Education

Education is a possible intervention as regards virtually all factors related to low birthweight. Spreading information may encourage women to book early at the antenatal clinic, to change habits thought to affect adversely the outcome of pregnancy, and to report at the first alarming sign. The systematic implementation of such a policy is considered to account for a major part for the improved perinatal results obtained by Papiernik's group [54].

Modification of Working Conditions

For women at greater risk of preterm birth because of their professional occupation and working conditions, several measures can be envisioned:

1. Reduction in the daily number of hours of work
2. Increased length of prenatal maternity leave
3. Change of work during pregnancy
4. Modification in the organisation of work places, to make them more suitable for pregnant women

This latter policy appears to be of real benefit to pregnant staff, while causing the least amount of inconvenience to other staff [18].

Prenatal Care

Prenatal care is an ill-defined and poorly understood health care commodity [31]. Lack of prenatal care is consistently associated with low birthweight; the reasons for this are unclear. Conventional prenatal care does little that could be expected to influence directly gestational length, or birthweight. Women of higher social and cultural level submit to prenatal care with greater regularity, and earlier, than women of lower status, yet when these factors are accounted for, it is the low-status women who benefit most from prenatal care [55].

Two short sentences of Stubblefield [55] sum it up nicely: "Prenatal care is the one intervention consistently associated with improved pregnancy outcome. This basic health care should be available to all women."

Administration of Beta-adrenergic Drugs

Despite extensive use of oral betamimetics in the prophylaxis of preterm labour, scientific evidence has not substantiated a beneficial effect of these drugs in terms of outcome of gestation, particularly perinatal mortality and later development of the child. Trials conducted in women with a history of previous preterm delivery, with untimely cervical dilatation, or with twin pregnancy did not show a positive effect [56,57].

It is possible that therapy was not applied to the right target population: the problem for clinicians is to begin treatment with tocolytic agents early enough to maximise the potential for success, while avoiding overtreating with potentially dangerous drugs [1,56]. It has been said [58] that prophylactic administration of tocolytics often serves to put the obstetrician's rather than the patient's mind at rest.

Administration of Progesterone

In six placebo-controlled trials, 17α-hydroxyprogesterone caproate was administered by intramuscular injections for prevention of preterm labour and delivery. Globally [57], the trial showed a statistically significant reduction in the incidence of preterm delivery, with a typical odds ratio of 0.50 and a 95% confidence interval between 0.30 and 0.85. A comparable decrease was noted in the occurrence of low birthweight, with a typical odds ratio of 0.46, and a 95% confidence interval of 0.27–0.80.

These effects on the rates of preterm delivery and low birthweight were not matched by any detectable lowering of the incidence of perinatal death or a significant decrease in the incidence of the respiratory distress syndrome [57].

Administration of Magnesium

Skajaa et al. [59] found no difference in the nutrient intake and muscle content of magnesium between normal pregnant women and women of similar gestational age who eventually went into preterm labour. Three prospective randomised trials of magnesium supplementation during pregnancy [60–62] have given conflicting results in terms of the potential benefit with regard to the incidence of preterm delivery and delivery of a low birthweight infant.

Administration of Antibiotics

The knowledge that germs are very likely involved in the aetiology of a certain number of cases of preterm labour has led several investigators to test whether antibiotic therapy might be a useful adjunct in its prevention. Although various studies have not demonstrated a beneficial effect, others have shown that, in the presence of some potential pathogens in the lower genital tract, the occurrence of preterm labour, preterm rupture of the membranes, and possibly fetal demise, could be lowered by the administration of erythromycin, particularly when given in the third trimester [29,63]. Although this is an interesting line of research, which deserves more scrutiny, the routine use of antimicrobial agents in pregnancies at risk cannot be recommended at this stage.

Cervical Cerclage

There is no good diagnostic test for cervical incompetence [64]. Most commonly, the decision to intervene surgically is based on past reproductive history and, in addition, on clinical assessment of the cervix during pregnancy. Testing cervical resistance in the interval between pregnancies by means of graduated dilators may allow a more objective assessment [65].

A variety of surgical techniques have been described for treatment of cervical incompetence; Shirodkar's and McDonald's methods are most frequently used [64,63].

Grant [65] reviewed the results of four randomised controlled trials of cervical cerclage [66–69] and concluded that the use of cerclage was associated with a greater frequency of (1) administration of tocolytics, (2) admission to hospital, (3) induction of labour, and (4) Caesarean section. However, interim results of the MRC/RCOG trial [69] suggest a modest beneficial effect of cerclage in women with singleton pregnancy, and a past history of second trimester miscarriage or preterm delivery. Women undergoing cerclage had significantly less deliveries before 33 weeks than control patients (8.2% versus 13.2%, $P=0.05$). Between 33 and 36 weeks, the number of deliveries was the same in both groups. Perinatal mortality was lower in the group treated.

Premature rupture of the membranes occurred more frequently after cerclage in one study [67] but not in another [66]. Puerperal sepsis appeared to be a real complication of the procedure [67,69].

Currently, there is no evidence in support of the use of cerclage on the basis of previous surgery to the cervix, multiple pregnancy, or other indications [64,65].

Intervention in Multiple Gestation

Presently, most births of triplets and quadruplets are the result of induction of ovulation. In England and Wales, the rate of triplet and quadruplet births was steady between 1939 and the late 1970s at 10 per 100000 deliveries. It gradually rose to 24.7 per 100000 in 1988 [70]. It is clear that induction of ovulation should be carried out with much more circumspection than is currently the case. Whether embryo reduction substantially prolongs gestation remains to be proven.

There is currently no good evidence that women with uncomplicated twin pregnancy should be coerced into resting in bed, at home or in hospital, from the beginning of the third trimester onwards. However, it may be useful to investigate by a controlled trial whether rest at an earlier stage of pregnancy (e.g. between 20 and 30 weeks' gestation) may be beneficial [71].

Sympathomimetic drugs and cervical cerclage have been of no benefit in twin pregnancy, and avoidance of coitus has not prolonged pregnancy either. However, giving information to the mother is important, and much attention must be devoted to signs of early preterm labour [27].

Concluding Remarks

Despite its many imperfections, the most important advance in the content of prenatal care has been risk assessment, and the formulation of appropriate interventions in response to each risk factor identified. A specific programme designed for a given population should bring about a substantial reduction in preterm births.

In France, between 1972 and 1981, births before 34 weeks' gestation were lowered by half, as were births of babies weighing less than 1500 g. In the city of Haguenau, implementation of a prevention programme was associated with a reduction of births before 34 weeks by two thirds, between 1971 and 1986 [70].

These facts speak for themselves. There is no place for complacency and no reason why the problem of preterm birth should not be tackled with the same energy, in other countries.

Acknowledgements. We are grateful to Ms Bea Pion for expert secretarial assistance.

References

1. Creasy RK. Preventing preterm birth. N Engl J Med 1991; 325:727–9.
2. Rush RW, Keirse MJNC, Howat P, Baum JD, Anderson ABM, Turnbull AC. Contributions of preterm delivery to peritnatal mortality. Br Med J 1976; 2:965–8.
3. Eastman NJ. Prematurity from the view-point of the obstetrician. Am Pract 1947; 1:343.
4. Hall MH. Incidence and distribution of preterm labour. In: Beard RW, Sharp F, eds. Preterm labour and its consequences. London: Royal College of Obstetricians and Gynaecologists, 1985; 5–13.
5. Turnbull AC, Lopez Bernal A. Human parturition and preterm labour. In: Beard RW, Sharp F, eds. Preterm labour and its consequences. London: Royal College of Obstetricians and Gynaecologists, 1985; 71–90.
6. Iams JD, Johnson FF, Creasy RK. Prevention of preterm birth. Clin Obstet Gynecol 1988; 31:599–615.
7. Papiernik-Berkhauer E. Coëfficient de risque d'accouchement prématuré. Press Méd 1969; 77:793–4.
8. Papiernik E, Kaminski M. Multifactorial study of the risk of prematurity at 32 weeks of gestation. I. A study of the frequency of 30 predictive characteristics. J Perinat Med 1974; 2:30–6.
9. Kaminski M, Papiernik E. Multifactorial study of the risk of prematurity at 32 weeks gestation. II.

A comparison between an empirical prediction and a discriminant analysis. J Perinat Med 1974; 2:37–44.

10. Papiernik E, Bouyer J, Dreyfus J. Risk factors for preterm births and results of a prevention policy – The Haguenau Perinatal Study 1971–1982. In: Beard RW, Sharp F, eds. Preterm labour and its consequences. London: Royal College of Obstetricians and Gynaecologists, 1985; 15–20.

11. Papiernik E, Bouyer J, Dreyfus J et al. Prevention of preterm births: a perinatal study in Haguenau, France. Pediatrics 1985; 76:154–8.

12. Hall MH, Carr-Hill RA. Impact of sex ratio on onset and management of labour. Br Med J 1982; 285: 401–3.

13. Bakketeig LS, Hoffman HJ, Harley EE. The tendency to repeat gestational age and birthweight in successive births. Am J Obstet Gynecol 1979; 135:1086–103.

14. Garn SM, Shaw HA, McGabe KD. Effects of socioeconomic status and race on weight-defined and gestational prematurity in the United States. In: Reed DM, Stanley FJ, eds. The epidemiology of prematurity. Baltimore: Urban and Schwarzenberg, 1977; 127–40.

15. Naeye RL, Peters EC. Causes and consequences of premature rupture of fetal membranes. Lancet 1980; i:192–4.

16. Saurel-Cubizolles MJ, Kaminski M, Garcia J. Conditions de travail des femmes enceintes et prématurité. In: Papiernik E, Bréart G, Spira N, eds. Prévention de la naissance prématurée. Paris: INSERM, 1986; 139–54.

17. Hogue CJR. Discussion. In: Papiernik E, Bréart G, Spira N, eds. Prévention de la naissance prématurée. Paris: INSERM, 1986; 175–9.

18. Kaminski M, Saurel-Cubizolles M-J. Les femmes enceintes travaillant à l'hôpital: projet de recherche pour l'évaluation d'une politique de modification des conditions de travail. In: Papiernik E, Bréart G, Spira N, eds. Paris: INSERM, 1986; 239–59.

19. Klebanoff MA, Shiono PH, Carey JC. The effect of physical activity during pregnancy on preterm delivery and birthweight. Am J Obstet Gynecol 1990; 163:1450–6.

20. Klebanoff MA, Shiono PH, Rhoads GG. Outcomes of pregnancy in a national sample of resident physicians. N Engl J Med 1990; 323:1040–5.

21. Sanjose S, Roman E, Beral V. Low birthweight and preterm delivery, Scotland, 1981–84: effect of parents' occupation. Lancet 1991; 338:428–31.

22. Katz VL, Jenkins T, Haley L, Bowes WA Jr. Catecholamine levels in pregnant physicians and nurses: a pilot study of stress and pregnancy. Obstet Gynecol 1991; 77:338–42.

23. Newton R. The influence of psychosocial stress in low birthweight and preterm labour. In: Beard RW, Sharp F, eds. Preterm labour and its consequences. London: Royal College of Obstetricians and Gynaecologists, 1985; 225–45.

24. Berg van den J, Oechsli FW. Prematurity. In: Bracken MB, ed. Perinatal epidemiology. New York: Oxford University Press, 1984; 69–85.

25. Andersen LF, Fuchs F. Sexual activity and preterm birth. In: Fuchs F, Stubblefield PG, eds. Preterm birth. New York: Macmillan, 1984; 112–20.

26. Carr-Hill RA, Hall MH. The repetition of spontaneous preterm labour. Br J Obstet Gynaecol 1985; 92:921–8.

27. Chamberlain G. Multiple pregnancy. Br Med J 1991; 303:111–15.

28. MacGillivray I, Campbell DM, Samphier M, Thompson B. Preterm deliveries in twin pregnancies in Aberdeen. Acta Genet Medicae Gemmellol (Roma) 1983; 31:207–11.

29. McGregor JA. Prevention of preterm birth; new initiatives based on microbial-host interactions. Obstet Gynecol Surv 1988; 43:1–14.

30. Armer TL, Duff P. Intraamniotic infection in patients with intact membranes and preterm labor Obstet Gynecol Surv 1991; 46:589–93.

31. Bragonier JR, Cushner IM, Hobel CJ. Social and personal factors in the etiology of preterm birth. In: Fuchs F, Stubblefield PG, eds. Preterm birth. New York: Macmillan, 1984; 64–85.

32. Whalley PJ. Bacteriuria of pregnancy. Am J Obstet Gynecol 1967; 97:723–38.

33. Polk F. Infectious processes and preterm labor. In: Fuchs F, Stubblefield PG, eds. Preterm birth. New York: Macmillan, 1984; 86–97.

34. Newcombe R, Federick J, Chalmers I. Antenatal identification of patients "at risk" of pre-term labour. In: Anderson A, Beard R, Brudenell JM, Dunn P, eds. Pre-term labour. London: Royal College of Obstetricians and Gynaecologists, 1977; 17–28.

35. Fedrick J. Antenatal identification of women at high risk of spontaneous pre-term birth. Br J Obstet Gynaecol 1976; 83:351–4.

36. Creasy RK, Gummer BA, Liggins GC. System for predicting spontaneous preterm birth. Obstet Gynecol 1980; 55:692–5.

37. Herron MA, Katz M, Creasy RK. Evaluation of a pre-term birth prevention program: preliminary report. Obstet Gynecol 1982; 59:452–6.
38. Eden RD, Sokoi RJ, Sorokin Y, Cook HJ, Sheeran G, Chik L. The mammary stimulation test – a predictor of preterm delivery? Am J Obstet Gynecol 1991; 164:1409–19.
39. Savitz DA, Blackmore CA, Thorp JM. Epidemiologic characteristics of preterm delivery: etiologic heterogeneity. Am J Obstet Gynecol 1991; 164:467–71.
40. Main DM, Gabbe SG. Risk scoring for pre-term labor: where do we go from here? Am J Obstet Gynecol 1987; 157:789–93.
41. Alexander S, Keirse MJNC. Formal risk scoring during pregnancy. In: Chalmers I, Enkin M, Keirse MJNC, eds. Effective care in pregnancy and childbirth, vol. 1. Oxford: Oxford University Press, 1989; 345–65.
42. Papiernik-Berkhauer E. Discussion. In: Anderson ABM, Beard R, Brudenell JM, Dunn P, eds. Pre-term labour. London: Royal College of Obstetricians and Gynaecologists, 1977; 29–39.
43. Amy JJ. In defence of the routine vaginal examination during pregnancy. In: Bréart G, Buekens P, eds. Evaluation of perinatal care – methodology and research proposals. Paris: Copédith, 1987; 87–90.
44. O'Donovan P, Gupta JK, Savage J, Lilford RJ. Should vaginal examination be recommended to all women in the antenatal booking clinic for reasons other than cervical smear? In: Bréart G, Buekens P, eds. Evaluation of perinatal care – methodology and research proposals. Paris: Copédith, 1987; 91–111.
45. Lenihan JP. Relationship of antepartum pelvic examination to premature rupture of the membranes. Obstet Gynecol 1984; 63:33–7.
46. Holbrook RH, Falcon J, Herron M, Lirette M, Laros RK, Creasy RK. Evaluation of the weekly cervical examination in a preterm birth prevention program. Am J Perinatol 1987; 4:240–4.
47. Heringa MP, Huisjes HJ. Routine vaginal examination (RVE): significance in prenatal care. In: Bréart G, Buekens P, eds. Evaluation of perinatal care – methodology and research proposals. Paris: Copédith, 1987; 113–21.
48. Newman RB, Godsey RL, Ellings JM, Campbell BA, Eller DP, Miller MC III. Quantification of cervical change: relationship to preterm delivery in the multifetal gestation. Am J Obstet Gynecol 1991; 165:264–9.
49. Rhoads GG, McNellis DC, Kessel SS. Home monitoring of uterine contractility. Am J Obstet Gynecol 1991; 165:2–6.
50. Lockwood CJ, Senyei AE, Dische MR et al. Fetal fribronectin in cervical and vaginal secretions as a predictor of preterm delivery. N Engl J Med 1991; 325:669–74.
51. Bréart G. Evaluation de l'efficacité de la surveillance prénatale et d'autres actions. In: Papiernik E, Bréart G, Spira N, eds. Prévention de la naissance prématurée. Paris: INSERM, 1986; 101–15.
52. Emmanuel I. Need for future epidemiologic research: studies for prevention and intervention. In: Reed DM, Stanley FJ, eds. The epidemiology of prematurity. Baltimore: Urban and Schwarzenberg, 1977; 339–47.
53. Rush D, Stein Z, Susser M. A randomized controlled trial of prenatal nutritional supplementation in New York City. Pediatrics 1980; 65:683–97.
54. Bouyer J, Papiernik E, Dreyfus J. Facteurs de risque de prématurité établis lors des consultations prénatales. In: Papiernik E, Bréart G, Spira N, eds. Prévention de la naissance prématurée. Paris: INSERM, 1986; 123–37.
55. Stubblefield PG. Causes and prevention of preterm birth: an overview. In: Fuchs F, Stubblefield PG, eds. Preterm birth. New York: Macmillan, 1984; 3–20.
56. Moutquin J-M. The limits of medical actions: betamimetics. In: Papiernik E, Bréart G, Spira N, eds. Prévention de la naissance prématurée. Paris: INSERM, 1986; 69–81.
57. Keirse MJNC, Grant A, King JF. Preterm labour. In: Chalmers I, Enkin M, Keirse MJNC, eds. Effective care in pregnancy and childbirth, vol. 1. Oxford: Oxford University Press, 1989; 694–745.
58. Keirse MJNC. Betamimetic drugs in the prophylaxis of preterm labour: extent and rationale of their use. Br J Obstet Gynaecol 1984; 91:431–7.
59. Skajaa K, Dørup I, Sandström B-M. Magnesium intake and status and pregnancy outcome in a Danish population. Br J Obstet Gynaecol 1991; 98:919–28.
60. Kovacs L, Molnar BG, Huhn E, Bodis L. Magnesiumsubstitution in der Schwangerschaft. Eine prospektive, randomisierte Doppelblindstudie. Geburtshilfe Frauenheilk 1988; 49:595–600.
61. Spätling L, Spätling G. Magnesium supplementation in pregnancy. A double-blind study. Br J Obstet Gynaecol 1988; 95:120–5.
62. Sibai BM, Villar MA, Bray E. Magnesium supplementation during pregnancy: a double-blind randomized controlled clinical trial. Am J Obstet Gynecol 1989; 161:115–19.

63. De Sutter P, Amy JJ. Macrolides in gynaecological practice. In: Bryskier A, Butzler JP, Neu HC, Tulkens PM, eds. Macrolides – chemistry, pharmacology and clinical uses. Paris: Arnette Blackwell, in press.
64. Charles D, Hurry DJ. Cervical incompetence. In: Fuchs F, Stubblefield PG, eds. Preterm birth. New York: Macmillan, 1984; 98–111.
65. Grant A. Cervical cerclage to prolong pregnancy. In: Chalmers I, Enkin M, Keirse MJNC, eds. Effective care in pregnancy and childbirth, vol 1. Oxford: Oxford University Press, 1989; 633–46.
66. Dor J, Shalev J, Mashiach G, Blankstein J, Serr DM. Elective cervical suture of twin pregnancies diagnosed ultrasonically in the first trimester following induced ovulation. Gynecol Obstet Invest 1982; 13:55–60.
67. Rush RW, Isaacs S, McPherson K, Jones L, Chalmers I, Grant A. A randomized controlled trial of cervical cerclage in women at high risk of preterm delivery. Br J Obstet Gynaecol 1984; 91:724–30.
68. Lazar P, Gueguren S, Dreyfus J, Renand R, Pontonnier G, Papiernik E. Multicentred controlled trial of cervical cerclage in women at moderate risk of preterm delivery. Br J Obstet Gynaecol 1984; 91:731–5.
69. MRC/RCOG Working party on cervical cerclage. Interim report of the Medical Research Council/Royal College of Obstetricians and Gynaecologists multicentre randomized trial of cervical cerclage. Br J Obstet Gynaecol 1988; 95:437–45.
70. Papiernik E. The very tiny baby, multiple births, and other questions about preterm deliveries. Curr Opinion Obstet Gynecol 1991; 3:4–7.
71. Crowther C, Chalmers I. Bed rest and hospitalization during pregnancy. In: Chalmers I, Enkin M, Keirse MJNC, eds. Effective care in pregnancy and childbirth, vol. 1. Oxford: Oxford University Press, 1989; 624–32.

Chapter 17

Inhibitors of Prostaglandin Synthesis for Treatment of Preterm Labour

M. J. N. C. Keirse

Agents which inhibit prostaglandin synthesis have been used clinically for the whole of this century [1]. Yet, before 1971 it was not realised that they exerted some of their known effects through inhibition of prostaglandin synthesis [2]. When this was discovered it had already been established, although not much earlier, that prostaglandins had contractile effects on the pregnant uterus powerful enough to use them for induction of labour and termination of pregnancy [3,4]. Considering the inventiveness of obstetricians in searching for new agents to control preterm labour (Table 17.1), one would have expected that inhibitors of prostaglandin synthesis – since they were freely available – would have been applied immediately to the problem of preterm labour. This did not happen, however [5,6]. The first English language report on the use of a prostaglandin synthesis inhibitor for treatment in preterm labour appeared only in 1974 [7]. This was after a retrospective study had shown prolongation of pregnancy in chronic aspirin users [8] and after it was demonstrated that inhibitors of prostaglandin synthesis prolonged the induction–abortion interval in women undergoing second trimester abortion by hypertonic saline [9]. In 1980, inhibitors of prostaglandin synthesis were not even mentioned in a questionnaire survey by Lewis et al. [5] which reported on tocolytic agents normally used by obstetricians in the UK for treatment of preterm labour. A similar survey in the Benelux countries, reported in 1984, showed that fewer than 2% of obstetricians would use an inhibitor of prostaglandin synthesis to arrest preterm labour [6].

On the other hand, the first reports on the use of inhibitors of prostaglandin synthesis in preterm labour contained little to differentiate them from a whole range of reports on other promising treatments whose success rates had been equally outstanding in uncontrolled observations (Table 17.1). From these reports it was impossible to ascertain whether the degree of success would have been smaller, equal, or even larger if no drug treatment had been applied

Table 17.1. Summary of approaches introduced since 1950 for the inhibition of preterm labour and their purported success rates in the first publication in the English language that documented their use

Agent	Year	Authors	No. of women	Criterion of success	Percentage success
Relaxin	1955	Abramson and Reid [11]	5	Delivery after 36 weeks	100
Isoxsuprine	1961	Bishop and Woutersz [12]	120	Contractions delayed 24h	82
Ethanol	1967	Fuchs et al. [13]	52	Delivery delayed 72 h	67
Orciprenaline	1970	Baillie et al. [14]	30	Delivery after 36 weeks	70
Mesuprine	1971	Barden [15]	17	Delivery delayed 24 h	53
Ritodrine	1971	Wesselius-De Casparis et al. [16]	43	Not delivered during treatment	80
Fenoterol	1972	Edelstein and Baillie [17]	28	Delivery delayed 1 week	71
Salbutamol	1973	Liggins and Vaughan [18]	88	Delivery delayed 24 h	85
Indomethacin[a]	1974	Zuckerman et al. [7]	50	Arrest of contractions	80
Sodium salicylate[a]	1974	Györy et al. [19]	50	Diminished uterine activity	100
Buphenine	1975	Castrén et al. [20]	43	Birthweight >2500 g	86
Terbutaline	1976	Ingemarsson [21]	15	Not delivered during treatment	80
Nifedipine	1977	Andersson [22]	10	Delivery delayed 3 days or more	100
Magnesium sulphate	1977	Steer and Petrie [23]	31	Contractions stopped 24 h	77
Flufenamic acid[a]	1978	Schwartz et al. [24]	18	Delivery delayed 24 h	83
Naproxen[a]	1979	Wiqvist [25]	10	Contractions reduced	100
Diazoxide	1984	Adamsons and Wallach [26]	118	Complete cessation of contractions	94
Utrogestan	1986	Erny et al. [27]	57	Decrease in contraction frequency	76
Oxytocin analogue	1987	Akerlund et al. [28]	13	Inhibition of contractions	100

Adapted from Keirse et al. [10].
[a] Inhibitor of prostaglandin synthesis.

[7,19,24,25]. Moreover, the definitions of success were not particularly robust in that arrest of contractions does not necessarily mean delay of delivery or prolongation of pregnancy, whereas the latter in turn does not necessarily imply that the outcome for the infant will be improved.

In the years that followed the first publications (Table 17.1) [7,19,24,25] many clinical studies (mostly uncontrolled) have testified to the effectiveness of inhibitors of prostaglandin synthesis in the arrest of preterm labour. Other, equally uncontrolled, reports testified to their "perinatal safety" disregarding the all-important question of whether babies would have been better off or worse off if no such treatment had been instituted during fetal life [29]. The possibility that babies could be worse off as a result of such treatment was soon suggested [30]. Although again based on uncontrolled observations and extrapolation of data from animal experimentation, this aspect soon dominated the literature on the use of prostaglandin synthesis inhibitors in preterm labour [31]. Consequently, obstetricians have probably been more reluctant to use inhibitors of prostaglandin synthesis than they were to use other agents, such as calcium antagonists and magnesium sulphate, although these have not been shown to be superior to either no treatment or alternative treatments, such as betamimetics [10].

Prostaglandin Synthesis Inhibitors: Agents and Mode of Action

Several drugs with widely different chemical structures and pharmacokinetic properties have the capacity to inhibit prostaglandin synthesis in vitro and in vivo. Those that have been used to treat preterm labour include naproxen [25], flufenamic acid [24], sodium salicylate [19] and acetylsalicylic acid (aspirin) [32,33] but the most widely used has been indomethacin [6,10]. These agents are sometimes referred to as prostaglandin synthetase inhibitors, but there is no such enzyme as prostaglandin synthetase. They are therefore, more appropriately described as inhibitors of prostaglandin synthesis. All of them act by inhibiting the enzyme prostaglandin H synthase, also known as cyclo-oxygenase, which converts a fatty acid precursor (most typically arachidonic acid) into prostaglandin endoperoxides (Fig. 17.1).

Since all the drugs act by inhibiting prostaglandin H synthase, they also suppress the production of prostacyclin and thromboxane in addition to that of the prostaglandins (Fig. 17.1). Little is known about the consequences of this in preterm labour, despite the fact that a great deal of data has now been gathered on prostacyclin and thromboxane production in pregnancy and in (preterm) labour [34–36].

Inhibition of prostaglandin H synthase does not always occur in the same way. Some inhibitors of prostaglandin synthesis, such as indomethacin, act by competing with arachidonic acid for the active site of the enzyme. The conse-

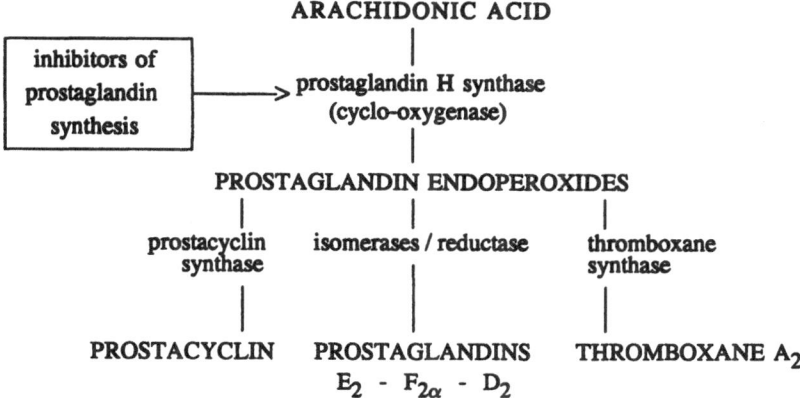

Fig. 17.1. Mode of action of inhibitors of prostaglandin synthesis.

quence of this is that inhibition of prostaglandin synthesis depends on the amount of drug available at the site of enzyme action; if it is high the enzyme will be inhibited; if drug concentrations decrease, the enzyme will resume activity. Other agents interfere with the enzyme in a more drastic manner. The most typical example thereof is acetylsalicylic acid (aspirin), which acetylates a site on the enzyme and thereby renders it permanently incapable of further production of prostaglandin endoperoxides. Inhibition of prostaglandin synthesis thereby becomes independent of drug levels and synthesis will only resume when new quantities of enzyme (a glycoprotein) have been made available through protein synthesis.

From a clinical point of view, it is important to realise that inhibitors of prostaglandin synthesis form a separate family among the tocolytic agents. Betamimetic drugs, for example, all act roughly in a similar manner with regard to both their desired and their undesired effects [10,37] but this is not so for inhibitors of prostaglandin synthesis. These compounds differ so much from each other, both chemically and pharmacologically, that it is not justified to assume that effects which have been observed with one particular compound can be extrapolated to another compound simply because both are known to suppress prostaglandin synthesis. For example, aspirin will readily acetylate any prosta-glandin H synthase that it encounters, but it is a weak acid that hydrolyses spontaneously soon after absorption. This means that it is then present in ionised form as sodium salicylate, which is only a weak inhibitor of prostaglandin H synthase [38]. These properties and the fact that platelets cannot synthesise new prostaglandin H synthase explain why a very low dose of aspirin may have marked effects on platelets (exposed to aspirin in the capillaries of the gut during absorption) whereas doses of as much as 6 g orally [32] and up to 10 g intravenously [33] have been required to obtain some tocolytic effect. There is, thus, ample reason not to use aspirin, when choosing an inhibitor of prostaglan-din synthesis for treatment of preterm labour.

All prostaglandin synthesis inhibitors are effective inhibitors of myometrial contractility, both in and outside pregnancy. From the comparative studies that have been conducted thus far, there is no doubt that they are more effective in this respect than any other class of agents currently known. No case has yet been reported in which another type of agent could suppress uterine contractility after inhibition of prostaglandin synthesis had failed. The reverse has repeatedly been observed [25,29,38]. It has also been shown that a single dose of the prostaglandin synthesis inhibitor, indomethacin, can either stop or prolong labour in a large proportion of women labouring at term [39].

Desired Effects in Preterm Labour: Evidence from Controlled Evaluations

Only one inhibitor of prostaglandin synthesis, indomethacin, has been subjected to controlled evaluations for the treatment of active preterm labour. For all other agents only anecdotal and observational data are available, which justify concern about whether alleged effects of treatment reported in such studies would not have been the same, or even better, if no treatment had been instituted.

Three types of controlled studies on the use of indomethacin in preterm labour have been conducted. The first relates to comparisons in which the effects of indomethacin were compared with no treatment or placebo treatment. The second involves studies in which indomethacin was either added or not added to other treatments believed to be effective in inhibiting preterm labour. The third concerns studies in which the use of indomethacin was compared with that of other active agents in preterm labour. The regimens of indomethacin administration in all these studies are shown in Table 17.2, as well as the number of women who participated in these studies and the nature of the control treatments used.

Three trials have been reported in which indomethacin was evaluated against placebo for the inhibition of preterm labour. Only an abstract is available for one

Table 17.2. Characteristics of controlled trials of indomethacin for treatment of preterm labour

Authors	No. reported/randomised		Treatment characteristics	
	Indomethacin	Control	Indomethacin	Control
Niebyl et al. [41]	15/17	15/15	50 mg orally → 6 × 25 mg (for 24 h)	Placebo, but 30% received betamimetics or ethanol
Zuckerman et al. [42]	18/18	18/18	100 mg suppository → 4 × 25 mg orally (for 24 h)	Placebo, but 44% received ritodrine
Spearing [44]	20/20	22/22	100 mg suppository × 2 first 24 h → 25 mg every 6 h for 48 h after cessation of contractions + ethanol	Ethanol intravenously
Katz et al. [45]	60/60	60/60	100 mg suppository → 4 × 25 mg orally at 6-hourly intervals + Ritodrine	Intravenous ritodrine followed by oral ritodrine for maintenance
Gamissans et al. [46–48]	148/148	149/149	50 mg suppositories every 8 h for 2 weeks + ritodrine until 35 weeks	Placebo + ritodrine continuously until at least 35 weeks
Morales et al. [49]	52/52	54/54	100 mg suppository → 25 mg orally every 4 h for 48 h	Ritodrine infusion up to 350 lg/min
Besinger et al. [50]	22/23	18/20	50 mg orally → 25–50 mg 4-hourly until contractions ceased → 25 mg every 4–6 h until 35 weeks of gestation	Ritodrine infusion followed by oral terbutaline for maintenance treatment until 35 weeks of gestation
Lumme et al. [51]	30/30	30/30	100 mg suppository on day 1, 3 × 50 mg orally on day 2+3	Nylidrine infusion up to 150 lg/min for 3 days
Morales and Madhav [54]	49/49	52/52	Indomethacin dose not reported	Magnesium sulphate dose not reported

of these trials and it contains no data on clinically important outcome measures [40]. The other two trials [41.42] were both small with fewer than 40 women each. Although they were both stated to have been conducted in a double-blind placebo-controlled manner, neither of them was entirely placebo-controlled since a number of women in whom treatment was thought to have failed received other tocolytic drugs (Table 17.2). In the study by Niebyl et al. [41] other tocolytic drugs were given to 30% of women in the placebo group and in the study by Zuckerman et al. [42] to 44% (Table 17.2).

Niebyl et al. [41] did not report whether and to what extent delivery was postponed; information on the failure rate only relates to whether or not cervical dilatation increased. Zuckerman et al. [42] found statistically significant differences in the delay of delivery for 48 h or more, in prolongation of pregnancy for more than 1 week, and in the incidences of preterm birth and low birthweight. All of these differences were in favour of indomethacin treatment. However, trials were too small to show differences in perinatal mortality and morbidity. It was reported by Niebyl et al. [41] that fewer infants in the treatment group had conditions that either caused death or were life threatening (3 of 16; 0.2 per infant) than in the "placebo" group (9 of 15; 0.6 per infant). Another publication on the same trial, however, states that there were two infants who died and three others who had major life-threatening problems in each of the two treatment groups [43]. It is impossible to know which of the two reports is correct.

In a second category of controlled studies, indomethacin was either given or not given to women treated with other labour-inhibiting drugs, such as ethanol or a betamimetic agent.

Spearing [44] assigned 42 women in sequence to a combined treatment with indomethacin and ethanol or to ethanol alone. Delivery was postoned for more than 48 hours in 16 of 20 women (80%) treated with indomethacin and in 12 of 22 women (55%) who received only ethanol.

In three trials indomethacin was either added or not added to treatment with a betamimetic agent. In all three trials ritodrine was used as the betamimetic agent. One of these trials alternately assigned 120 women in labour before 35 weeks' of gestation to treatment with intravenous ritodrine or to intravenous ritodrine in combination with indomethacin [45]. All women also received oral ritodrine for maintenance treatment up to 35 weeks' gestation. The other two trials, one in women with intact membranes and one in women with ruptured membranes, were conducted by Gamissans et al. [46–48]. Women participated in these trials up to 34 weeks' gestation, if they had ruptured membranes, and up to 36 weeks if the membranes were intact. They all received ritodrine intravenously followed by intramuscular or oral maintenance treatment up to 35 (ruptured membranes) or 38 (intact membranes) weeks of pregnancy. In addition, either placebo or 50 mg indomethacin suppositories were added to the treatment and administered every 8 h for 2 weeks. Unfortunately, a number of internal inconsistencies in the three reports of these trials make one wary of drawing firm conclusions from these data. For example, in the first report on women with ruptured membranes only 12 of 55 women reached a gestational age of 37 weeks or more at delivery [47]. At the time of the later report, a further 19 women had been entered, but an additional 42 women (54 of 74) had now reached 37 weeks or more at delivery [48]. There are other aspects that are difficult to comprehend. For instance, the incidence of delivery within 10 days in women with intact membranes was 37% in the 1982 report of this trial [47]; but this had dropped to 13% in the 1984 report of the same trial [48].

More recently, a third category of controlled studies has been reported in which the use of indomethacin was compared with that of other active agents in preterm labour (Table 17.2). These studies have involved control groups treated intravenously with the betamimetic agents, ritodrine [49,50] and nylidrine [51–53], or with magnesium sulphate [54]. Using sealed envelopes Morales et al. [49] randomly allocated 52 women in labour before 32 weeks' gestation to receive indomethacin for 48 h and 54 to receive intravenous ritodrine. A similar approach was followed by Besinger et al. [50] for women in preterm labour between 23 and 34 weeks, but these authors continued indomethacin treatment after the cessation of contractions giving 25 mg indomethacin every 4–6 h up to 35 weeks' gestation. Lumme et al. [51] reported a placebo-controlled trial of indomethacin treatment for 3 days versus treatment with the betamimetic agent nylidrine in women in labour between 25 and 34 weeks. Women randomised to nylidrine treatment received placebo suppositories and tablets, whereas those randomised to indomethacin received a placebo infusion. The same group has reported Doppler fetal echocardiography changes [52] and changes in maternal plasma hormone levels [53] in women randomised to indomethacin and nylidrine treatment, but the women on whom data are presented in these reports have also been included in the report of the clinical data presented by Lumme et al. [51]. A randomized trial of indomethacin versus magnesium sulphate in 101 women with intact membranes and preterm labour before 32 weeks' gestation was conducted by Morales and Madhav [54] but only limited information on this trial has been reported thus far.

When all these trial reports [41–54] are analysed, there would seem to be little doubt that indomethacin is more effective than any other tocolytic agent used in these trials, whether it be placebo, ethanol, magnesium sulphate, or a betamimetic drug, in terms of inhibiting uterine contractions preterm. This conclusion cannot be reached from each individual trial since many of them have been either too small or not reported completely enough to detect important differences in outcomes that are less likely to be biased than subjective measures, such as changes in frequency or intensity of contractions. None of the trial reports is inconsistent with this conclusion, however.

Despite reservations about the heterogeneous nature of these trials, about selective reporting of outcomes that are available for some trials but not for others, and about potential bias in some of the trials, the data that could be extracted reliably from the various reports have been amalgamated in Tables 17.3–17.6.

Thus, all five trials [42,44,49,50,54] that provide data on the incidence of delivery within 48 h of starting treatment reported that this occurred less frequently in women treated with indomethacin than in women receiving the alternative treatment irrespective of the nature of the alternative treatment (Table 17.3). The same applied for the four trials [42,48–50] providing data on the incidence of delivery within 7 or 10 days after starting treatment and to the three trials [42,48,51] which provide data on the incidence of preterm delivery (Table 17.4). In each of the reports indomethacin was associated with the better outcome.

Data on fetal and neonatal death were only available in seven of the nine trials (Table 17.5). It is noteworthy that in all except one in which no deaths occurred,

Table 17.3. Incidence of delivery within 48 h after starting treatment in controlled trials of indomethacin treatment for inhibition of preterm labour

Authors	No. with outcome/total		Odds ratio and (95% confidence interval)
	Indomethacin	Control	
Zuckerman et al. [42]	1/18	14/18	0.06 (0.02–0.21)
Spearing [44]	4/20	10/22	0.33 (0.09–1.16)
Morales et al. [49]	3/52	9/54	0.34 (0.10–1.13)
Besinger et al. [50]	2/22	3/18	0.51 (0.08–3.27)
Morales and Madhav [54]	5/49	7/52	0.73 (0.22–2.44)
Typical odds ratio and (95% confidence interval)			0.29 (0.16–0.53)

Table 17.4. Incidence of preterm delivery in controlled trials of indomethacin treatment for inhibition of preterm labour

Authors	No. with outcome/total		Odds ratio and (95% confidence interval)
	Indomethacin	Control	
Zuckerman et al. [42]	3/18	14/18	0.09 (0.03–0.34)
Gamissans et al. [48]	69/148	94/149	0.52 (0.33–0.81)
Lumme et al. [51]	9/30	17/30	0.34 (0.12–0.95)
Typical odds ratio and (95% confidence interval)			0.41 (0.28–0.61)

Table 17.5. Fetal and neonatal deaths in controlled trials of indomethacin treatment for inhibition of preterm labour

Authors	No. of deaths/infants		Odds ratio and (95% confidence interval)
	Indomethacin	Control	
Niebyl et al. [41]	2/16	2/15	0.93 (0.12–7.35)
Zuckerman et al. [42]	1/18	2/18	0.49 (0.05–5.07)
Spearing [44]	4/20	5/23	0.90 (0.21–3.87)
Katz et al. [45]	0/60	0/60	1.00
Gamissans et al. [48]	11/148	20/149	0.53 (0.25–1.11)
Morales et al. [49]	2/47	3/50	0.70 (0.12–4.21)
Besinger et al. [50]	1/25	1/20	0.79 (0.05–13.34)
Lumme et al. [51]	no data available		
Morales and Madhav [54]	no data available		
Typical odds ratio and (95% confidence interval)			0.62 (0.35–1.09)

Table 17.6. Cumulative incidence of measures of poor outcome across trials comparing indomethacin with other treatments (including placebo) for inhibition of preterm labour

Outcome	No. of trials (ref.)	Numbers (%)		Odds ratio and (95% confidence interval)
		Indomethacin	Control	
Delivered <48 h	5 [42,44,49,50,54]	15/161 (9.3)	43/164 (26.2)	0.29 (0.16–0.53)
Delivered <7–10 days	4 [42,48–50]	56/240 (23.3)	92/239 (38.5)	0.49 (0.33–0.72)
Delivered <37 weeks	3 [42,48,51]	81/196 (41.3)	125/197 (63.5)	0.41 (0.28–0.61)
Fetal and neonatal death	7 [41,42,44,45,48–50]	21/334 (6.3)	33/335 (9.9)	0.62 (0.35–1.09)
Respiratory distress syndrome	4 [41,42,45,48]	8/242 (3.3)	12/242 (5.0)	0.62 (0.25–1.58)

the mortality rate was lower in infants whose mothers had received indomethacin than in infants of mothers who had received the control treatment (Table 17.5). However, this effect is still compatible with chance because the 95% confidence interval of the typical odds ratio across trials still includes unity (Table 17.5). Very few reports provide categorical data on measures of infant morbidity and information on the occurrence of respiratory distress syndrome, the most frequent serious morbidity condition of preterm infants, is only available for four trials. In one of them [45] not a single case of respiratory distress syndrome occurred. The overall incidence of respiratory distress syndrome in the trials for which this information is available was even lower than the overall incidence of mortality in the trials that provided information on mortality (Table 17.6). This testifies to the fact that caution is necessary in the interpretation of the amalgamated data from all of these trials.

Undesired Effects: Evidence from Controlled and Uncontrolled Evaluations

Inhibitors of prostaglandin synthesis are not innocuous. Four points need to be considered. First, there are numerous potential side effects because of the ubiquitous nature of the prostaglandins. Second, in the doses that are used for inhibition of preterm labour these agents also suppress prostacyclin and thromboxane synthesis. Third, all inhibitors of prostaglandin synthesis that are currently in use cross the placental barrier from mother to fetus [55–57]. Fourth, the drugs are both chemically and pharmacologically so different from each other that they should not be considered as interchangeable. They may roughly fulfil the same function, but, as mentioned earlier, this does not mean that they will all have the same effects and ill-effects.

The most serious potential side effects are peptic ulceration, gastrointestinal and other bleeding, thrombocytopenia and allergic reactions. Gastrointestinal irritation is common with the use of prostaglandin synthesis inhibitors, and it can occur irrespective of the route of administration. With indomethacin it is less frequent with rectal than with oral administration and, as the bioavailability of the drug is identical with both routes of administration [58,59], the rectal route offers some advantage. Nausea, vomiting, dyspepsia, diarrhoea and allergic rashes have all been observed in women treated, even briefly, with prostaglandin synthesis inhibitors in preterm labour. Headache and dizziness are also reported and they may occur at the very start of treatment. Gamissans et al. [46–48] reported systematically on the incidence of headache; maternal tachycardia above 120 beats per minute, vomiting, epigastric pain and rectal intolerance in their trials comparing indomethacin with placebo in association with ritodrine treatment. Only two of these side effects were observed more frequently in the indomethacin-treated group. Epigastric pain was observed in six (4%) and rectal intolerance in seven (5%) of 148 indomethacin-treated women; these symptoms occurred in only two of 149 women in the control group [48].

On the other hand, the four trials which compared indomethacin with either a betamimetic agent or magnesium sulphate all indicated a much lower rate of side effects with indomethacin than with the alternative treatment, irrespective of whether the latter consisted of ritodrine, nylidrine, or magnesium sulphate. For three of these trials [49,51,54] the total number of women experiencing side effects is reported; among them side effects occurred in only 13.7% of indomethacin-treated women as compared with 71.2% in women receiving the alternative treatment (Table 17.7). Besinger et al. [50] did not report the overall number of women who experienced side effects, but all individual side effects except gastrointestinal symptoms occurred more frequently in women treated with ritodrine than with indomethacin. They observed gastrointestinal side effects in 54% of 22 indomethacin-treated women and in 44% of 18 ritodrine-treated women [50].

Table 17.7. Incidence of maternal side effects in controlled comparisons of indomethacin versus betamimetics (ritodrine [49] and nylidrine [51]) or magnesium sulphate [54] for inhibition of preterm labour

Authors	Side effects/total		Odds ratio and (95% confidence interval)
	Indomethacin	Control	
Morales et al. [49]	6/52	39/50	0.07 (0.03–0.15)
Lumme et al. [51]	6/30	25/30	0.08 (0.03–0.23)
Morales and Madhav [54]	6/49	30/52	0.14 (0.06–0.32)
Typical odds ratio and (95% confidence interval)			0.09 (0.06–0.15)

It is generally believed that signs of infection may be masked by administration of prostaglandin synthesis inhibitors. It is not known, however, whether this would hamper or postpone the diagnosis of incipient intrauterine infection if it occurs.

Indomethacin crosses from the mother to the fetus [55] and may influence several fetal functions. A great deal of information has been gathered on the fetal effects of prostaglandin synthesis inhibition in experimental animals. The results are not always easy to interpret, however, because of the variety of species studied, differences in the type of drug used and in the dose, route and duration of its use. Apart from a prolonged bleeding time, which is a constant feature in infants born with detectable levels of such drugs, data on effects in human fetuses and neonates are mostly based on anecdotal reports. The most consistent observations relate to the cardiopulmonary circulation and to renal, cerebral and haemostatic functions.

The Fetal Ductus Arteriosus

The greatest worries about the use of such drugs for the inhibition of preterm labour have resulted from their influence on the ductus arteriosus. Closure of the ductus after birth consists of an initial functional closure by muscular contractions followed by definitive anatomical closure, which is a much slower process. In most term neonates the ductus arteriosus is closed functionally by 2 days after birth, but anatomical closure is rarely accomplished within the first week of life [60]. The effects of products of endoperoxide metabolism in the prenatal and postnatal regulation of the ductus arteriosus have been studied extensively. In vitro and in vivo experimental manipulation of the cyclo-oxygenase pathway has significant effects on ductus vasoactivity. Thus, PGE_2, PGI_2, and PGE_1 each cause vasodilatation of the ductus arteriosus. This provides the rationale for the use of PGE_1 to maintain ductus patency in several forms of congenital heart disease with severe pulmonary or systemic outflow obstruction in neonatal medicine. On the other hand, prostaglandin synthesis inhibitors cause constriction of the ductus arteriosus in the neonate, an effect that has been demonstrated conclusively in placebo controlled trials of neonatal indomethacin administration [61]. Autopsy and cardiac catheterisation data from infants who presented with congestive heart failure at or after birth, have suggested that severe constriction of the ductus may also occur before birth in association with inhibition of prostaglandin synthesis [31,62,63].

Constriction of the ductus during fetal life probably has little effect on fetal oxygenation in the short term, as effective shunting can be maintained through the foramen ovale. In experimental animals even complete surgical ligation is compatible with intrauterine survival for a considerable length of time [64]. Levin et al. [31,65,66] showed experimentally that constriction of the ductus arteriosus in utero causes a marked increase in pulmonary arterial pressure, which results in increased smooth muscle development in the wall of pulmonary arterial resistance vessels. These morphological changes, which were also observed in human fetuses [30], are similar to those seen in the clinical syndrome of persistent pulmonary hypertension of the newborn. Further experimental evidence has indicated that the increase in both pulmonary and ductal vascular resistance could, by increasing right ventricular and diastolic pressure, produce subendothelial ischaemia, particularly in the papillary muscles of the tricuspid valve [31]. Prolonged prenatal constriction of the ductus arteriosus could thus lead to both persistent pulmonary hypertension and tricuspid insufficiency in the newborn.

Eronen et al. [52] studied systolic and diastolic velocities in the fetal ductus arteriosus in 27 women randomised to either nylidrine or indomethacin treatment in preterm labour. Indomethacin treatment was found to constrict the ductus arteriosus in 9 of 14 fetuses exposed to indomethacin and tricuspid valve regurgitation was observed in three of them. Fetal echocardiograms returned to normal patterns within 3 days after cessation of treatment, however. These authors also observed that ductal constriction was more likely to occur with increasing gestational age [52]. Although others found no relationship between ductal constriction and gestational age [67], this finding would be consistent with data indicating that the ductus of the immature infant is more sensitive to the dilating effects of prostaglandins than the ductus of the near-term infant [61,68]. This would suggest that the risk of ductal closure is likely to be greater at gestational ages at which benefit from delay of delivery is least likely.

Only five cases of pulmonary hypertension were encountered in the trials reviewed. Three of these occurred among 25 infants born to mothers who had received indomethacin [50]. It should be noted, however, that indomethacin treatment was maintained for exceptionally long times in this trial (Table 17.2) and this is likely to have increased the risk. A further two cases of pulmonary hypertension, one in the placebo group and one in the indomethacin treated group, occurred in Gamissans' trial in women with ruptured membranes [47,48]. Earlier compilations of cases from both controlled and uncontrolled clinical studies in which careful paediatric examination of the newborn had been carried out after the use of inhibitors of prostaglandin synthesis in preterm labour have estimated the risk of pulmonary hypertension to be in the range of 1.5–2.3% [10,25,48]. Whether or not this is more frequent than it would have been without inhibition of prostaglandin synthesis is impossible to determine from such data, which include a whole range of gestations as well as widely varying doses and durations of treatment. The large majority of these infants eventually recover, but they may require intensive treatment to overcome their initial problems.

Other Effects

Indomethacin treatment may alter both fetal and neonatal renal function. Renal dysfunction and reduced urinary output have repeatedly been noted in infants treated with indomethacin to close a patent ductus arteriosus [69–71]. The effect is apparently dose related and transient. Renal function usually returns toward pretreatment values within 24 h after stopping the treatment [71]. Several reports have indicated impaired renal function in fetuses and in neonates at birth after administration of prostaglandin synthesis inhibitors to the mother [72–74]. Long-term maternal treatment may influence fetal urine output enough to alter amniotic fluid volume [52]. The effect appears to be dose dependent and has been employed to reduce excessive amniotic fluid volumes. There is no evidence from either maternal or neonatal indomethacin treatment, however, that the use of indomethacin in preterm labour would lead to permanent impairment of renal function in the infant [71].

There is also some concern about fetal cerebrovascular effects of indomethacin treatment [75]. Indomethacin interferes with platelet function and could thus potentially increase the risk of periventricular haemorrhage, already a major worry in very preterm infants. Another concern is that decreases in cerebral blood flow reported after indomethacin administration could result in ischaemic brain injury [76]. Thus far, it would appear that, with judicious use of indomethacin, these risks are more theoretical than real. There is no information on ischaemic brain injury in the controlled trials of indomethacin usage in preterm labour, and only limited information on the incidence of intraventricular haemorrhage. Even in the trial by Besinger et al. [50] with prolonged indomethacin usage up to 35 weeks' gestation there were only three cases of intraventricular haemorrhage among 25 infants (12%) born after indomethacin exposure as opposed to two cases among 20 infants (10%) whose mothers had received ritodrine. The concern about cerebral damage secondary to either changes in cerebral blood flow or increased risks of periventricular haemorrhage is not supported by the data available from neonatal indomethacin treatments. Horbar [77] recently analysed the results of nine trials in which indomethacin had been administered within the first 24 h after birth and in which cranial ultrasonography was used to assess periventricular haemorrhage. Indomethacin given within 24 h after birth was associated with a statistically significantly decreased risk both of periventricular haemorrhage overall and of severe periventricular haemorrhage. These data are not necessarily relevant to the fetal situation, since indomethacin may exert protective effects in the newborn infant through its influence on the ductus arteriosus. However, in the absence of controlled data to suggest increased cerebral risks in the fetus, anecdotal reports should be seen in the light of the totality of the evidence that is available. Thus far, it would seem that judicious indomethacin treatment in preterm labour at early gestational ages is more likely to decrease than to increase perinatal mortality from whatever causes (Table 17.5).

Inhibitors of the cyclo-oxygenase enzyme all inhibit platelet aggregation and prolong bleeding time. They do so in the mother, in the fetus and in the neonate [39,78]. Since nenoates, and particularly preterm neonates, eliminate these drugs far less efficiently than their mothers [38], these effects will be of longer duration in the baby than in the mother. There are major differences in this respect between different inhibitors of prostaglandin synthesis. Aspirin is particularly troublesome in this respect. As mentioned earlier it acetylates the cyclo-oxygenase enzyme and incapacitates it permanently. Unlike most cells in the body, blood platelets cannot manufacture new enzyme and this implies that not only the enzyme, but that also the platelets themselves are rendered permanently non-functional. For normal function to resume they must be replaced by new platelets.

Conclusions

The overall quality of the controlled research that has been reported on the use of inhibitors of prostaglandin synthesis for the treatment of active preterm labour is not particularly high and all of this research relates to only one agent: indomethacin. This implies that, except for rare circumstances, only indomethacin should be considered for treatment of preterm labour in clinical practice. This does not mean that other inhibitors of prostaglandin synthesis have no effects. It merely implies that there is currently no justification for using other inhibitors of prostaglandin synthesis in preterm labour outside the context of well-controlled clinical research.

The lasting effect of aspirin on platelet function, the fact that salicylates are less efficient prostaglandin synthesis inhibitors than other such inhibitors, and the ensuing need for very high doses, provide a strong case for not using any of the salycylates in the treatment of preterm labour.

Despite reservations about the quality of the evidence, it is clear that indomethacin can be a useful drug for prolonging pregnancy beyond the stage at which neonatal mortality and morbidity are likely to be unacceptably high. More, and better controlled data will be needed, however, before the usefulness of prostaglandin synthesis inhibition in preterm labour can be assessed more adequately.

Because there are wide variations in the half-life of indomethacin between individuals [38], indomethacin is better administered in smaller doses at 4-hourly intervals rather than in a larger dose which is given less frequently. Doses of 50–100 mg would seem to be the most appropriate for obtaining early arrest of contractions whereas doses as low as 12.5–25 mg may be sufficient to maintain uterine quiescence for as long as is necessary.

Despite the lack of clear evidence in the literature, two aspects deserve special mention. First, the responsiveness of the ductus arteriosus to indomethacin is likely to be lower at lower gestational ages. Data relating to the human fetus are not unanimous in this respect, but there is strong support for this concept from data in experimental animals and in human neonates. This would imply that the risk of ductus constriction and its potential sequelae are smallest when most gain can be expected from arresting preterm labour, and largest at gestational ages at which inhibition of labour is probably no longer justified. Second, although this too cannot be demonstrated with certainty from the controlled and uncontrolled studies reviewed, it is likely that both drug doses and duration of treatment have an influence on the frequency and severity of fetal side effects. The longer prostaglandin synthesis inhibition is continued, the lower the gain and the greater the risk is likely to be. On balance, however, judicious use of indomethacin in very preterm labour is likely to confer more benefit than harm to the mothers and babies treated.

References

1. Smith MJH, Smith PK. The salicylates. A critical bibliographic review. New York: Wiley, 1966.
2. Vane JR. Inhibition of prostaglandin synthesis as a mechanism of action for aspirin-like drugs. Nature 1971; 231:232–5.
3. Karim SMM, Trussell RR, Patel RC, Hillier K. Response of pregnant human uterus to prostaglandin $F_{2\alpha}$ – induction of labour. Br Med J 1968; 4:621–3.
4. Karim SMM, Filshie GM. Use of prostaglandin E_2 for therapeutic abortion. Br Med J 1970; 3:198–200.
5. Lewis PJ, de Swiet M, Boylan P, Bulpitt CJ. How obstetricians in the United Kingdom manage preterm labour. Br J Obstet Gynaecol 1980; 87:574–7.
6. Keirse MJNC. A survey of tocolytic drug treatment in preterm labour. Br J Obstet Gynaecol 1984; 91:424–30.
7. Zuckerman H, Reiss U, Rubinstein I. Inhibition of human premature labor by indomethacin. Obstet Gynecol 1974; 44:787–92.
8. Lewis RB, Schulman JD. Influence of acetylsalicylic acid, an inhibitor of prostaglandin synthesis, on the duration of human gestation and labour. Lancet 1973; 2:1159–61.
9. Waltman R, Tricomi V, Palav A. Aspirin and indomethacin: effect on installation/abortion time of mid-trimester hypertonic saline induced abortion. Prostaglandins 1973; 3:47–58.
10. Keirse MJNC, Grant A, King JF. Preterm labour. In: Chalmers I, Enkin M, Keirse MJNC, eds. Effective care in pregnancy and childbirth. Oxford: Oxford University Press, 1989; 694–745.
11. Abrahamson D, Reid DE. Use of relaxin in treatment of threatened premature labor. J Clin Endocrinol 1955; 15:206–9.

12. Bishop EH, Woutersz TB. Isoxsuprine, a myometrial relaxant – a preliminary report. Obstet Gynecol 1961; 17:442–6.
13. Fuchs F, Fuchs A-R, Poblete VG, Risk A. Effect of alcohol on threatened premature labor. Am J Obstet Gynecol 1967; 99:627–37.
14. Baillie P, Meehan FP, Tyack AJ. Treatment of premature labour with orciprenaline. Br Med J 1970; 4:154–5.
15. Barden TP. Inhibition of human premature labor by mesuprine hydrochloride. Obstet Gynecol 1971; 37:98–105.
16. Wesselius-De Casparis A, Thiery M, Yo Le Sian A et al. Results of double-blind, multicentre study with ritodrine in premature labour. Br Med J 1971; 3:144–7.
17. Edelstein H, Baillie P. The use of fenoterol (Berotec) as compared with orciprenaline (Alupent) in the treatment of premature labour. A comparative study. Med Proc 1972; 18:92–6.
18. Liggins GC, Vaughan GS. Intravenous infusion of salbutamol in the management of premature labor. J Obstet Gynaecol Br Commonw 1973; 80:29–33.
19. Györy G, Kiss C, Benyo T, Bagdany S, Szalay J, Kurcz M, Virag S. Inhibition of labour by prostaglandin antagonist in impending abortion and preterm and term labour. Lancet 1974; ii:293.
20. Castrén O, Gummerus M, Saarikoski S. Treatment of imminent premature labour. A comparison between the effects of nylidrin chloride and isoxuprine chloride as well as of ethanol. Acta Obstet Gynecol Scand 1975; 54:95–100.
21. Ingemarsson I. Effect of terbutaline on premature labor. A double-blind placebo-controlled study. Am J Obstet Gynecol 1976; 125:520–4.
22. Andersson KE. Inhibition of uterine activity by the calcium antagonist nifedipine. In: Anderson A, Beard R, Brudenell JM, Dunn PM, eds. Pre-term labour. Proceedings of the fifth study group of the Royal College of Obstetricians and Gynaecologists. London: Royal College of Obstetricians and Gynaecologists, 1977; 101–14.
23. Steer CM, Petrie RH. A comparison of magnesium sulfate and alcohol for the prevention of premature labor. Am J Obstet Gynecol 1977; 129:1–4.
24. Schwartz A, Brook I, Insler V, Kohen F, Zor U, Lindner HR. Effect of flufenamic acid on uterine contractions and plasma levels of 15-keto-13,14-dihydro-prostaglandin $F_{2\alpha}$ in preterm labor. Gynecol Obstet Invest 1978; 9:139–49.
25. Wiqvist N. The use of inhibitors of prostaglandin synthesis in obstetrics. In: Keirse MJNC, Anderson ABM, Bennebroek Gravenhorst J, eds. Human parturition. The Hague: Leiden University Press, 1979; 189–200.
26. Adamsons K, Wallach RC. Diazoxide and calcium antagonists in preterm labor. In: Fuchs F, Stubblefield PG, eds. Preterm birth: causes, prevention and management. New York: Macmillan, 1984; 249–63.
27. Erny R, Pigne A, Prouvost C, Gamerre M, Malet C, Serment H, Barrat J. The effects of oral administration of progesterone for premature labor. Am J Obstet Gynecol 1986; 154:525–9.
28. Akerlund M, Strömberg P, Hauksson A, Andersen LF, Lyndrup J, Trojnar J, Melin P. Inhibition of uterine contractions of premature labour with an oxytocin analogue. Results from a pilot study. Br J Obstet Gynaecol 1987; 94:1040–4.
29. Van Kets H, Thiery M, Dermon R, Van Egmond H, Baele G. Perinatal hazards of chronic antenatal tocolysis with indomethacin. Prostaglandins 1979; 18:893–907.
30. Levin DL, Fixler DE, Morriss FC, Tyson J. Morphologic analysis of the pulmonary vascular bed in infants exposed in utero to prostaglandin synthetase inhibitors. J Pediatr 1978; 92:478–83.
31. Levin DL. Effects of inhibition of prostaglandin synthesis on fetal development, oxygenation, and the fetal circulation. Semin Perinatol 1980; 4:35–44.
32. Dornhöfer W, Mosler KH. Prostaglandine und β-Stimulatoren. In: Jung H, Klöck FK, eds. Th 1165a (Partusisten) bei der Behandlung in der Geburtshilfe und Perinatologie. Stuttgart: Georg Thieme, 1975; 196–202.
33. Wolff F, Berg R, Bolte A. Klinische Untersuchungen zur wehenhemmenden Wirkung der Azetylsalizylsäure (ASS) und ihre Nebenwirkungen. Geburtshilfe Frauenheilkd 1981; 41:96–100.
34. Noort WA. Prostanoid excretion in human term and preterm gestation. PhD thesis, Leiden University, The Netherlands, 1989.
35. Keirse MJNC. Eicosanoids in human pregnancy and parturition. In: Mitchell MD, ed. Eicosanoids in reproduction. Boca Raton; CRC Press, 1990; 199–222.
36. Erwich JJHM. Placental eicosanoids – arachidonic acid metabolism in the human placenta. PhD thesis, Leiden University, The Netherlands, 1991.
37. King JF, Grant A, Keirse MJNC, Chalmers I. Beta-mimetics in preterm labour: an overview of the randomized controlled trials. Br J Obstet Gynaecol 1988; 95:211–22.

38. Keirse MJNC. Potential hazards of prostaglandin synthetase inhibitors for management of preterm labour. J Drug Res 1981; 6:915–19.
39. Reiss U, Atad J, Rubinstein I, Zuckerman H. The effect of indomethacin in labour at term. Int J Gynaecol Obstet 1976; 14:369–74.
40. Ridgway L, Wright J, Newton E. The effect of indomethacin on fetal heart biometry. Am J Obstet Gynecol 1991; 164:349.
41. Niebyl JR, Blake DA, White RD, Kumor KM, Dubin NH, Robinson JC, Egner PG. The inhibition of premature labor with indomethacin. Am J Obstet Gynecol 1980; 136:1014–19.
42. Zuckerman H, Shalev E, Gilad G, Katzuni E. Further study of the inhibition of premature labor by indomethacin. Part II. Double-blind study. J Perinat Med 1984; 12:25–9.
43. Blake DA, Niebyl JR, White RD, Kumor KM, Dubin NH, Robinson JC, Egner EG. Treatment of premature labor with indomethacin. Adv Prostaglandin Thromboxane Res 1980; 8:1466–7.
44. Spearing G. Alcohol, indomethacin and salbutamol. A comparative trial of their use in preterm labour. Obstet Gynecol 1979; 53:171–4.
45. Katz Z, Lancet M, Yemini M, Mogilner BM, Feigl A, Ben-Hur H. Treatment of premature labor contractions with combined ritodrine and indomethacine. Int J Gynaecol Obstet 1983, 21:337–42.
46. Gamissans O, Canas E, Cararach V, Ribas J, Puerto B, Edo A. A study of indomethacin combined with ritodrine in threatened preterm labor. Eur J Obstet Gynecol Reprod Biol 1978; 8:123–8.
47. Gamissans O, Cararach V, Serra J. The role of prostaglandin-inhibitors, beta-adrenergic drugs and glucocorticoids in the management of threatened preterm labor. In: Jung H, Lamberti G, eds. Beta-mimetic drugs in obstetrics and perinatology. Stuttgart; Georg Thieme, 1982; 71–84.
48. Gamissans O, Balasch J. Prostaglandin synthetase inhibitors in the treatment of preterm labor. In: Fuchs F, Stubblefield PG, eds. Preterm Birth: Causes, Prevention and Management. New York: Macmillan, 1984; 223–48.
49. Morales WJ, Smith SG, Angel JL, O'Brien WF, Knuppel RA. Efficacy and safety of indomethacin versus ritodrine in the management of preterm labor: a randomized study. Obstet Gynecol 1989; 74:567–72.
50. Besinger RE, Niebyl JR, Keyes WG, Johnson TRB. Randomized comparative trial of indomethacin and ritodrine for the long-term treatment of preterm labor. Am J Obstet Gynecol 1991; 164:981–8.
51. Lumme R, Kurki T, Pyorala T, Ylikorkala O. Indomethacin is more effective than nylidrine in arresting preterm labor. In: Keirse MJNC, Noort WA, eds. Prostaglandins in reproduction. Proceedings of 2nd European Congress on Prostaglandins in Reproduction, The Hague, Netherlands, 1991; 202.
52. Eronen M, Pesonen E, Kurki T, Ylikorkala O, Hallman M. The effects of indomethacin and a beta-sympathomimetic agent on the fetal ductus arteriosus during treatment of premature labor: a randomized double-blind study. Am J Obstet Gynecol 1991, 164:141–6.
53. Kurki T, Laatikainen T, Salminen-Lappalainen K, Ylikorkala O. Maternal plasma cortico-trophin-releasing hormone – elevated in preterm labour but unaffected by indomethacin or nylidrin. Br J Obstet Gynaecol 1991; 98:685–91.
54. Morales W, Madhav H. Efficacy and safety of indomethacin vs. magnesium sulfate in the management of preterm labor: a randomized study. Am J Obstet Gynecol 1991; 164:280.
55. Traeger A, Nöschel H, Zaumseil J. Zur Pharmakokinetik von Indomethazin bei Schwangeren, Kreissenden und deren Neugeborenen. Zentralbl Gynäkol 1973; 95:635–41.
56. Turner G, Collins E. Fetal effects of regular salicylate ingestion in pregnancy. Lancet 1975; ii:338–9.
57. Wilkinson AR. Naproxen levels in preterm infants after maternal treatment. Lancet 1980; ii:591–2.
58. Alvan G, Orme M, Bertillson L, Strand REK, Palmèr L. Pharmacokinetics of indomethacin. Clin Pharmacol Ther 1975; 18:364–73.
59. Wallusch WW, Novak H, Leopold G, Netter KJ. Comparative bioavailability: influence of various diets on the bioavailability of indomethacin. Int Clin Pharmacol 1978; 16:40–4.
60. Gittenberger-de Groot AC. Persistent ductus arteriosus: most probably a primary congenital malformation. Br Heart J 1977; 39:610–18.
61. Nehgme RA, O'Connor TZ, Lister G, Bracken MB. Patent ductus arteriosus. In: Sinclair JC, Bracken MB, eds. Effective care of the newborn infant. Oxford: Oxford University Press. in press.
62. Arcilla RA, Thilenius OG, Ranniger K. Congestive heart failure from suspected ductal closure in utero. J Pediatr 1969; 75:74–8.

63. Kohler HG. Premature closure of the ductus arteriosus (P.C.D.A.): a possible cause of intrauterine circulatory failure. Early Hum Dev 1978; 2:15–23.
64. Haller JA, Morgan W, Rodgers B, Gengos D, Margulies S. Chronic hemodynamic effects of occluding the fetal ductus arteriosus. J Thorac Cardiovasc Surg 1967; 54:770–6.
65. Levin DL, Hyman AI, Heymann MA, Rudolph AM. Fetal hypertension and the development of increased pulmonary vascular smooth muscle: a possible mechanism for persistent pulmonary hypertension of the newborn. J Pediatr 1978; 92:265–9.
66. Levin DL, Mills LJ, Parkey M, Garriott J, Campbell W. Constriction of the fetal ductus arteriosus after administration of indomethacin to the pregnant ewe. J Pediatr 1979; 94:647–50.
67. Moise KJ, Huhta JC. Sharif DS, Ou CH, Kirshon B, Wasserstrum N, Cano L. Indomethacin in the treatment of preterm labor. Effects on the fetal ductus arteriosus. N Engl J Med 1988; 319:327–31.
68. McCarthy JS, Zies LG, Gelband H. Age-dependent closure of the patent ductus arteriosus by indomethacin. Pediatrics 1978; 62:706–12.
69. Heymann MA, Rudolph AM, Silverman NH. Closure of the ductus arteriosus in premature infants by inhibition of prostaglandin synthesis. N Engl J Med 1976; 295:530–3.
70. Betkerur MV, Yeh TF, Miller K, Glasser RJ, Pildes RS. Indomethacin and its effect on renal function and urinary kallikrein excretion in premature infants with patent ductus arteriosus. Pediatrics 1981; 68: 99–102.
71. Gleason CA. Prostaglandins and the developing kidney. Semin Perinatol 1987; 11:12–21.
72. Cantor B, Tyler T, Nelson RM, Stein GH. Oligohydramnios and transient neonatal anuria. A possible association with the maternal use of prostaglandin synthetase inhibitors. J Reprod Med 1980; 24:220–3.
73. Itskovitz J, Abramovice H, Brandes JM. Oligohydramnion, meconium and perinatal death concurrent with indomethacin treatment in human pregnancy. J Reprod Med 1980; 24:137–40.
74. Veersema D, deJong PA, VanWijck JAM. Indomethacin and the fetal renal nonfunction. Eur J Obstet Gynecol Reprod Biol 1983; 16:113–21.
75. Baerts W, Fetter WPF, Hop WJ et al. Cerebral lesions in preterm infants after tocolytic indomethacin. Dev Med Child Neurol 1990; 32:910–18.
76. Van Bel F, Van de Bor M, Stijnen T et al. Cerebral blood flow velocity change in preterm infants after a single dose of indomethacin: duration of its effect. Pediatrics 1989; 84:802–8.
77. Horbar JD. Prevention of periventricular–intraventricular hemorrhage. In: Sinclair JC, Bracken MB, eds. Effective care of the newborn infant. Oxford: Oxford University Press. in press.
78. Friedman Z, Whitman V, Maisels MJ, Berman WJr, Marks KH, Vessell ES. Indomethacin disposition and indomethacin-induced platelet dysfunction in premature infants. J Clin Pharmacol 1978; 18:272–9.

Discussion

Nathanielsz: As I understand it, PGHS is a "suicide enzyme" and it kills itself off after two or three cyclings through its substrate. Is one of the problems of inhibiting it the fact that the way to control its activity might be to inhibit its synthesis rather than to block it?

Keirse: If that could be done it would be a far better way. But I would not know how to do it. It is a glycoprotein and how does one stop a glycoprotein being synthesised? Not with protein synthesis inhibitors because they are likely to be toxic.

Nathanielsz: I was trying to look at what we know about the things that regulate its production, and attack the role of prostaglandins from that angle.

To follow up on that, could the reason that we get such variable responses be related to this mode of action of the NSAID? There is a lot of patient variability when one gives indomethacin, and I wondered if that might be related to the fact that this is not the usual method of enzyme activity.

Keirse: No. It is just drug levels, at 5–6 h. It is not necessarily related to their action. Indomethacin has a very short action in vivo. It probably works for no longer than 6 h in virtually everyone.

Elder: How would one detect the fetal fibronectin?

Amy: It is an immunoassay. It is assessed in the vaginal fluid and then in the cervical mucous plug. The study to which I referred is a study where the presence of fibronectin was looked for in women who had uterine contractions. It has not yet been shown that fibronectin will appear in women who may be at increased risk but who are not having uterine contractions.

The method, as I have discussed it, means that we get in too late. We should have the means to predict objectively an increased risk of preterm delivery at a much earlier stage than the stage where the woman is already experiencing uterine contractions that can be assessed clinically.

Keirse: That was published recently in *New England Journal of Medicine*.

Nathanielsz: There is a company in California selling the test. One takes a Q-tip type swab, introduces it into the cervix, breaks it off and sends it up to them and they measure by radioimmunoassay.

Rees: A Japanese company is selling a dot test. One can take some fluid from the vagina and do it as a blue dot test.

MacKenzie: We have heard that perhaps 50% of preterm labours are associated with intra-uterine infection. If one adds 5% or 10% congenital abnormalities, and a proportion with antepartum haemorrhage, can we expect tocolysis to have much of an impact on reducing preterm delivery?

Keirse: I think that there are between 10% and 20%, depending on the population, where one could perhaps do something about it, given safe and effective agents. But not more than that.

Smith: Can I address the issue of rest and prevention of preterm labour? Obviously it is quite important. On the one hand there are the consequences for people going into preterm labour, and on the other there is the considerable amount of Health Service resource put into patients sitting around on antenatal wards.

My understanding is that nobody has ever shown that hospital bed rest makes any difference to preterm labour.

Amy: I agree. Preterm labour is a condition that is multivariate, so when one implements the correction of a single risk factor, not much of an effect will be observed. To coerce people to stay in bed in hospital is a tremendous cost to society and is of very limited effect. For those women who, for instance, have a profession that involves many hours standing and strenuous activity that is physically, emotionally and/or intellectually demanding, their working conditions should be adjusted but they should not necessarily be made to rest. It was demonstrated several years ago in women with multiple pregnancy that only when the whole issue of the multiple pregnancy was addressed – which might involve putting the woman to rest at an early stage, giving vitamin and iron supplementation and adding other corrective measures – could any discernible effect be seen in terms of perinatal mortality and perinatal results.

Drife: What about the mechanism? I find it interesting that on the one hand we are getting very detailed discussions of the exact enzymes involved in the process of initiation of labour, and on the other hand such a non-specific phenomenon as rest and relaxation should produce such an improvement. How does that work?

Amy: But I do not think it has been demonstrated that rest is of any benefit in women who do not belong to that small group of women at increased risk because of their profession or some other physical activity. In other women at risk I do not think that rest will improve the perinatal results.

Husslein: There was a question about how we might get people to accept antenatal care. Austria has started a programme that is extremely effective in getting people to antenatal care although it is very expensive. We pay our patients to come to antenatal care, and by this means we have achieved 99% antenatal coverage.

What we did, and it is not that bad an idea, was to start by paying them a lot of money, and to cut down the amount of money over the years, since by now the population understands that antenatal care is a normal activity and that they must go to antenatal care if they want to have a healthy baby. It is a controversial policy in terms of reaching the population, but a very efficient one.

There have been several studies of cost effectiveness but it is difficult to judge. One can put whatever one wants on one side or the other. Those in favour of the system argue that they are preventing much damage and that it is extremely cost effective. What it does, is alert people to their responsibility and to health as being something they have to take care of.

Fraser: Why does there seem to have been so much emphasis on the use of indomethacin as a prostaglandin inhibitor in premature labour when other PGSIs, such as the fenamates, may have fewer side effects and may be somewhat more effective?

Keirse: It may be a matter of availability. In the Netherlands we do not have one single fenamate on the market. For some countries there is the problem of availability.

Fraser: Is there anything in the literature on other prostaglandins?

Keirse: Yes. There is a study on flufenamic acid and a study on naproxen. But they are all uncontrolled. There are no controlled trials.

Drife: Is there general agreement that this is the direction that the treatment of premature labour should take?

Amy: When we address the issue of preterm labour and decreasing the incidence of preterm delivery, then, when we think in terms of tocolysis, we are getting in at a late stage of the manifestation of the syndrome. If further data should show that infection is indeed present, as has been said, in about 50% of preterm labours, then to use antibiotics may be a reasonable approach.

I did not go into this in my chapter; I should have done so. Many clinicians have used erythromycin, because it is effective both on *Chlamydia* and on *Ureaplasma*, both of which have been implicated in the aetiology of preterm labour. Some studies have not shown a beneficial effect and some studies have shown a clear beneficial effect particularly when the erythromycin was given during the third trimester. The reasoning is that when erythromycin is given during the third trimester, there is less chance of the woman being contaminated again by a regular sexual partner than when it is administered during the first two trimesters of pregnancy.

Drife: What about the idea of manipulating vaginal pH with Aci-jel or with yogurt?

Amy: Alteration of the vaginal pH is a consequence of a certain microbial infestation rather than the cause.

Elder: I do not think we know.

Index